Meal Preparation and Traini

The Health Professional's

Meal Preparation and Training

The Health Care Professional's Guide

Judith Lannefeld Klinger, OTR, MA

Foreword by Mathew H. M. Lee, MD, FACP

**With the Howard A. Rusk Institute of Rehabilitation Medicine
New York University Medical Center**

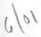

Publisher: John H. Bond
Editorial Director: Amy E. Drummond
Creative Director: Linda Baker
Editorial Assistant: Viktoria Kristiansson

Printed in the United States of America

Klinger, Judith Lannefeld.
    Meal preparation and training: the health care professional's guide/Judith Lannefeld Klinger.
        p. cm.
        Includes bibliographical references and index.
    ISBN 1-55642-343-8
    1. Cookery for the physically handicapped. I. Title.
    [DNLM: 1. Occupational Therapy--methods. 2. Disabled-rehabilitation. 3. Aged. 4. Cookery--methods. 5. Cooking and
    Eating Utensils. 6. Home Care Services. WB 555 K65m 1997]
TX652.K4688 1997
641.5'087--dc21
DNLM/DLC
for Library of Congress   97-16055

This book is a companion to *Mealtime Manual for People with Disabilities and the Aging*. Anyone who wishes to obtain a copy can contact the publisher listed below.

Published by: SLACK Incorporated
               6900 Grove Road
               Thorofare, NJ 08086-9447 USA
               Telephone: 609-848-1000
               Fax: 609-853-5991
               World Wide Web: http://www.slackinc.com

Contact SLACK Incorporated for more information about other books in this field or about the availability of our books from distributors outside the United States.

Last digit is print number: 10 9 8 7 6 5 4 3 2 1

DEDICATION AND ACKNOWLEDGMENTS

This professional guide is dedicated to all health care workers who seek with their clients to reach the highest level of which they are capable and to those who find joy in their work. Ours is a field that always has new challenges and delights. The book is especially dedicated to Muriel Zimmerman, MA, OTR, FAOT, who was my mentor first when I was a student, then as a colleague, and who set that standard of being aware of possibilities for patients about which others might only dream. We are still reaching for the stars!

Deep thanks and appreciation go to those who have assisted in the preparation of this guide: Lucy Beck, MA, CHE, at the Howard A. Rusk Institute of Rehabilitation Medicine, New York University Medical Center, for her input and reading of the manuscript; Sophie Chiotelis, OTR, MA, Occupational Therapy Director at the Howard A. Rusk Institute of Rehabilitation Medicine for her unwavering support; Sharon Wright, ASID, formerly at the Rusk Institute and at Harmarville Rehabilitation Center for sharing ideas; Kathleen Culler, MS, OTR, at the Rehabilitation Institute of Chicago and Lynn Yasuda, MSEd, OTR, FAOT, at Rancho Los Amigos Medical Center for sharing materials; Nancy Tate at AT&T for her guidance and computer wisdom; Greg Klinger for his illustrations; and to my husband Herb for his support and patience.

Judith Lannefeld Klinger, OTR, MA

CONTENTS

SECTION ONE
WORKING WITH THE PERSON WITH A DISABILITY

ASSESSING THE SITUATION

THE DISABILITIES

SECTION TWO
IN AND AROUND THE KITCHEN AND THE HOME

SECTION THREE
KITCHEN TOOLS, APPLIANCES, AND TECHNIQUES

SECTION FOUR
HELP FOR THE HEALTH CARE PROFESSIONAL AND THE CAREGIVER

FOREWORD

We are very pleased to see the publication of *Meal Preparation and Training: The Health Care Professional's Guide* in the year of the 50th anniversary of the Howard A. Rusk Institute of Rehabilitation Medicine. As the first rehabilitation program in our nation, we have strived to be at the forefront of rehabilitation, helping individuals achieve independent lives.

With the revision of the classic *Mealtime Manual* and this accompanying *Professional's Guide*, practitioners will have a complete reference work to guide them in planning functional activities to assess and retrain individuals in the tasks of daily living. Practitioners, whether occupational therapists, physical therapists, or social workers, need as much practical information as possible in order to focus treatment and be effective within the shorter treatment time frames in today's health care environment.

Mrs. Klinger has provided an eclectic range of treatment approaches and resources that cannot fail to be of help to the concerned therapist, whether in hospital, home, or community practice.

As Dr. Rusk wrote in the foreword to the second edition of *Mealtime Manual*, "...just as men and women everywhere yearn to be free, so do they want to be as self-sufficient and productive as possible." With this book, we can help them to be so.

Mathew H. M. Lee, MD, FACP
Professor and Acting Chairman
Howard A. Rusk Institute of Rehabilitation Medicine
New York University Medical Center

INTRODUCTION

Meal Preparation and Training: The Health Care Professional's Guide is designed to be used with *Mealtime Manual for People with Disabilities and the Aging*. The purpose of the guide is twofold: one, to give recommendations for training and specific adaptations; two, to provide additional references on funding and resources that will help you provide assistance to your clients.

Mealtime Manual for People with Disabilities and the Aging is written for both the consumer and health care professionals. It provides information for direct application to the kitchen and food preparation. Some of our clients, however, need graded programs to attain independence. *Meal Preparation and Training: The Health Care Professional's Guide* gives sources for developing homemaking activities geared to varied physical and cognitive needs. As with *Mealtime Manual for People with Disabilities and the Aging*, addresses for equipment and helpful organizations are listed in Section Four. (A few addresses may be limited to use by professionals.)

In the 22 years since *Mealtime Manual for People with Disabilities and the Aging* was first published, there has been a marked change in the field of homemaking rehabilitation and home modification. In the 1960s and early 1970s, most patients were seen in rehabilitation centers, hospital stays were longer, and an individual often came home well-prepared to handle daily routines and tasks.

Now, hospital stays are shorter. Many patients are admitted for only a few days; staffs are overloaded with documentation. Rather than an on-site evaluation with the family, both the home visit and discharge planning are frequently hospital-based. Home care must shoulder a bigger burden. Stroke patients are hardly stabilized, often unable to ambulate, before they come home. Chronic health problems limit the activities of 32 million Americans, many of whom live at home but need help.

Acceptance of the rights and needs of people with disabilities was recognized with the passage of the Americans with Disabilities Act. As a civil rights law, compliance is a gradual, but expanding, process. Transportation is the main area that remains and is expected to take up to 30 years to complete. Small changes are already being seen, such as city and town curb ramps, more accessible public buildings, wider doors that wheelchairs can pass through, and an increasing number of new buses with lifts. Telecommunications must be accessible for people with and without language skills. As health care professionals, we will be called upon to help implement some of these changes. Appendix F as well as Chapter 25 include resources for adapting housing and transportation.

Advances in the field of rehabilitation continue to grow. Self-help and support groups are more regularly a part of follow-up from a hospital stay. Some equipment, such as wheelchair cushions, has evolved to be more functional and protective. Wheelchairs are more adaptable and streamlined. More products are available to assist with home modifications.

Evaluation of a client cannot be limited to one area or concern. Tasks of daily living interconnect. Our focus is on homemaking and meal preparation. To do this independently or with minimal help, however, means that the individual must be able to communicate and understand, respond to an emergency, bathe and dress, handle toileting needs, have a means of mobility, and be able to move around the home and community.

Feeling good about one's appearance increases health and the feeling of well-being. Depression leads to lack of caring. This may extend to poor nutrition, the "it's too much trouble" syndrome, or to overeating. Aids to make self-care easier allow the individual to move on to family-oriented activities, homemaking, and social and community interaction. Firms like Aviano USA (65B), Fashion-Ease (202), J.C. Penney (289), Laurel Designs (314), and Very Special Clothing, Inc. (559) provide clothing that is easier to put on and wear. See addresses in Appendix E and publications on adapted clothing in Appendix F under Self-Help Aids.

The Guide is divided into several sections. Section One assesses the situation, the types of patients, as well as the caregivers and family, then focuses on specific disabilities and problems. Section Two is involved with the kitchen and the home, from safety and modifications to transporting items. Section Three narrows in on equipment, appliances, nutrition, shopping, and includes a guide to teaching recipes. Section Four provides help for the health care professional and caregivers with extensive support materials. These include funding, agencies and organizations, sources, general references, and forms and plans for making equipment. The forms and plans may be photocopied, enlarged if desired, and are designed for use with clients. The materials in this guide are to be combined with *Mealtime Manual for People with Disabilities and the Aging* to offer you a solid base for home management and meal preparation training.

We look forward to your comments and suggestions, and wish success and joy to both you and your clients.

HOW TO FIND WHAT YOU NEED

Each of the products described in the *Professionals Guide* is followed by a list of numbers indicating the manufacturers and sources of the product. These numbers are keyed to the addresses listed under Appendix E, Sources for Equipment and Materials. Companies and addresses were current as of the date of publication.

We hope you do not find the numbering system confusing, as it saves many pages of repetition. Most of the toll-free numbers given here are for out-of-state calls; if the company or organization is within your state, call information for the local number.

Whenever possible, you should purchase the item from a local retailer or mail-order firm. If you cannot locate one, then contact the manufacturer for your nearest retail source. If you have no luck locating an item, write to us on the Tear-Out Suggestion Card, and we will try to help.

Section One

WORKING WITH THE
PERSON WITH A DISABILITY

The Older Client

People older than 85 years are the fastest growing segment of the population in the United States. Today, there are more than 2.5 million in this group. This number is expected to increase to almost 13 million in the next 50 years. As professional health care workers, the elderly are an expanding percentage of our patient load. Those with chronic diseases often live long lives, though they are sometimes disabled and frequently need care.

The ratio of adult children to parents has decreased dramatically. In 1900, there were 13.6 adults between the ages of 18 and 64 for each person 65 or older. Today, that ratio is less than 4.8 to 1. With the high level of mobility within our country, many adult children no longer live nearby, so their parents are left to subsist on their own. For those who do have extended families or are close, there is the stress of being a caretaker. This has been called the Sandwich Generation, people caught between bringing up their own children and caring for their aging parents. With increasing longevity, it may be just the time the adult child has brought up his or her own family and is ready for relaxation or retirement. Chapter 6 discusses helpful agencies and resources.

The values that elder members add to an extended family should be emphasized whenever possible. Although more care may be required, the opportunity for children to share the duties and to reap both the present love and the feeling of life's continuation cannot be minimized. To help "accentuate the positive," several books on grandparenting are listed in this chapter's Resources section. Sharing these with family members may ease the burdens, even let a little of the rainbow shine through. Sharing traditional or favorite recipes may rekindle interest in food for the grandparent and create not only a wider nutritional base but lasting memories for the youngster.

PROBLEMS TO CONSIDER IN EVALUATION

Factors affecting our aging clients range from lowered energy and increasing physical limitations to the cognitive inability to handle activities of daily living. Specific problems for assessment include loss of hearing, difficulty remembering, impaired balance, reduced vision, poor nutrition, and lack of safety awareness. Some of these disabilities are covered more fully in the chapters that follow.

According to the National Association for the Visually Handicapped, 97% of people living to age 80 have a visual impairment not correctable by standard lenses. This can result in the inability to read controls or labels, define where steps begin, and see open cabinet doors. Painting the top and bottom steps a different color than the rest of the stairs or highlighting the edges with tape helps prevent falls.

Proper lighting becomes more important for people as they grow older. Lighting should be even and produce minimal glare. Adding light to meal preparation areas makes it possible to carry out a wider range of tasks more safely. Increased illumination is easily and inexpensively added with undercabinet lights.

Loss of hearing is a common problem of aging, but one a client may not be as aware of as visual difficulties. Amplified signals for telephones and doorbells help. See Chapter 20.

Safety is a major concern. The statistics on falls among older adults is alarming. One-third to two-thirds of individuals older than 65 sustain one or more falls per year. These falls often result in serious injury, such as hip fracture. Falls are the sixth leading cause of death overall after age 65, with one-third to just more than one-half of the deaths due to accidents among older people caused by falls. Factors that contribute to an elderly client's risk of falling include changes in the nervous system resulting in slowed reaction time, reduced vision involving both disturbances in depth and figure-ground perception, diminished mental status, and hearing. Other elements relate to psychosocial effects, such as depression, lowered self-esteem, and even life satisfaction. In a controlled study by Fisher, Bonder, and Falconnier, the most important risk was found to be medical conditions that also involve the side effects of medication that interferes with function. The only statistically significant contributor was the number of medications an individual was taking. However, all factors must

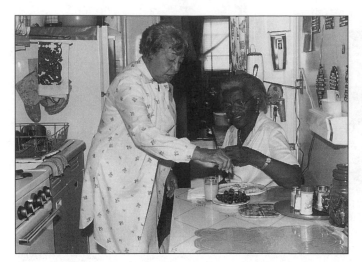

Figure 1-1. This senior companion assists her charge with a meal. (Senior Companion Program. Photo courtesy of ACTION®, Washington, DC.)

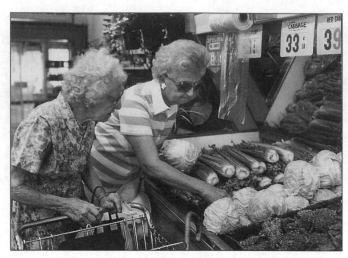

Figure 1-2. A volunteer helper assists with shopping. (Senior Companion Program. Photo courtesy of ACTION®, Washington, DC.)

be considered together in a treatment plan to increase safety and decrease the number of falls.

When working with an older client, it is not possible to isolate homemaking or meal difficulties. If an individual is not eating, the reasons may be the physical inability to shop or prepare the meals, lack of interest in food due to loss of taste, depression or social isolation, or a budget that does not include food as a priority.

A senior companion can assist his or her charge with meals, reading, and other tasks (Figure 1-1). Having a helper allows this elderly woman's daughters to work during the day then take over the supervision at night.

Getting to and from one's home for shopping and medical or other appointments is made easier with a volunteer helper (Figure 1-2).

Simple aids may make it possible for your patient to function more safely and easily. Often a can opener is a barrier to preparing quick meals. Weakened, arthritic hands cannot handle a standard manual opener and often cannot operate an older electric one. Test the patient's model. If your client has short-term memory loss, you may have to repeat the lesson of using a new can opener.

Problems extend to opening other kinds of containers. Even the plastic top that covers a yogurt or cottage cheese container is hard to release with weakened hands until you show the patient how to use ingenuity. In this case, use the edge of the counter to release the top. See sections on container opening in *Mealtime Manual for People with Disabilities and the Aging*.

When memory and physical limitations make using a regular stove unsafe, a microwave oven may be substituted and the stove disconnected (Figure 1-3). A heat-proof cover placed over the turned-off burners creates extra counter space. Digital and push-button controls are sometimes confusing to the older homemaker. A chart shows times for heating water, milk, frozen vegetables, and soups. Burner covers and mats cost about $10 per set and up from department stores and mail-order firms. **Sources:** 109, 241, 262, 361, 561B.

A treatment program may include teaching older clients methods and employment of aids to help memory retention. A large-

print calendar for appointments and social activities is an initial step. If a free calendar is not available locally, one source is 326. This firm also carries large-print address books for recording numbers of family and friends. Emergency numbers should be posted by the telephone in large print. If reading or remembering a telephone number is difficult, place the photo of the person right next to the number on a sheet or use a small photo album with the photo and number. Memory message recording cards allow an individual to record memos for later recall on a small, battery-operated unit. Cost is about $20 and up from office supply firms and mail-order firms. **Sources** include 235.

Medication is remembered more easily when organized in a holder (Figure 1-4). A small, one-week holder is about $1.50 from drugstores. When medication must be taken several times a day, a holder with three or four compartments for each day may be used. **Sources** include 53, 53B, 250, 361.

An ice cube tray may be converted into a holder for pills with days written across the top and times along the narrow edge (Figure 1-5). A cross piece of styrofoam or cardboard divides the day into sections.

The American Association of Retired Persons (AARP) offers a free video or slide show on common aids for the older person. See this chapter's Resources. Detailed information on a variety of aids and sources may be obtained through the computerized listing services. See Appendix C. Funding for assistive devices is often a problem. A limited number of items are covered by Medicare and insurance companies. These usually have to do with ambulation or bed mobility. Obtaining a prescription from the physician may increase the chance of reimbursement. If reimbursement is not possible and the patient cannot afford the cost, contact specialized funding agencies. In Connecticut, for example, the local chapter of the Arthritis Foundation has a fund to cover a limited amount of homemaking assistance and equipment for a person with rheumatoid arthritis.

The majority of elderly Americans live in their own homes. This means they have to handle upkeep, repair, and utility costs. Not only does the physical ability to take on maintenance jobs

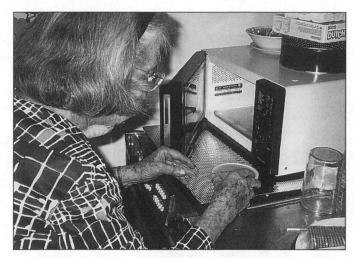

Figure 1-3. When memory and physical limitations make using a regular stove unsafe, a microwave oven may be substituted and the stove disconnected. (Friends House, Sandy Spring, MD. Photo by J.K.)

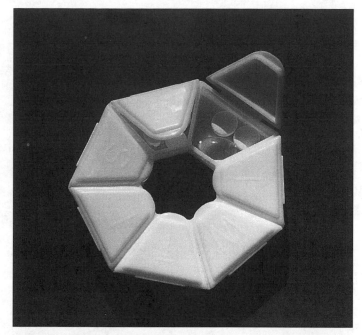

Figure 1-4. Medication is remembered more easily when organized in a holder. (Photo by J.K.)

become more difficult, unsafe, and sometimes impossible, but costs of hiring help continue to rise. Programs to assist with fuel costs and with chore services may allow your patient to stay at home. See Chapter 25 for a reference on home modification and repairs with a state-by-state listing.

When finances are a problem, a social worker or other health care worker should sit down with the older patient and explain some of the new options available. Two of these are the reverse mortgage program and the federally funded Congregate Housing Services Program (CHSP). The CHSP provides non-medical support to frail, low-income tenants as an alternative to living in an institution. A reverse mortgage may be discussed with a local bank. The AARP has a Home Equity Information Center with publications for both the consumer and professional. Address is in Appendix C. The AARP publication *The DoAble Renewable Home* gives ideas for retrofitting a home for the elderly. See Resources in Chapter 25. Knowing about alternative types of residences in the area helps when a patient must make a change. Again, the AARP has a video that defines different kinds of housing options. The organization is also involved in a program called AARP Connections for Independence, which links AARP members with agencies that need volunteers to assist individuals who are 60 and older and wish to remain in their own homes.

Lack of socialization decreases interest in life, and this includes maintaining good nutrition. A therapist or other professional can offer new ideas to isolated older patients. Community activities are the first choice, but when the person is housebound or lives in a rural area with few amenities, alternates should be sought. One idea is SeniorNet®. This non-profit, nationwide computer network, designed for adults over 55, has developed as an "electronic community for older people." The second are computer programs designed to let the individual record incidents throughout an entire life span. A guide asks questions and gives an outline for spurring ideas. It increases mentation, reduces depression, and is a way of renewing positive communication with other family members.

SeniorNet® teaches individuals how to communicate by computer with keyboard friends across the country (Figure 1-6). The training site gathers participants together. When conversing by computer, members share greetings, day-to-day activities, even recipes from home or a central computer setup. **Source:** 471. See this chapter's Resources.

ALZHEIMER'S DISEASE

More than 1.5 million Americans suffer from Alzheimer's disease. It is the fourth leading cause of death among the elderly. As the patient continues to deteriorate, treatment goals change. In early stages, the individual, under supervision, may continue to do light household tasks, such as setting the table, preparing salad, and mixing batter. In later stages, activities focus on safety, control of the wandering syndrome, self feeding, and then assisted feeding as apraxia increases.

The health care worker assists the caregiver, assessing the home for safety, teaching ways for the patient to maintain dignity in self-care and other activities, and counseling for handling stress and for the transition to institutional care. As a health care professional, becoming aware of support programs extends your effectiveness and energy. Finding respite programs and a support group for the caregiver, locating day care facilities for the patient, and providing nutritional information and adapted equipment are all facets of the treatment plan. Both the Alzheimer's Disease and Related Disorders Association and the NIA Alzheimer's Disease Education and Referral Center distribute information. Addresses are in Appendix C. Some services of your local chapter may include free literature, evaluation centers, information on legal and financial resources, support groups, seminars, respite care, home care aides, day care, nationwide referrals, and telephone support link programs.

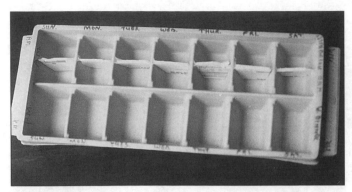

Figure 1-5. An ice cube tray may be converted into a holder for pills. (Photo by J.K.)

Contact the local Office of Aging; get their listing of services. Two national organizations that offer information and free referrals are Children of Aging Parents and the National Association of Area Agencies on Aging.

RESOURCES

Addresses for publications, periodicals, and organizations are given in Section Four.

PUBLICATIONS

Aging and Vision. Making the Most of Impaired Vision. (1987). New York: The American Foundation for the Blind, and Washington, DC: the American Association of Retired Persons. Discusses causes of vision loss, suggestions for lighting and color contrast, devices for daily life, travel, and resources. Free from both organizations.

The American Academy of Orthopaedic Surgeons brochures of interest to older clients include *Arthritis*, *Common Foot Problems*, *Low Back Pain*, *Sprains and Strains*, *Scoliosis*, *Total Joint Replacement*, and *Osteoporosis*. Single copies are free by sending a self-addressed, stamped, business-size envelope (one for each brochure) to the AAOS.

The American Association of Retired Persons distributes a wide range of information and services. Publications relating to general questions as well as housing, homemaking, and meal preparation include *Home-Made Money: Consumer Information on Home Equity Conversions*, #D12894, free; *Questions and Answers About Counseling Needs and Resources*, #D13932, free; *Reminiscence: Finding Meaning in Memories*, #D13186, free; *The Rights of Older Persons*, #D14225, 413 pages, $9.45; *Your Home, Your Choice: A Workbook for Older People and Their Families*, #D12143, free. Includes checklists for determining need; assistance for staying in own home; types of housing options including housesharing, ECHO housing, congregate, and supportive housing; and resources.

Aspen Reference Group. (1991). *Geriatric Patient Education Resource Manual*. Frederick, MD: Aspen. $247. Medical conditions, drugs, nutrition, communication, adaptive aids, caregivers, family. Charts, checklists, practical tools. Annual supplements sent for 30-day no-risk evaluation.

Beers, M. H., & Urice, S. K. (1992). *Aging in Good Health: A*

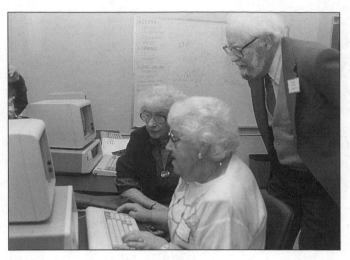

Figure 1-6. SeniorNet® teaches individuals how to communicate by computer with keyboard friends across the country. (Photo of SeniorNet® site in Orinda, CA., courtesy of SeniorNet®, San Francisco, CA. Site sponsor: Pacific Bell. Photo by F. Middleton/SeniorNet®.)

Complete, Essential Medical Guide for Older Men and Women and Their Families. New York: Pocket Books, Simon & Schuster. $22. Normal aging, effects of medication, body systems, health problems, legal issues.

Bortz, W. M. (1991). *We Live Too Short and Die Too Long.* New York: Bantam Doubleday Dell. $19.95. Enhancing aging instead of trying to prevent it.

Brenton, M., & *Prevention* Magazine Staff. (1984). *Aging Slowly.* Emmaus, PA: Rodale Press. $17.95.

Carlin, V. F., & Mansberg, R. (1984). *If I Live To Be a Hundred: Congregate Living for Later Life.* Crystal Lake, IL: Parker Publishing Co. $17.95.

Cheney, W. J., et al. (1992). *The Second 50 Years: A Reference Manual for Senior Citizens.* New York: Paragon. $21.95. Large-print book covers assistance programs, health issues, nutrition, consumerism, and living alone.

Chernoff, R. (1991). *Geriatric Nutrition: The Health Professional's Handbook.* Frederick, MD: Aspen. $72. Nutritional assessment, intervention, support, and health promotion programs for elderly.

Cohen, D., & Eisendorfer, C. (1993). *Seven Steps to Effective Parent Care: A Planning and Action Guide for Adult Children with Aging Parents.* New York: Putnam Berkley. $21.95.

Cox, B. J., & Walker, L. I. (1991). *Bridging the Communication Gap with the Elderly: Practical Strategies for Caregivers*, AHPI. $25.95.

Davis, L. J., & Kirkland, M. (Eds.). (1996). *The Role of Occupational Therapy with the Elderly (ROTE)*. Bethesda, MD: American Occupational Therapy Association. #1600, 3-ring binder, $50 AOTA member, $61 non-member. Core gerontological knowledge for working with the elderly. Four modules cover cognitive, nutritional and physiological changes associated with aging; roles and functions of occupational therapy in geriatric practice; assessment, treatment planning, and continuity of care; activity programming; preventive treatment approaches; care for the terminally ill; and service management issues.

Deichman, E. S., & Kocieki, R. (Eds.). (1989). *Working with the Elderly: An Introduction*. Buffalo, NY: Golden Age Books, Prometheus. $29.95. Maintaining integrity, independence, and individuality of older people.

Design for Aging: Strategies for Collaboration Between Architects and Occupational Therapists. (1993). Bethesda, MD: American Occupational Therapy Association. #1801, $5 AOTA member, $8 non-member.

Developing Respite Services for the Elderly. Seattle, WA: University of Washington Press. $8.95. Establishing and operating respite programs, introducing patients and families to respite services.

Discharge Planning Fact Sheet. Summarizes key aspects of discharge planning to familiarize aging-network providers with this hospital service. *A Plan for Developing a Program to Improve Discharge Planning*. 6-step blueprint for creating aging-network programs that enhance continuity of health care. Both free from the Long Term Care National Resource Center at UCLA/USC.

Di Domenico, R. L., & Zieglet, W. Z. (1994). *Practical Rehabilitation Techniques for Geriatric Aides* (2nd ed.). Frederick, MD: Aspen. $88. Restorative techniques, understanding medical problems. Anticipating everyday problems.

Dychtwald, K., & Flower, J. (1990). *Age Wave*. New York: Bantam Doubleday Dell.

Emlet, C. A., et al. (1995). *In-Home Assessment of Older Adults: An Interdisciplinary Approach*. Frederick, MD: Aspen. $49. MSW, OTR, PHN, and PT. Case studies, charts, checklists, resources to photo copy.

Evans, W., & Rosenberg, I. (1991). *Biomarkers*. New York: Simon and Schuster. Premise: as people age, they do not have to lose their fitness if they have proper nutrition and exercise.

Finding Legal Help: An Older Person's Guide, and an AARP Handbook covering Social Security issues, guardianship, the right to refuse medical treatment, age discrimination, and civil service issues are available from LCE, Inc. $2. **Source:** 315.

Fire Safety Tips for Older Adults. (1993). Quincy, MA: National Fire Protection Association. Free, large-print brochure listing techniques for protection and planning escape if fire occurs.

Fisher, A., Bonder, B., & Falconnier, L. Falls in older persons; a multifactorial study. *Gerontologist, 28*, 208A.

Fry, P. S., & Caprio-Prevette, M. D. (1995). *Memory Enhancement for Older Adults*. Frederick, MD: Aspen. $79. Intervention program integrating cognitive restructuring and traditional memory training.

Furlong, M., & Kearsley, G. (1990). *Computers for Kids Over 60*. San Francisco, CA: SeniorNet®. $14.95. Large print. Explains the computer revolution, concepts of software and hardware, invites reader to join the excitement. **Source:** 471.

Furlong, M., & Lipson, S. (1996). *Young at Heart: Computing for Seniors*. New York: McGraw Hill. $22.95

Geriatric Practice in OT. (1991). Bethesda, MD: American Occupational Therapy Association. #1940, $8 AOTA member, $10 non-member. Resources for conducting inservice and staff development programming. Professional organizations, journals, articles, audiovisuals, databases.

Gallo, J. J., et al. (1995). *Handbook of Geriatric Assessment* (2nd ed.). Frederick, MD: Aspen. $44. Mental status testing; func-

tional, values history, economic, and physical assessments; health maintenance schedules; geriatric assessment programs and practice.

Golub, S., & Freedman, R. J. (Eds.). (1985). *Health Needs of Women As They Age*. New York: Haworth. $14.95. Status of health and position of aging women in America. Societal needs and approaches, specific clinical problems, such as Alzheimer's disease, hypertension, eye problems, osteoporosis, reproductive cancer.

Gordon, B. (1995). *Remembering and Forgetting in Everyday Life*. New York: MasterMedia Ltd.

Growing Older in Your Home: Modifications for Your Changing Needs. (1995). Bethesda,. MD: American Occupational Therapy Association. Three packets: #5072, Kitchen Modifications; #5073, Bedroom Modifications; #5074, Bathroom Modifications. Units of 25 per packet: $5.50 AOTA member, $7.50 non-member. Handouts for clients with suggestions to ease activities and increase safety.

Gumbrium, J. F. (1993). *Speaking of Life: Horizons of Meaning for Nursing Home Residents*. Hawthorne: NY: Aldine de Gruyter.

Hartke, R. (1991). *Psychological Aspects of Geriatric Rehabilitation*. Rehabilitation Institute of Chicago Publication Series. Frederick, MD: Aspen. $52. Practical sourcebook on role of psychology in successful rehabilitation of the aging.

Health Promotion and Wellness in Older Adults. (1991). Bethesda, MD: American Occupational Therapy Association. #1950, $8 AOTA member, $10 non-member. Curriculum resources, journals, articles, professional organizations, educational and training resources for facilitating training in geriatric wellness.

Heart to Heart: Older Women and Heart Disease: A Guide for Program Planners and Volunteer Leaders. Washington, DC: Health Advocacy Services, American Association of Retired Persons. Free.

Johns Hopkins Medical Letter, *Health Over 50* (Eds.). (1992). *The Johns Hopkins Medical Handbook: The 100 Major Medical Disorders of People Over the Age of 50*. New York: Random House.

Kiernat, J. M. (1991). *Occupational Therapy and the Older Adult: A Clinical Manual*. Frederick, MD: Aspen. $45. Practical information on educating patients, treating the whole person, preventing disability, treating physical and cognitive problems, home care, adult day care, terminally ill.

Levy, M. T. (1991). *Parenting Mom and Dad: A Guide for Older Children Who Care*. New York: Prentice Hall. $10.95.

Lewis, C. B. (1989). *Improving Mobility in Older Persons: A Manual for Geriatric Specialists*. Frederick, MD: Aspen. $56. Causes of dysmobility, goal setting, sitting, standing, bed mobility, gait, balance, sensory environment, drugs, resources.

Lewis, C. B. (1995). *Aging: The Health Care Challenge* (3rd ed.). Philadelphia: F.A. Davis. $39.95.

Lewis, S. C. (1989). *Elder Care in Occupational Therapy*. Thorofare, NJ: SLACK Inc. $36. Review of the aging process, pragmatic guide with variety of modalities for working with later-life adults.

McIlwain, H. H., Bruce, D. F., Silverfield, J. C., Burnette, M. C., & Germain, B. F. (1993). *Winning With Osteoporosis*. New York: Wiley. $12.95.

The National Institute on Aging Public Information office distributes free publications, including *Health Resources for Older Women*; *Older and Wiser: The Baltimore Longitudinal Study of Aging* (information packet); *Special Report on Aging 1990*; *Talking with Your Doctor: A Guide for Older People; Age Pages on Diabetes, Osteoporosis, Stroke Prevention and Treatment*; *Finding Good Medical Care for Older Americans, When You Need a Nursing Home, Accidents and the Elderly, Preventing Falls and Fractures, Hints for Shopping, Cooking and Enjoying Meals, Nutrition: A Lifelong Concern*. NIA publications may be reproduced without obtaining copyright permission; excellent hand-outs for patient education.

Older Adult Services: Resource Guide. (1995). Bethesda, MD: American Occupational Therapy Association. $10 AOTA member, $20 non-member. Bibliographies, audiovisuals, resource personnel.

Options for Elderly Homeowners: A Guide to Reverse Mortgages and Their Alternatives. Free from U.S. Department of Housing and Urban Development, Single Family Development Div.

Orr, A., & Casablanca-Hilton, J. *Helping an Older Visually Impaired Parent*. New York: American Foundation for the Blind. Ways in which people can cope and adjust, services and options available for the elderly visually impaired person.

Paige, J., & Gordon, P. (1991). *Choice Years: Health, Happiness, and Beauty Through Menopause and Beyond*. New York: Villard, Random House. $22.50. Section on nutrition for women, with implications of proper diet, a month's menu plan and recipes.

Product Safety for Older Consumers: What Manufacturers/ Designers Need to Consider. (1991). Washington, DC: U.S. Product Safety Commission. CPSC Publication 702.

Resources for Elders with Disabilities (3rd ed.). (1996). Lexington, MA: Resources for Rehabilitation. $48.95.

Schmall, V., et al. *Depression in Later Life*, #PNW 347, $1.50; *Alcohol Problems in Later Life*, PNW342, $1; *Sensory Changes in Later Life*, $1; *Helping Memory-Impaired Elders: A Guide for Caregivers*, PNW314, $1; and *Living Arrangements in Later Life*, PNW318, $1. Oregon State University, Pacific Northwest Extension Service has a number of helpful publications related to aging.

Seeing Well as You Grow Older. Free booklet from the American Association of Ophthalmology.

Singer, G., & Singer, L. (1994). *Towards the Greater Enjoyment of Later Life*. Pequannock, NJ: Maddak, Inc. Workbook for clients discusses changes we face as we age and provides a coping exercise. **Source:** 343.

Skala, K. (1992). *American Guidance for Seniors*. Falls Church, VA: American Guidance. $15.95 plus $3 shipping. How to navigate maze to receive help, benefits, or service from federal, state, and county agencies. **Source:** 40.

Sleep As We Grow Older. (1995). Rochester, MN: American Sleep Disorders Association. Free.

VHI™ Geriatric Kit. Gays Mills, WI: Country Technology. 377 reproducible cards for customizing rehabilitation include transfer techniques, stress and relaxation, exercises, back care, arthritis, stroke, Parkinson's, osteoporosis, more, $230.

Werner, A., & Firman, J. *Home Care for Older People: A Consumer's Guide*. Washington, DC: United Seniors Health

Cooperative. $12.

West, R. (1990). *Memory Fitness Over 40*. Gainesville, FL: Triad. $14.95. Practical strategies to improve memory. Changes that occur with age, how to minimize memory loss. Self-test for assessing memory ability.

Alzheimer's Disease

For information on Alzheimer's disease and related disorders, write to the NIA Alzheimer's Disease Education and Referral (ADEAR) Center and the Alzheimer's Disease and Related Disorders Association. The Association runs a program called Safe Return designed to help identify, locate, and return individuals who are memory impaired due to Alzheimer's disease or a related disorder. The program provides an identity bracelet or necklace, clothing labels and wallet cards, registration of individual's description in a national database, a 24-hour, toll-free number to contact when an individual is lost or found, plus access to the National Crime Information Computer of 17,000 law enforcement agencies and a network of more than 220 Alzheimer's Association chapters. Cost is $25. Contact chapter nearest you.

Alzheimer's Disease: Unraveling the Mystery. Washington, DC: Alzheimer's Disease Education and Referral Center, National Institute on Aging. Free, 48-page booklet for professionals, caregivers, and family.

Aronson, M. K. (Ed.). (1988). *Understanding Alzheimer's Disease: What It Is, How to Cope With It, Future Directions*. New York: Alzheimer's Disease and Related Disorders Association, Scribners. $16, available from the Alzheimer's Association.

Carroll, D. (1990). *When Your Loved One Has Alzheimer's: A Caregiver's Guide*. New York: HarperCollins. $17.95 How-to book to lighten load and assist psychological survival of caregiver; resources.

Cohen, D., & Eisendorfer, C. (1987). *The Loss of Self: A Family Resource for the Care of Alzheimer's and Related Disorders*. New York: NAL, Penguin. $12.95.

Coping and Caring: Living with Alzheimer's Disease. Washington, DC: American Association of Retired Persons. Free.

Coughlan, P. B. (1993). *Facing Alzheimer's: Family Caregivers Speak*. New York: Ballantine, Random House. $4.99.

Danna, J. *When Alzheimer's Hits Home*. (1996). Briarwood, NY: Palomino Press. $14.95.

Greutzner, H. (1992). *Alzheimer's: A Caregiver's Guide and Sourcebook*. New York: Wiley.

Hinnefeld, J. (1994). *Everything You Need to Know When Someone You Love Has Alzheimer's Disease*. New York: Rosen. $15.95. Helps pre-teenagers to teenagers understand changes, and provides suggestions for helping family.

Hodgson, H. (1995). *Alzheimer's: Finding the Words—A Communication Guide for Those Who Care*. Minneapolis: Chronimed. $12.95.

Lawson Keller, J. (Ed.). (1992). *The Male Caregiver's Guidebook: Caring for Your Loved One with Alzheimer's at Home*. Alzheimer's Association, Iowa Golden Chapter. Write national chapter for information.

Mace, N. L., & Rabins, P. V. (1991). *The Thirty-Six Hour Day: A Family Guide to Caring for Persons with Alzheimer's Disease*,

Related Dementing Illnesses and Memory Loss in Later Life. New York: Johns Hopkins University Press. $10, available from the Alzheimer's Association.

McGowin, D. F. (1993). *Living in the Labyrinth: A Personal Journey Through the Maze of Alzheimer's*. Elder Books. Addresses early onset, gives coping experiences from patient's perspective. $12, available from the Alzheimer's Association.

Oakley, F. (1993). *Understanding the ABCs of Alzheimer's Disease: A Guide for Caregivers*. Bethesda, MD: American Occupational Therapy Association. #1980, $4.50 AOTA member, $5.50 non-member.

Powell, L. S., & Courtice, K. (1992). *Alzheimer's Disease: A Guide for Families*. Reading, MA: Addison-Wesley. $10.95. Guide for professionals, family, and caregivers. Making communication with patient easier, handling your own emotions, finding resources, handling unpredictable behavior.

Roberts, D. J. (1991). *Taking Care of Caregivers: For Families and Others Who Care for People with Alzheimer's Disease and Other Forms of Dementia*. Palo Alto, CA: Bull Pub.

United States Congress, Office of Technology Assessment. Special Care Units for People with Alzheimer's and Other Dementias: Consumer Education, Research, Regulatory, and Reimbursement Issues: Summary; GPO Stock No. 0520003-01296-1. (1992). Washington, DC: U.S. Government Printing Office.

Useful Information on Alzheimer's Disease. (1991). Rockville, MD: National Institute of Mental Health, Department of Health and Human Services. DHHS Publication No. (ADM) 90-1696. Brief overview, references, sources for help. Free.

Wall, F. A. (1996). *Where Did Mary Go? A Loving Husband's Struggle with Alzheimer's*. Amherst, NY: Prometheus. Day-to-day road map of the problems, frustrations, solutions as well as the development of a caregiver's courage.

Wilkinson, B. (1995). *Coping When a Grandparent Has Alzheimer's Disease*. New York: Rosen. $15.95. Advice to teenagers on how to deal with complex problems posed by this disease.

Also see audiovisuals in this chapter, on the family and caregivers in Chapter 6 of this guide, and the listing of books for caregivers in the preface of *Mealtime Manual*, under Going Further.

Grandparenting

Cherlin, A. J., & Furstenberg, F. F., Jr. (1992). *The New American Grandparent: A Place in the Family, A Life Apart*. New York: Basic Books, HarperCollins. $14.95. New roles faced by today's grandparents who live longer, often have more education, and are called upon to assist in more crises.

de Toledo, S., & Brown, D. E. (1995). *Grandparents as Parents*. New York: Guilford. $16.95. A survival guide for raising a second family.

Doucette, D. D., & LaCure, J. (1996). *Raising our Children's Children*. Minneapolis: Fairview.

Kornhaber, A., & Woodward, K. L. (1991). *Grandparents/Grandchildren: The Vital Connection*. New York: Anchor Press, Bantam Doubleday Dell. $21.95. Explores emotional attachments between grandparents and grandchildren, the loss of those attachments, and how to establish bonds.

Le Shan, E. (1984). *Grandparents: A Special Kind of Love*. New York: Macmillan. $15. For children, discusses good relationships and what happens when a grandparent is ill or dies.

PERIODICALS

See Appendix D for addresses and rates.

Aging. Washington, DC: United States Administration on Aging, U.S. Department of Health and Human Services. Innovative programs in communities.

Alzheimer's Disease and Associated Disorders—An International Journal.

American Journal of Occupational Therapy. American Occupational Therapy Association.

Focus on Geriatric Care and Rehabilitation. Aspen Publishers. Practical monthly newsletter edited by practicing geriatric specialists. Each issue focuses on one clinical topic with background, assessment, therapeutic approaches, models of treatment, and caregiving concerns.

The Gerontologist. Gerontological Society of America.

Gerontology Special Interest Newsletter. American Occupational Therapy Association. Quarterly, $10 AOTA members, $15 non-members.

Health Report. United Seniors Health Cooperative. Focus on health care and financial matters. Address in Appendix C.

Journal of the American Geriatrics Society. Baltimore: Williams & Wilkins.

Journal of Gerontological Nursing. Thorofare, NJ: SLACK Inc.

Journal of Housing for the Elderly. 2 issues per year, $160. Haworth Press. **Source:** 247.

Modern Maturity. American Association of Retired Persons.

See Periodicals in *Mealtime Manual*.

Topics in Geriatric Rehabilitation. Aspen Publishers. Focuses on one specific area each quarterly issue.

Wiser Now. Better Directions. Monthly.

AUDIOVISUALS

The Alzheimer's Disease and Related Disorders Association has films for distribution. Contact them for the latest list. Some of these include: *Caring: Families Coping with Alzheimer's Disease*; *Do You Remember Love?*; *Living with Grace*; *Someone I Once Knew*; *Whispering Hope*; *You Are Not Alone*.

Dempsey-Lyle, S., & Hoffman, T. L. *Into Aging: Understanding Issues Affecting the Later Stages of Life* (2nd ed.). Thorofare, NJ: SLACK, Inc. $46. Simulation game. A "walk through" the aging process to experience daily living as an elderly individual acquiring physical disabilities, the social and financial setbacks and losses associated with aging.

Ethics Committees: Allies in Long-Term Care. American Association of Retired Persons and the American Association of Homes for the Aging. Interdisciplinary approach: what one does when a patient rejects treatment, refuses to eat, requires restraints. 30 minute video, Facilitator's Manual, up to 25 guidebooks without charge. In bulk, 25 copies are $2.75. #D14172. Free loan; allow 90 days for delivery. To borrow, write AARP, Dept/ER, Program Scheduling Office.

Films and videos on Aging and Sensory Change: Annotated Resource List (3rd ed.). The Lighthouse, Inc. More than 80 resources to educate consumers and professionals about age-related hearing and vision losses, and sensory impairments, $5. **Source:** 326.

Fit After Fifty. Three J Productions, Ltd., $39.95. Exercise VHS tape for the elderly and people who lead a sedentary life. Developed by three women who wanted a workout, not a "wipe-out." Equipment required consists of a chair, a 24-inch loop of 1-inch elastic and a frisbee. **Source:** 526.

Gadgets, Gizmos & Thingamabobs. Serif, Center for the Study of Aging. 19-minute VHS video. 28-minute tape also available. Each comes with a copy of both the *Resource Directory* and the *Presenter's Guide,* $49.95. Makes seniors aware of how self-help devices can improve their lives. Gives hints on how to assess for need, suggests sources for purchase of aids. **Source:** 472.

Home Care for People with Alzheimer's Disease. (1995). Aspen Patient Education Video Series. Frederick, MD: Aspen. $215. Three, 13-minute VHS videos and booklets (activities of daily living, communication, and home safety) will help develop education program for caregivers.

Making Life a Little Easier: Self Help Tools for the Home. Washington, DC: American Association of Retired Persons, Dept/ER. Free loan video. Must request 90 days in advance. Comes with hand-outs listing principles to decide if an aid is needed, sources, publications, and helpful agencies.

Morris, A, & Hunt, G. *A Part of Daily Life: Alzheimer's Caregivers Simplify Activities and the Home.* (1994). Bethesda, MD: American Occupational Therapy Association. 16-minute VHS video and 27-page *Resource Book,* #1122. $25 AOTA members, $35 non-members. Conversations with caregivers and vignettes for use with families.

Senior Exercise Program. Y13 Productions. Gradually paced, 40-minute exercise program with physical therapist leading group through controlled regimen. Accompanied by classical and swing music, $99 plus $6 handling and shipping. **Source:** 588.

CONTINUING EDUCATION

Larson, K. O., Pedretti, L. W., Stevens-Ratchford, R. G., & Crabtree, J. (Eds.). (1996). *Self-Paced Clinical Course, ROTE: The Role of Occupational Therapy with the Elderly.* Bethesda, MD: American Occupational Therapy Association. #3009. $240 AOTA members, $290 non-members. Four modules: 1) geriatric occupational therapy, 2) occupational therapy in health care and community settings, 3) occupational therapy intervention process, and 4) service management issues. Completion gives 24 contact hours. The Association also sponsors frequent continuing education workshops on topics including needs of the elderly and Alzheimer's disease.

Also see Resources in Chapter 3.

AGENCIES CONCERNED WITH NUTRITION

See Appendix C.

2

The Parent Who Has a Disability and the Younger Client

WHEN THE PARENT HAS A DISABILITY

Mothers or fathers who just happen to have a disability raise and enjoy the same active children as anyone else.

Young children are curious and prone to falls. The parent who has a disability needs to prepare with gates, screens, careful storage of dangerous household materials, and other safety precautions. Safety belts and slings add extra protection when moving an infant from one place to another by carriage, cart, or wheelchair. Safety precautions during meal preparation are discussed in *Mealtime Manual*, Chapter 26.

When a parent is using a wheelchair or has upper extremity limitations, highchairs and other equipment should be at the parent's optimal level for feeding, transferring, or lifting the child (Figure 2-1). Make sure that closures on the highchair tray, safety gates, and crib are operable by the parent and that they lock securely.

The self-storing, Wing™ tablet arm tray fits down at the side of the wheelchair while moving, then flips up to allow a parent to carry the child safely (Figure 2-2). A safety belt or sling holder holds the child securely if the parent has weak upper extremities. The Wing™ attaches to all sport or lightweight wheelchairs, three-wheel scooters, and power and manual chairs. Tray is 12 inches wide and 24 inches long and comes with right or left mount. It may be removed by turning one knob. To order, specify side plus type of mobility aid, i.e., wheelchair, manual or powered, three-wheeled power scooter, or sport chair. Cost is about $200. **Sources:** 9, 14, 21, 140, 383, 461, 553.

Nursery equipment should be carefully selected. Adaptations may be made, such as a modified, gated, or side-opening crib that lets the parent slide rather than lift an infant. Deaf parents require non-auditory signals to know when a child is calling or crying; controls attached to a fan or bright light is one solution. Another answer is a hearing ear dog to alert or fetch the parent when needed. See Chapter 20. A baby-view video monitor allows the parent in another room to see a child while he or she is sleeping, even when the bedroom is dark. Cost is about $200 and up from department stores.

Commercially available household safety aids include cabinet locks, toilet lid lock, drawer and appliance latches, lamp and appliance cord keepers to keep items from being pulled over by a child, door knob cover with lock guard to prevent being locked in bathroom, patio door stop set, corner guards, Break-Thru window tassel cords that separate if a child gets entangled in the cords, outlet and plug protector covers, a digital thermometer with no glass, and a baby medi-spoon, which holds liquid in a tubular handle rather than in the bowl of a spoon. **Source** for many items: 457.

When taking the child in an automobile, he or she should always sit in the back seat, secured in a car seat. Finding a car seat with fastenings which the parent with a disability can handle may take some time and modifications. *Parenting with a Disability,* published by Through the Looking Glass, can offer some tested solutions. See Resources.

Articles on parents with various disabilities raising children frequently appear in family service magazines as well as in periodicals for people with disabilities. Check *Accent on Living*, *Spinal Network*, and *Rehabilitation Gazette*. See Periodicals in *Mealtime Manual*. Several resources are listed at the end of this chapter and in Chapter 9.

WHEN THE CHILD HAS A DISABILITY

When a child has a disability, the whole family is involved. A full assessment and evaluation of the child is required. There is also the added dimension of teaching parents the importance of letting the child become as independent as possible. This is true whether working with a young diabetic, who will become responsible for his or her own insulin testing and schedule, or a child with cerebral palsy, muscular dystrophy, or arthrogryposis, who wants to do as much as possible and may require adapted equipment and training to become independent.

You may be working with the child at school, home, or in the hospital. No matter what the locale, communication with staff and family members is paramount to helping the child achieve desired goals.

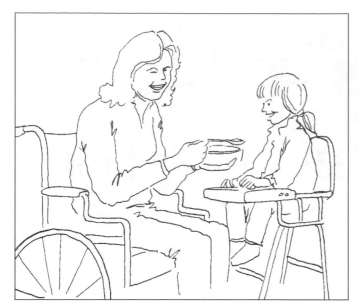

Figure 2-1. When a parent is using a wheelchair or has upper extremity limitations, highchairs and other equipment should be at the parent's optimal level for feeding, transferring, or lifting the child. (Illustration by G.K.)

When teaching meal planning and self-feeding skills, there is an opportunity to instill good nutritional habits while your patient is young. Many materials have been developed to teach children about nutrition. Check publications from the U.S. Consumer Information Center.

Teaching the family is as important as training the patient. It is the family that must carry out and reinforce the techniques and skills throughout each day. Setting up charts, goals, programs, and finding new ways to involve the whole family increase chances of success and are more effective than simply giving verbal suggestions.

Suggesting ways to increase the child's nutritional intake is part of the family's education. Some of the suggestions for the hospice client may be adapted for young clients, such as double-milk shakes. Children will eat vegetables that are part of a soup or casserole more easily than when served separately. Broccoli, carrots, zucchini, and spinach may be grated or chopped and added to spaghetti sauce or lasagna fillings. Adding applesauce or pureed zucchini to cakes and cookies raises nutrition and makes the finished product moister, thus easier to swallow.

When a child is severely disabled, parents have a heavier duty as caregivers and may need encouragement to take respite periods. Mutual self-help or support groups become important reinforcements for the whole family.

As part of a family activity, a child can use an adapted switch to operate an electric mixer (Figure 2-3). **Source:** 4.

See Resources and additional switches in Chapter 9, Chapter 11, and Chapter 27.

Evaluation for a wheelchair must take into account use of the chair at home, in the school, and socially as well as the growing patterns of the child. Just as with adults, modifications may be made in the home to accommodate a wheelchair. For children who use a chair at school, a power chair may be considered, depending on the ability of the child and the school policies. In

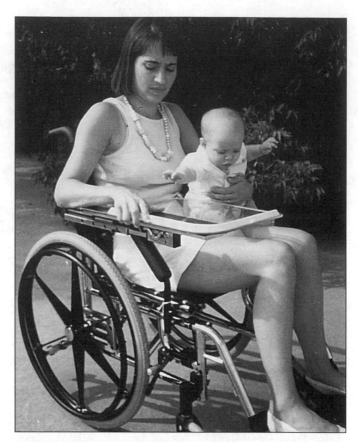

Figure 2-2. The self-storing Wing™ tablet arm tray fits down at the side of wheelchair while moving, then flips up to let this mother with paraplegia carry her child safely and hold her while feeding or playing. (Photo courtesy of Consumer Care Products, Inc., Sheboygan, WI.)

many cases, not having to propel a chair frees an aide for another activity.

A young child who is profoundly involved or ambulatory within a limited range but cannot walk long distances on family or other outings may require the use of a lightweight buggy. The mobile unit should provide comfortable and correct positioning of the trunk, head, and extremities. Accessories include head supports, canopies for sun or rain, and detachable trays. Some units are designed to grow with the child. **Manufacturers** of compact, folding strollers include 145, 395, 499. In the car, a special safety belt that is easy to put on a child who has a disability and allows the child to lie or sit in the back seat is made by 196.

A stander lets a child take a fuller role in family activities and chores (Figure 2-4). The market for standing systems for children is expanding, with several companies making units for children, some for children as young as nine months, the age when children normally begin to pull themselves up to a standing position. Standing systems allow the school-age child to interact more easily at home and school. Some of these are stationary, others mobile. Prices range from about $600 and up, depending on features and size. **Manufacturers** include Consumer Care Products, Inc. (140); Etac USA, Inc. (191); Kayes Products, Inc. (302); Mulholland (372B); Permobil Inc. (408); Rifton (445); Stand Aid of Iowa, Inc. (493); TherAdapt (516B); and TumbleForms (537).

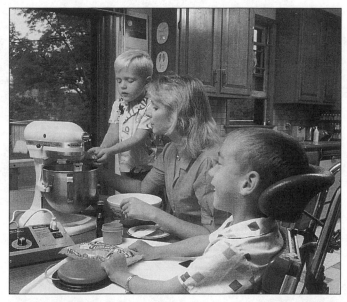

Figure 2-3. As part of a family activity, this child uses an adapted switch to operate the electric mixer. (Photo courtesy of AbleNet®, Inc., Minneapolis, MN.)

A lift allows the parent or child in a wheelchair to be part of family and community activities, without the stress of transfers or lifting of a chair in and out of a vehicle (Figure 2-5). The half lift shown permits passage in and out of the vehicle while the lift is folded. This is helpful when other riders need to come or go or to reach and assist the passenger while in the vehicle. **Source:** 155. Other lifts are discussed in Chapter 30.

DEVELOPING EATING SKILLS

Children with developmental or congenital disabilities may present challenges at mealtime. Immature upper neurosensimotor development, perceptual and cognitive dysfunction, intellectual limitations, and behavior problems create barriers to self-feeding. Correct positioning of the child maximizes function as well as swallowing skills.

When working on feeding skills with a young child, the body must be positioned for maximum function and ease of eating (Figure 2-6). This may be achieved from method of holding by the caregiver to various types of adaptive equipment.

A sling to position or keep a child elevated while in the crib is **manufactured** by 536.

A hand-held nurser encourages self-feeding during infancy, freeing the mother with a disability from holding bottle (Figure 2-7). The open design is also easier to clutch for a child with limitations in hand function, promoting grasping skills and bringing hands to midline. Lightweight plastic with nipple and cap, dishwasher and sterilization safe. **Manufacturer:** 51. **Source:** 14. Cost is about $2.30 each and up from housewares stores and self-help supply firms.

Feeding the child with severe cerebral palsy or aiding an older patient with marked incoordination or spasticity may require stabilization of the body to reduce overflow movements (Figure 2-8). Hand-positioning cones help maintain the hands and fingers in a functional position and prevent deformity. Used in combination

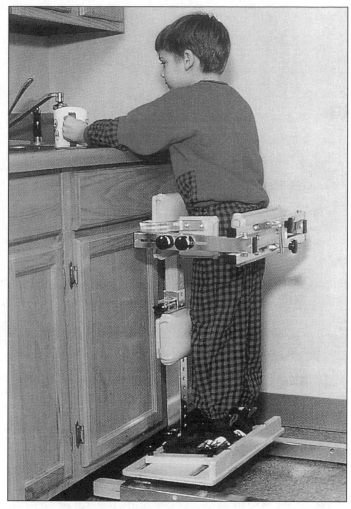

Figure 2-4. A stander lets a child take a fuller role in family activities and chores. (Photo courtesy of Kayes Products, Inc., Hillsborough, NC.)

with surface anchors, they assist in body alignment by stabilizing the shoulders and neck through hand and arm control. Wood cones have a cushioned Plastazote surface. Anchor base may be mounted either vertically or horizontally, with Poly-Lock® hook and loop fastener. **Sources:** 14, 140.

Fashioning an appropriate feeding utensil paired with attractive foods and calm persevering training with the child and caregiver results in success. See Chapter 4, Chapter 11, Chapter 21, and Chapter 22.

Special eating utensils help when teaching feeding skills (Figure 2-9). The maroon spoon has a narrow, shallow bowl. It is designed for feeding therapy with children who have poor lip closure, hypersensitivity, and tongue thrust. Cost is about $17 for a set of 25 small spoons, $21 for a set of 25 large spoons. A Flexi-cup is helpful for early cup training because you control the shape of the rim by gently squeezing the sides. Cost is $12 for a set of five. **Sources** for both items: 1, 132, 140, 294.

A Scooper™ bowl or plate aids children in feeding themselves (Figure 2-10). The curved rim guides food into the spoon, while the suction base keeps it in place. Bowl with the ring removed is top-shelf dishwasher safe and may be sterilized. **Manufacturer:**

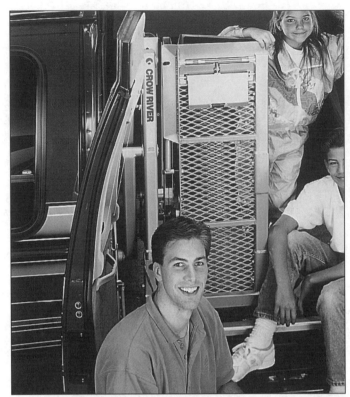

Figure 2-5. A lift allows the individual in a wheelchair to be part of family and community activities, without the stress of transfers or lifting of a chair in and out of the vehicle. (Photo courtesy of Crow River Industries, Inc., Minneapolis, MN.)

531. Cost is about $4 from housewares stores.

An L-shaped spoon may let a child with severe developmental delay or cerebral palsy eat independently after initial training (Figure 2-11). Unlike using a regular built-up spoon, which requires wrist motion, this adapted utensil requires the child just to flex the elbow and slightly supinate the forearm to bring it to his or her mouth. Spoon bowl may be angled to catch the food. It should be used with a scoop dish or plate guard. The angled handle keeps the hand from contacting the food, maintaining concentration on the feeding process.

Handling liquid medicines with an infant who has normal or abnormal excess motions or when the parent has hand limitations is easier with an oral syringe or bulb-type dosage dropper (Figure 2-12). To use the syringe, an adaptor is placed into the mouth of the medicine bottle, the tip of the dispenser is fitted into it, and the plunger pulled. Markings on the side give volume in milliliters or fractions of a teaspoon. Liquid is released through the tip, right into the child's mouth, far enough back to make swallowing easier than with a spoon. Syringe is top-shelf dishwasher safe. **Manufacturers:** 53, 53B, 250. Cost is about $1.50 each and up from pharmacies.

RESOURCES

Addresses for publishers, periodicals, and organizations are given in Section Four. For additional resources, see Going Further in *Mealtime Manual*, Chapter 26.

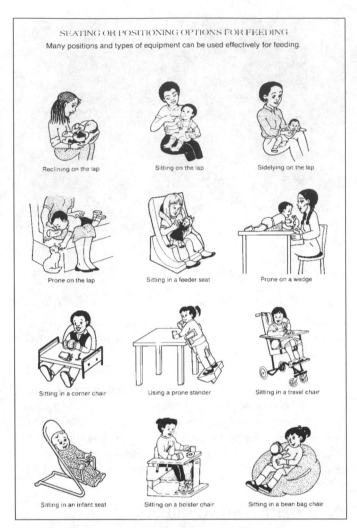

Figure 2-6. When working on feeding skills with a young child, the body must be positioned for maximum function and ease of eating. (From *Pre-Feeding Skills*, copyright 1987, Therapy Skill Builders, San Antonio, TX. Reprinted with permission.)

PUBLICATIONS

Adaptive Parenting Equipment, Idea Book I. See *Mealtime Manual*, Chapter 26.

American Heart Association Kids' Cookbook. Thirty recipes geared for 8- to 12-year-olds include pizza, chicken nuggets, pasta, microwave food, and snacks. AHA approved, kid-tested. Includes safety and nutrition basics. A great way to start parent and child cooking together. $15 plus $2 shipping from the American Heart Association.

Batshaw, M. L., & Perret, Y. (1992). *Children With Disabilities—A Medical Primer*. Baltimore: Brookes. $28.

Batshaw, M. L. (1991). *Your Child Has a Disability: A Practical Guide to Daily Care*. Boston: Little Brown. $18.95.

Bauman, C., & Fishman, S. E. *The Child Chart: Childhood Inventory of Language and Development (CHILD)*. Vero Beach, FL: The Speech Bin. $8.50. Comprehensive wall chart includes skills in language, gross and fine motor skills, and social behavior. **Source:** 488.

Bernstein, J., & Fireside, B. J. (1991). *Special Parents/Special*

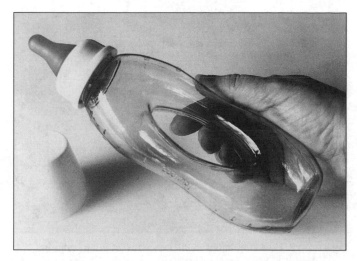

Figure 2-7. This hand-held nurser encourages self-feeding during infancy, freeing the mother with a disability from holding bottle. (Bottle by Ansa® Bottle Co., Inc., Muskogee, OK. Photo by J.K.)

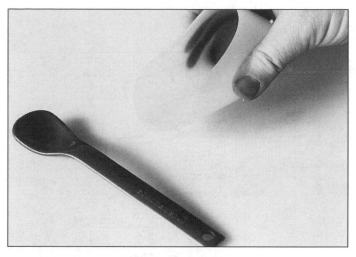

Figure 2-9. Special eating utensils help when teaching feeding skills. (Photo by J.K.)

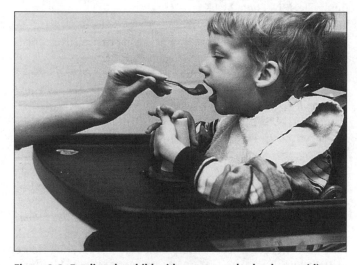

Figure 2-8. Feeding the child with severe cerebral palsy or aiding an older patient with marked incoordination or spasticity may require stabilization of the body to reduce overflow movements. (Photo courtesy of Consumer Care Products, Inc., Sheboygan, WI.)

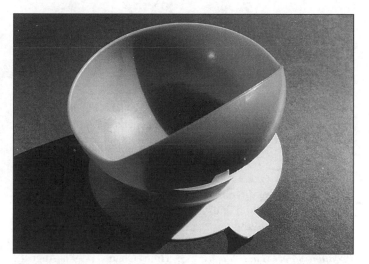

Figure 2-10. A Scooper™ bowl or plate aids child in self-feeding. (Photo by J.K.)

Children. Morton Grove, IL: A. Whitman. $12.95. Four families with handicapped parents, grades 3 to 7.

Blackman, J. (1989). *Medical Aspects of Developmental Disabilities in Children Birth to Three* (2nd ed.). Frederick, MD: Aspen. $43. Revised classic reference summarizes 39 medical conditions and treatments. Each receives description, course, management, educational implications.

Brewer, E. J., & Angel, K. C. (1995). *Parenting a Child with Arthritis: A Practical, Empathetic Guide to Help You and Your Child Live with Arthritis.* Los Angeles: Lowell House. $15.00.

Briggs, M. H. (1996). *Building Early Intervention Teams: Working Together for Children and Families.* Frederick, MD: Aspen. $48. Helps early intervention professionals establish, maintain, and grow more effective teams for young clients and their families.

Buscaglia, L. *The Disabled and Their Parents* (3rd. ed.). Thorofare, NJ: SLACK, Inc. $22.95.

Campion, M. J. (1990). *The Baby Challenge: A Handbook on Pregnancy for Women with a Physical Disability.* New York: Routledge. $15.95.

Children's Disability Bookshop Catalog. The Disability Bookshop, Vancouver, Wash. Shop-by-mail catalog listing hard-to-find titles covering a wide range of health topics for children including asthma, cerebral palsy, deafness, Down Syndrome, learning disabilities, head and brain injury, resource directories, $4 postage and handling. **Source:** 169.

Cohen L. R., et al. (1996). *Child Development, Health, and Safety: Educational Materials for Home Visitors and Parents.* Frederick, MD: Aspen. $59. Reproducible parent education sheets, checklists, forms, and instructions. Includes tools, development and health, safety, parenting, visit ideas, cues to child maltreatment. Safety, for example, covers baby walkers, the kitchen, fire prevention, car seats, etc.

Cole, D. J. (1990).Feeding Programs for Children Who Refuse to Eat—A Case Study. *Occupational Therapy Forum*, 5 (41), Developmental delay.

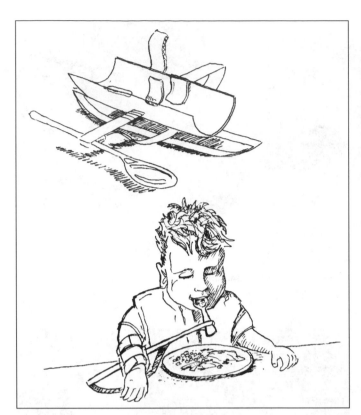

Figure 2-11. An L-shaped spoon may let a child with severe developmental delay or cerebral palsy eat independently after initial training. (Illustration by G.K.)

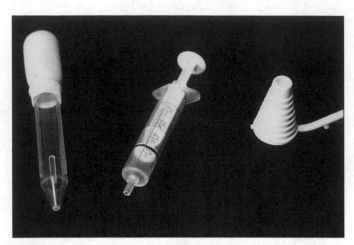

Figure 2-12. Handling liquid medicines with an infant who has normal or abnormal excess motions or when the parent has hand limitations is easier with an oral syringe or bulb-type dosage dropper. (Bulb-type oral syringe from Health Enterprises, Inc., North Attleboro, MA; syringe-type from Apothecary Products, Burnsville, MN. Photo by J.K.)

Consumer's Guide to Therapeutic Services for Children with Disabilities. Cambridge, MA: Human Services Research Institute with United Cerebral Palsy Associations. Order from Human Services. **Source:** 269.

Crib Safety—Keep Them on the Safe Side (1985, October). *Product Safety Fact Sheets,* 43. High Chairs (1990, August). *Product Safety Fact Sheets,* 70. Washington, DC: U.S. Consumer Product Safety Commission. Free.

Dickson, I., & Gordon, S. (1993). *One Miracle at a Time: Getting Help for a Child with a Disability* (rev. ed.). New York: Fireside, Simon & Schuster.

Dunn, W. W. (Ed.). (1990). *Pediatric Occupational Therapy: Facilitating Effective Service Provision.* Thorofare, NJ: SLACK Inc. $46. Theoretical and clinical applications for assessment and treatment of pediatric service delivery. Case studies, evaluation charts, family perspective, federal and local laws governing referral, assessment, and treatment.

Feeding Position Stickers. (1987). San Antonio, TX: Therapy Skill Builders. $11.95. Illustrates 13 positions recommended to help physically handicapped children maximize oral motor skills for eating. **Source:** 522.

Garee, B. (Ed.). (1989). *Parenting: Tips From Parents (who happen to have a disability) on Raising Children.* Bloomington, IL: Accent. $7.95. **Source:** 8.

Gartner, A., et al. (1991). *Supporting Families with a Child with a Disability.* Baltimore: Brookes. $25. Discusses the significance that various cultures and their values play in defining disability and types of treatment offered or accepted. Professionals as facilitators

assist family in developing expertise and competence; gives strategies for implementing program of support.

Holzberg, R., & Walsh-Burton, S. (1995). *The Parental Voice: Problems Faced by Parents of the Deaf-Blind, Severely and Profoundly Handicapped Child.* Springfield, IL: Charles C. Thomas. $37.95.

Jaeger, D. L. (1989). *Transferring and Lifting Children and Adolescents: Home Instruction Sheets.* San Antonio, TX: Therapy Skill Builders. $39. Physical therapist gives parents and caregivers instruction sheets for 10 categories of transfers. 74 loose-leaf reproducible sheets in tabbed binder.

Hanson, M. J. (1977). *Teaching Your Down's Syndrome Infant: A Guide for Parents.* Originally published by University Park Press. Order code 324.008, $20 from the National Clearing House of Rehabilitation Training Materials. Program for the child from birth to two years. Suggestions for scoring the level of response in each skill area to determine when to begin the next level.

Klein, M. D., & Delaney, T. A. *Feeding and Nutrition for the Child With Special Needs: Handouts for Parents.* San Antonio, TX: Therapy Skill Builders. $97. Integrated feeding and nutrition tips for family and caregivers of infants and children of all ages. 195 reproducible hand-outs cover nutrition guidelines, tube feedings, independent feeding, breast and bottle feeding, introduction of spoon feeding, cup and straw drinking, oral-motor treatments, nutrition treatment strategies, conditions affecting feeding and nutrition, family mealtime interactions, and communication.

Learning to Live with Disability: A Guidebook for Families. National Rehabilitation Information Center.

Magination Press, Brunner/Mazel, publishes books to help children understand their disabilities: *Putting on the Brakes: Young People's Guide to Understanding Attention Deficit Hyperactivity Disorder,* by Patricia O. Quinn and Judith M. Stern, 1991, $10; *You Can Call Me Willy: A Story for Children About AIDS,* by Joan C. Verniero, 1995, $9; *Sarah and Puffle: A Story for Children About Diabetes,* by Linnea Mulder, 1992, $12. **Source:** 99.

Marsh, J. B. (Ed.). (1995). *From the Heart: On Being the Mother of a Child With Special Needs*. Bethesda, MD: Woodbine House. $14.95. Narratives by nine mothers on raising children with special needs, relationships with professionals, family, and schools. Helps understanding by professionals and teachers who do not understand the role they endure.

McAnaney, K. D. (1992). *I Wish...Dreams and Realities of Parenting a Special Needs Child*. United Cerebral Palsy Association of California. $8.95. Contact United Cerebral Palsy Associations.

Miller, N. B. (1994). *Nobody's Perfect: Living and Growing with Children Who Have Special Needs*. Baltimore, MD: Brookes, $21.

Moore, C. B., & Morton, K. G. *A Reader's Guide for Parents of Children with Mental, Physical, or Emotional Disabilities*. Washington, DC: National Center for Education in Maternal and Child Health.

Morris, S. E., & Klein, M. D. *Pre-Feeding Skills: A Comprehensive Resource for Feeding Development*. San Antonio, TX: Therapy Skill Builders. $55. Framework for developing therapy plan, from anatomy and normal development to assessment and treatment, from birth to adolescence.

National Information Center for Children and Youth with Disabilities, Minneapolis. Write for list of publications.

National Research & Training Center on Families of Adults with Disabilities. Clearinghouse of bibliographies and other materials pertaining to parenting with a disability, national database of parents with disabilities, assistive technology and parenting project that develops and studies the impact of equipment to assist parents with a disability, training of and consultation to parents and professionals. Produce newsletter, *Parenting with a Disability,* three times a year free of charge. See Periodicals in *Mealtime Manual.*

Pediatrics: Resource Guide. (1994). Bethesda, MD: American Occupational Therapy Association. #4230. $10 AOTA members, $20 non-members. Bibliographies, audiovisuals, resource personnel.

Queen, P. M., & Lang, C. E. (1992). *Handbook of Pediatric Nutrition*. Frederick, MD: Aspen. $70. Growth, nutritional assessment pre-term through adolescence.

Ratto, L. L. (1991). *Coping with Being Physically Challenged*. New York: Rosen. For teenager who has physical disabilities as well as anger and depression, shows how to cope on a day-to-day basis.

The Safe Nursery. (1989). Washington, DC: U.S. Consumer Product Safety Commission. Publication No. 202. Free. Discussion and checklists help any parent purchase safe equipment for a child.

Tips for Your Baby's Safety. (1985). Washington, DC: U.S. Consumer Product Safety Commission. Free.

What Everyone Should Know About Child Safety. (1983). South Deerfield, MA: Channing L. Bete Co. $1.25 per copy. Illustrated booklet reviewing prevention of accidents in traffic, fire, home storage, selection of equipment, and teaching of babysitters. **Source:** 114.

Wolff, L. S., & Glass, R. P. (1992). *Feeding and Swallowing Disorders in Infancy: Assessment and Management*. San Antonio, TX: Therapy Skill Builders. $63. Information on sucking, swallowing, and breathing to aid in evaluation of infants ages birth to one year.

PERIODICALS

Addresses and rates in Appendix D.

Child. See *Mealtime Manual. The Organized Parent* from publishers of *Child* provides an excellent outline for working with the new mother.

Closer Look. Free quarterly newsletter with articles, news, and suggestions for parents of physically or mentally handicapped children. Project of Parents' Campaign for Handicapped Children and Youth.

Directions: Technology in Special Education, DREAMMS for Kids. Newsletter for parents and educators of young students and children with special needs. Technology tips, easing home instruction, software and hardware reviews.

Down Syndrome Amongst Us. Published by young mother of son with Down Syndrome. For information call 718-834-2055.

The Exceptional Child.

The Exceptional Parent: The Magazine for Families and Professionals. Also have website, the Family Education Network (FEN): http://families.com.

Infants and Young Children. Interdisciplinary Journal of Special Care Practices. Aspen.

Parenting. See *Mealtime Manual.*

Parents. See *Mealtime Manual.*

Through the Looking Glass. Parenting with a Disability. See *Mealtime Manual.*

AUDIOVISUALS

Disability and Motherhood. Fanlight Productions. 25-minute VHS video, CL-192. $195 purchase. Three women with disabilities including cerebral palsy, blindness, and use of a wheelchair confront viewers with the reality that love and caring are the most important "abilities" to be a good parent. **Source:** 200.

Don't Cry for Me. Oak Tree, Inc., 54-minute VHS video, CK-095. Also Kondrat, M. *Embers of the Fire*. 28-minute VHS video, CK-098. And Weinrich, J. *Heartland*. Red Motel Pictures. 60-minute VHS video, CK-114. And *Keeping the Balance*. University of Calgary and the Alberta Lung Association. 23-minute VHS video, CK-089. Four videos on children with cystic fibrosis, $99 each. Write Fanlight Productions for descriptions. **Source:** 200.

In the Middle. Child, Youth & Family Services, Fanlight Productions. 28-minute VHS video, CL-011. $99. Child with spina bifida, her family, teachers, and classmates document problems and joys during her first year mainstreamed in Head Start program. **Source:** 200.

Kaufman, T. *See What I'm Saying*. Fanlight Productions. 31-minute VHS video, CL-090. $195. Follows deaf child from a speaking family through first year at elementary school at Gallaudet University. Demonstrates acquisition of communications skills. Program is close-captioned, dubbed, and signed. **Source:** 200.

Mortola, P., & Walsh, P. (Producers). (1991). *Children with Cerebral Palsy: A Look into Techniques for Parents and Professionals*. Bethesda, MD: American Occupational Therapy Association. VHS video, 25 minutes. #8030V (for purchase only), $75 AOTA members/$95 non-members. "Bridges the gap" between clinic and home, educating parents on basic concepts and techniques that OTs use in clinical settings.

Nelson, C. A. From *Clinician's View: Issues in Cerebral Palsy*. Three videos: assessment; application of focused treatment; and positioning for promotion of functional skill. Also Magrun, W. M. *Somatic Application in Cerebral Palsy: Linking Assessment with Treatment* and *Feeding as a Process of Accommodation*. And Nolan, C. A. *Effective Intervention for Self-Feeding Success*. Write for full catalog descriptions and costs. **Source:** 124.

Satter, E. *Feeding with Love and Good Sense*. San Antonio, TX: Therapy Skill Builders. Series, $177, single tapes $59 each. Four 15-minute color VHS videos cover basics of feeding at different ages: infant, older baby, toddler, and preschooler. **Source:** 522.

Uzes, P. *They Don't Come With Manuals*. Fanlight Productions. 29-minute, VHS video, CL-038. $145. Coping techniques of raising a child with a disability from parents' perspective. Interviews several families about their quests for knowledge, experiences with professionals, the rewards as well as the stresses. **Source:** 200.

Also see *Caring for Persons with Developmental Disabilities: A Training Program for Respite Care Providers* in Chapter 21 and Resources in Chapter 4.

CHAPTER 3

The Client Who Lives Alone

Individuals of any age with disabilities who live alone have specific requirements based on their social and health needs. Factors for the health care worker to assess include safety within the home and its environment, fire plans and the emergency system, nutrition, social support, and general health.

Encouraging your clients to share a meal at a senior center or other group setting adds spice to life and increases interest in nutrition (Figure 3-1). Churches and local organizations provide lunches on a daily or special-occasion basis.

A telephone reassurance service is a safety net that should be available in every community for people who live alone, are permanently or temporarily homebound, or are frail and elderly (Figure 3-2). This automatic, daily call at a pre-selected time checks on the client's welfare; if the call is not answered, the service summons help by calling a pre-selected neighbor, relative, health care worker, or the fire or police department. It provides security to the client, family, and health care system.

If a telephone reassurance program is not accessible to your clients, you might help set one up. It may be done locally through a visiting nurse service, nursing home, police or fire department, or other reliable organization. For information on starting a program, see Resources. A national telephone reassurance subscriber service is available through TeleAssure™. You may call a DemoLine. Cost is about $1 a day; two calls plus a message for the day are provided. The client must be able to press a specific button (which may be highlighted) to let the caller know contact has been made; the client may also speak to the service. The time of the next call is given. This is an opportunity to let the service know if the recipient will be away. **Source:** 511.

Several types of telephones, such as a push-button phone with big numbers and emergency contacts highlighted, allow an individual with physical or cognitive difficulties to more easily call for help. See *Mealtime Manual*, Chapter 11. One phone unit, the Voiceprint, dials an individual when the name is said. Up to 20 names may be stored. It also works as a speakerphone. **Source:** 256. Cost is about $200. Other phones have headsets built in. The person who tires when holding a receiver or cannot grasp a receiver may prefer a headset. Cost is about $50 and up. **Sources** include 235, 256.

Cordless phones can travel with the person in an apartment or house for use in case of emergency. Cost is about $45 and up. A holster or pocket to carry the phone on a belt or attached to a walker or wheelchair may be easily devised or purchased from mail-order firms. **Sources:** 241, 361, 508, 561B.

An emergency response system travels with the client and allows immediate contact if the subscriber should fall or have an emergency (Figure 3-3). A wireless, water-resistant pendant is worn around the neck. Pushing a button allows a call to be sent to a central board. Various organizations within an area provide back-up operator service. These include hospitals, fire, ambulance, and police departments, or an independent agency. See *Mealtime Manual*, Chapter 11, for an example of a national company. National **sources** include 281, 323. Some units have special features, such as a medication or memory jogger up to four times a day, a programmable activity monitor that reports if no activity has been detected within a selected period of time and summons help, door/window sensors, and optional fire and temperature safety (if heat goes off or rises too quickly) sensors. The medical history of the individual is kept on a computer database so it can be communicated to an emergency team while they are en route to the person's assistance.

When cost is a major factor, one can purchase a personal assistance system not connected to a central board but pre-programmed with an alarm to alert neighbors and four pre-selected numbers (which may include neighbors, relatives, and the fire department), that are called in rotation until a human response is achieved. The unit then plays a pre-recorded voice message; the listener can push a button to get more information or, failing to obtain a response, summon help. Cost is about $140. **Sources:** 59, 98, 235.

Security systems for a home may also be considered and are discussed in Chapter 24.

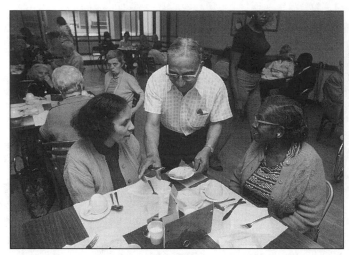

Figure 3-1. Encouraging your clients to share a meal at a senior center or other group setting adds spice to life and increases interest in nutrition. (Photo courtesy of ACTION®, Washington, DC.)

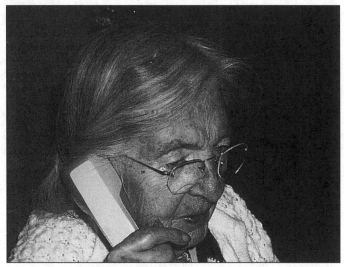

Figure 3-2. A telephone reassurance service is a safety net for people who live alone, are permanently or temporarily homebound, or are frail and elderly. (Photo by J.K.)

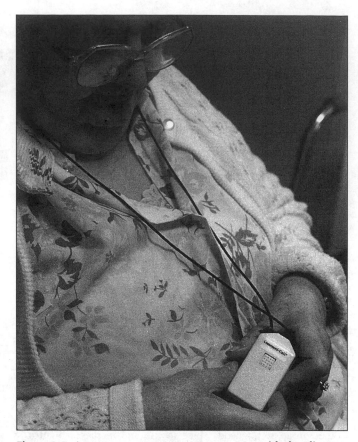

Figure 3-3. An emergency response system stays with the client and allows immediate contact if the subscriber should fall or have an emergency. (Photo by J.K.)

(Figure 3-4). Lighter in weight and lower in cost, they may, with homemaking training, encourage your client to better nutrition. Recommendations of menus or recipes designed for one or two servings can also stimulate your patient's eating desire. **Manufacturer:** 530. Handle removes for washing. Cost is about $35 from department stores and mail-order firms including 273, 295, 558.

PETS

Studies have documented the contribution of pets to better mental health and overall well-being for older people and those who live alone. If you have a patient who would benefit from the added security and companionship of a dog or cat, contact Purina Pets for People. Sponsored by the Ralston-Purina Company, the program will bring together your client with a pet that needs a home. Address is in Appendix C. Other pet programs, including service dogs, are discussed in Chapter 20 and Chapter 30.

APPLIANCES

Appliances designed for use when cooking for one or two include mini-food processors, crockery cookers, and skillets

RESOURCES

Addresses for publishers, periodicals, and organizations are given in Section Four.

PUBLICATIONS

Better Homes & Gardens Great Cooking for Two. (1992). Des Moines, IA: Meredith. $16.95. More than 200 easy-to-prepare recipes that often rely on fruit- or yogurt-based sauces to provide flavor without added fat. Larger-print book includes streamlined preparation techniques, photos, and nutritional breakdowns.

Bustad, L. K. (1981). *Animals, Aging, and the Aged.* Minneapolis: University of Minnesota Press. Out-of-print, check with local library. Overview by veterinarian of contributions of companion animals to the elderly with guidelines on selecting a pet.

Care-Ring Information Sheet, San Pedro Hospital, 1300 W. Seventh Street, San Pedro, CA 90732. How to start a volunteer telephone reassurance service.

Oliver, M. (1990). *Marge Oliver's Good Food for One* and *Marge Oliver's Cookbook for Seniors*. Bellingham, WA: Self-Counsel Press. $9.95 each. Larger-print, easy recipes to meet single-serving requirements as well as the needs of two or more people.

The Delta Society and Therapet Press, **Source:** 519, both offer materials on the therapeutic value of pets for the elderly or isolated individual.

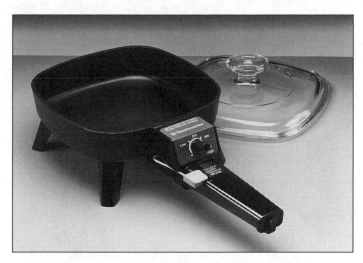

Figure 3-4. This mini-electric skillet is designed for the single cook. (Photo courtesy of Toastmaster®, Inc., Columbia, MO.)

4

The Client with Eating Difficulties

Feeding oneself is one of the first skills we seek to master as children. Self-feeding soon becomes a social as well as a personal activity.

The problems that clients face in this area vary widely. Complete evaluation and assessment of neck and trunk stability, swallowing patterns, and upper extremity function should be done by an occupational therapist and speech therapist. As a health care provider, you may find the needs of your client to be physical, as well as emotional. Sometimes, you may be asked to teach a patient how to transfer from gastronomy tube to oral feeding. You may be the individual with whom a hospice or ALS patient discusses fears of a future change to tube feeding. The person with whom you are working may have a complete lack of interest in food due to loss of taste, reactions from medications, dementia, or eating disorders, such as anorexia nervosa or bulimia. Our focus in the guide is on physical disabilities, but some references to other eating disorders and problems are given in the Resources at the end of this chapter.

Physical limitations in grasp and range of motion may be overcome with adapted cutlery. Inability to see the plate or control motions is helped by scoop-shaped containers and plate guards against which to push the eating utensil. Added weight may reduce incoordination in cases where strength is not affected. Devices are described and illustrated in Chapter 22 in *Mealtime Manual*.

EATING ASSESSMENT KIT

If working with physical limitations, an assessment kit permits efficient evaluation of needs. Recommended items might include the following:
- Dycem®, **Source:** 178; Medi Grip®, **Source:** 554; Posey Grip®, **Source:** 413; or Neotex® protective mesh matting, **Source:** 442; for stabilizing plates and dishes.
- Scoop dish or plate.
- Plate guards for large and small plates.

- Cylindrical foam or varied sizes of foam curlers to make built-up handles.
- Utensils with built-up handles.
- Swivel spoon.
- Fold-up extension holder.
- Universal cuff with palmar pocket.
- Cock-up splint with palmar pocket.
- Rocker knife.
- Mug with large handle.
- Covered mug with large handle.
- Flexible cup.
- Long straws.
- Short straws with flexible necks.
- Small, sharp knife with large handle.

Optional aids might include the following:
- Bibs for adults and children.
- Octopus holders.
- Rubber spoon.
- Weighted spoon.
- Cushion grip tape.
- Dycem® pressure sensitive tape.
- Quad-Quip™ meat cutter knife, **Source:** 383.
- Glass holder.
- T-handle mug.
- Mug or cup with spout.
- T-handle knife.

A basic feeding evaluation kit costs about $100 from **source:** 461.

Additional aids might include:
- Balanced forearm orthoses and/or overhead slings if working with individuals with severe physical handicaps.
- Food processor, blender, or manual strainer/food mill for mashing and pureeing, if working with patients with swallowing difficulties. Hand-held blenders allow mixing of soups or powdered drinks directly in cup or bowl. See Chapter 5.

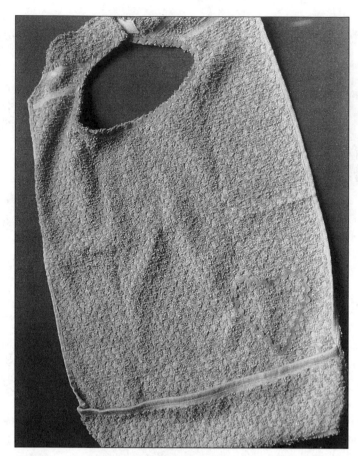

Figure 4-1. A regular hand towel may be quickly adapted as here. A four-inch deep tray at the bottom catches crumbs. Velcro® tabs at the back fasten the bib securely. (Photo by J.K.)

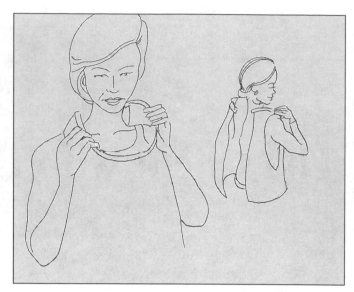

Figure 4-2. A flexible plastic headband threaded through a casing around the neck allows the client to put the bib on independently. (Illustration by G.K.)

EATING SURFACE

The height of the table or lapboard from which the individual takes his or her food can affect performance. Poor posture reduces the ability to use utensils safely and efficiently. Check both the seating and height. Add lateral supports if trunk muscles are weak, and also consider them if your patient tires quickly.

A chair with arms provides lateral support and is easier to sit down in and get up from when lower extremities are unsteady or weak. An office swivel chair with the casters removed lets a person with limited mobility, such as caused by Parkinson's disease or arthritis, comfortably get into a close enough position at the table. If reaching is difficult, eating training may start while seated in a wheelchair with a lapboard that allows close placement of the food or a pull-up table that fits between the arms of the chair. See the Matilda Walking Table in Chapter 13.

BIBS

If a client has marked difficulty handling food, a bib helps preserve dignity. Adult cloth and vinyl bibs that provide full-front protection and come with Velcro® closures are available through hospital supply firms, or a pattern may be drawn and volunteers or even another patient as part of his or her therapy enlisted to make up several. Cost of a commercially available

bib is about $7 and up. **Sources:** 21, 171, 176, 198, 202, 383, 461, 553.

An adult sized bib may be made of single-thickness terrycloth or of double-thickness, machine washable material with terrycloth on one side and cotton or lightweight vinyl on the other (Figure 4-1).

A flexible plastic headband threaded through a casing around the neck allows the client to put the bib on independently without having to reach the back of the neck (Figure 4-2).

EATING AIDS

Eating aids are described and illustrated in *Mealtime Manual*, Chapter 22. The therapist may add to his or her eating evaluation kit with materials to build up utensils that the patient has at home and include a can of non-skid coating to apply to bases of dishes and bowls. The spray lasts from three to six months and is easily removed with rubbing alcohol. **Source:** 205.

Note: Eating utensils that combine a spoon/fork with a cutting blade are not recommended.

Eating utensils with built-up handles are widely available from hospital and self-help supply firms (Figure 4-3). See *Mealtime Manual*, Chapter 22.

Materials for building up handles of eating and other utensils are available from therapy supply firms (Figure 4-4). Dyna-Form-It® is a custom molding rubber reinforced with Kevlar® in a putty-like form. It dries in 24 hours, is non-toxic, washable, and waterproof when dry. **Sources:** 33, 334, 461. Cost is about $12 per can.

The Handi-Cuff was designed by a person with hand limitations (Figure 4-5). It may be used on the right or left hand for holding utensils for eating, cooking, writing, brushing teeth, and operating a typewriter or computer. Small springs secure the tool. **Manufacturer:** 300. **Source:** 279. Cost is about $11.

A turn-round universal holder rotates 360° for optimal positioning (Figure 4-6). This flexibility makes it a good assessment tool as well as a permanent multi-use device. It is designed to

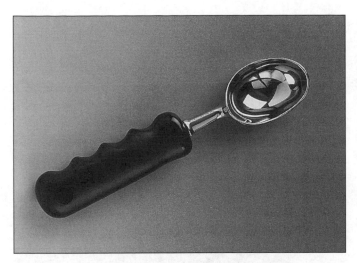

Figure 4-3. Eating utensils with built-up handles are widely available from hospital and self-help supply firms. (Photo courtesy of Lifetime Hoan.)

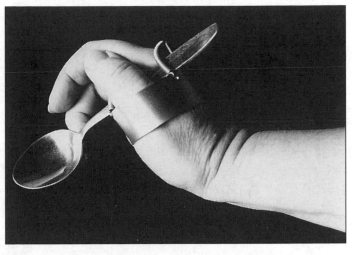

Figure 4-5. The Handi-Cuff, from K&S Enterprises, was designed for a person with hand limitations. (Photo by J.K.)

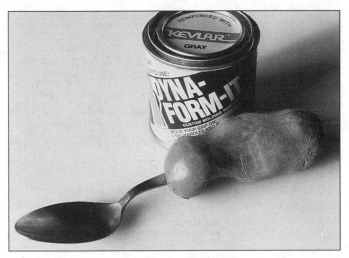

Figure 4-4. Dyna-Form-It® is a custom molding rubber reinforced with Kevlar® in a putty-like form. (Photo by J.K.)

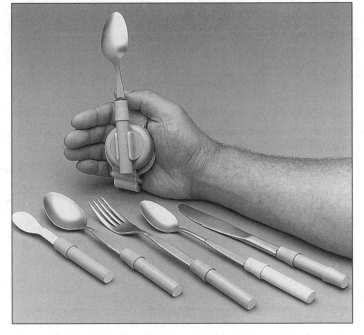

Figure 4-6. This turn-round universal holder rotates 360° for optimal positioning. (Photo courtesy of Smith & Nephew Rolyan, Inc., Germantown, WI.)

assist a person with loss of grasp from quadriplegia, muscular dystrophy, Guillain-Barré, arthritis, and other diseases where grip is weak. The high density cuff with holder attaches to either hand with Velcro® and comes with a variety of accessories that are dishwasher safe. These include a fork, iced tea spoon, soup spoon, cartridge razor, toothbrush, hairbrush, and other holders. **Source:** 481. Cost is about $14 for the holder and $5.50 to $16 for each accessory from self-help equipment firms.

EATING AIDS FOR USE WITH SEVERE LOSS OF UPPER EXTREMITY FUNCTION

Occasionally, it becomes necessary to design an eating aid to overcome limited motion as with severe rheumatoid arthritis or arthrogryposis. Extension handles or L-shaped handles on utensils may compensate for limited range. If commercially available

utensils are not appropriate, aids may be custom-designed so even the most severely limited can eat independently.

Overhead slings and ball-bearing forearm orthoses permit patients with severe loss of muscle power in the upper extremities to eat independently. This includes quadriplegics and individuals with multiple sclerosis, post-polio paralysis, amyotrophic lateral sclerosis, muscular dystrophy, and cerebral palsy. In cases of marked ataxia, friction adaptations to the feeder arms compensate for overflow motion. **Sources:** 14, 33, 292, 383, 461. See Chapter 9.

A forearm support allows gravity reduced, self-feeding when working with a temporary weakness such as Guillain-Barré (Figure 4-7). The unit may stand independently or be attached to

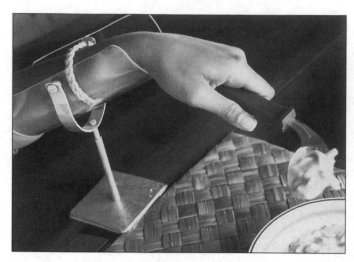

Figure 4-7. This forearm support allows gravity-reduced self-feeding when working with a temporary weakness such as Guillain-Barré. (Photo by J.K.)

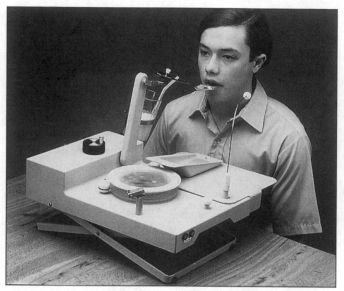

Figure 4-8. The Winsford feeder aids the person with complete loss of arm function. (Photo courtesy of Winsford Products, Pennington, NJ.)

the eating surface with a clamp. Cost is about $40 from rehabilitation firms. **Sources:** 33, 383, 461.

Occasionally, a patient with no functional use of his or her upper extremities will be motivated to feed himself or herself. Battery-powered feeders permit self-feeding.

The Winsford feeder allows the person with complete loss of arm function to eat soup and cereal, as well as solid food, select spoon contents, and sip liquids at his or her own pace with a normal dish and spoon (Figure 4-8). It is battery-operated for flexibility of location. The user must be able to sit in an upright position and have reasonable control of head motion.

Operation is by a hand/foot or chin switch. Pushing the switch in one direction moves food onto the spoon and raises the spoon to the mouth. Repeating that motion returns the utensil to the plate. Pressing the switch in the other direction rotates the plate to place the food in front of the pusher. Some foods must be cut to spoon size. A slight head motion to the right permits drinking liquids from a glass, cup, or milk carton with aid of a bendable straw. Cost including fitted carrying case is about $2453 through medical equipment dealers in the U.S. and Canada. **Manufacturer:** 582. **Sources:** 383, 461, 582. A similar unit is available from **source** 362.

DRINKING AIDS

One-way straws are helpful for patients, such as those with Parkinson's disease, who have difficulty sucking. A one-way valve stays filled with liquid after removing it from the lips, eliminating sucking in air and reducing the energy required. The straw may be washed normally or sterilized by boiling. A clip on the side stabilizes it on a glass or cup. A package of two straws, one seven-inch and one 10-inch, is about $5.50 from hospital suppliers. **Sources:** 205, 383.

The translucent Flexi Cut-Out cup for infants or people with feeding difficulties lets the therapist or caregiver visually monitor the flow of fluid (Figure 4-9). It is flexible enough to shape to the mouth

and has a wide cut-out to reduce neck extension. **Sources:** 132, 294, 302. Cost is about $3.50 each; a set of five is $8. The child being fed is supported by roll bolsters, available from **source** 132.

A gravity-assisted drinking cup assists the client who has difficulty drinking independently. The therapist or patient controls the flow of liquid intake by adjusting the position of the cup or by blocking the opening. An eight-ounce cup with six straws costs about $9. Replacement straws are available. **Source:** 383.

Also see the dose cup in Chapter 5.

The person who must increase or maintain fluid intake needs to have water or other liquid close at hand. In a wheelchair, this may be done by attaching a small tray or cup holder to the arm of the chair. **Sources:** 8, 21, 198, 383, 461. Cost is about $6 and up from self-help equipment firms.

An over-arm chair tray has an adjustable clamp for use with furniture or wheelchair arms (Figure 4-10). The 13-inch by 9½-inch surface has inserts for beverages, plate, television remote control, and more. Of ABS plastic, it may be used indoors and out. Stable for lightweight items, it is not designed for heavy weights, such as bowls for meal preparation. Cost is about $20. **Sources:** 361, 476, 508, 545, 561B.

For the person not using a wheelchair, a mug, easy-to-handle pitcher, or other container must be accessible and the patient able to use it (Figure 4-11A). The travelling juice cup is dishwasher safe. **Manufacturer:** 480. Cost is about $2.50 from housewares stores. Sipper jugs are also **manufactured** by 57, 538.

A covered mug with a built-in straw in the handle aids the client who has difficulty sucking (Figure 4-11B). The cup can be held horizontally, simulating gravity, and providing controlled flow. **Manufacturer:** 57. Cost is about $1 from children's departments of variety stores. Additional adaptations for drinking aids are shown in Chapter 22 in *Mealtime Manual*.

For the person who drinks very slowly yet desires a warm beverage, a mug-activated warmer may be indicated. Unit turns on

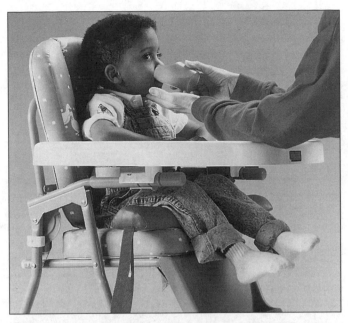

Figure 4-9. The translucent Flexi Cut-Out cup for infants or people with feeding difficulties lets the therapist or caregiver visually monitor the flow of fluid. (Photo courtesy of Communication Skill Builders, San Antonio, TX.)

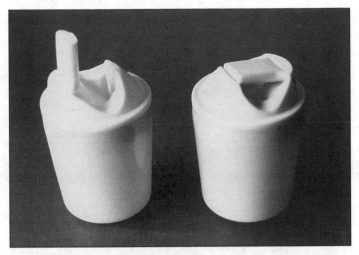

Figure 4-11A. The traveling juice cup is sealed for leak-proof carrying when the spout is down, then snaps open for drinking. (Cup from SmileTote, Inc., Los Angeles, CA. Photo by J.K.)

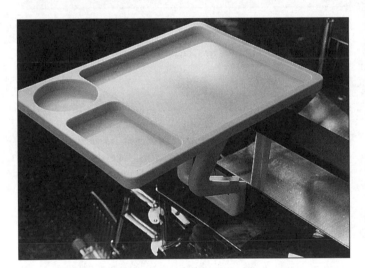

Figure 4-10. This over-arm chair tray has an adjustable clamp for use with furniture or wheelchair arms. (Photo by J.K.)

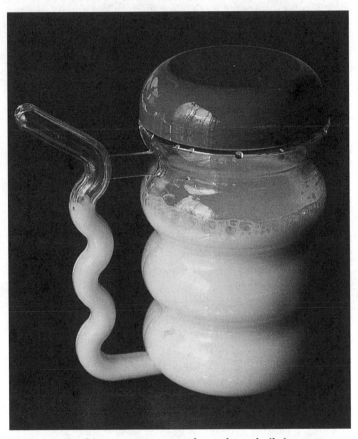

Figure 4-11B. This 14-ounce covered mug has a built-in straw. (Arrow Plastics Mfg. Co., Elk Grove, IL. Photo by J.K.)

when mug is in place, off when removed. It has an indicator light and an automatic 30-minute shut-off when mug is in place. **Manufacturers:** 372, 460. Cost is about $15 from department and housewares stores. See Chapter 20, *Mealtime Manual*.

SWALLOWING DIFFICULTIES

An individual may have difficulty swallowing due to dysphagia, the effects of amyotrophic lateral sclerosis, Parkinson's disease, cerebral palsy, stroke, chemotherapy and radiation, or a glomus tumor.

A dysphagia cup, designed for people with swallowing difficulties, is contoured to allow for sufficient nose clearance without

tilting the head back (Figure 4-12). Cup shape directs the flow of liquids to the center of the mouth. The large handle accommodates an extended hand or weak grasp. Eight-ounce capacity, dishwasher safe. Cost is about $17 from rehabilitation and self-help equipment firms. **Sources:** 98, 383, 461, 522.

A patient who has difficulty swallowing may find that semisolid foods go down more easily. A neutral tasting thickener

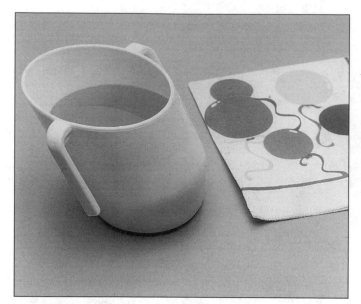

Figure 4-12. A dysphagia cup, designed for people with swallowing difficulties, is contoured to allow for sufficient nose clearance without tilting the head back. (Photo courtesy of North Coast Medical, Inc., San Jose, CA.)

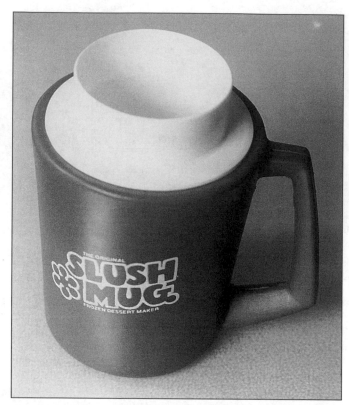

Figure 4-13. Clients with amyotrophic lateral sclerosis and others with swallowing difficulties often find that frozen slush is easier to swallow than liquid. (Mug by Glacierware, Easthampton, MA. Photo by J.K.)

added to liquid foods increases swallowing control. Several products are on the market including Puree Entrees and Nutra Thik by Menu Magic®, Thick-It® by Diafood, and Thick & Easy®.

Modified food starch thickeners may be added to hot or cold foods without cooking. They add calories to food and are available in regular or maximum thickening to produce mixtures ranging from the consistency of apricot nectar to pudding. For additional information and costs, write or call for local distributor. **Sources:** Menu Magic®, 356 (carried by Bruce, 98); Thick-It® by Milani Foods, 360 (carried by 98). Before trying, discuss needs with a dietitian, nutritionist, nurse, or physician. See Chapter 5 for soft eating utensils and suggestions, and for the *Non-Chew Cookbook* (under Resources), which gives recipes for easy-to-swallow dishes.

The Department of Defense has developed liquid meals for injured soldiers who can't eat solid foods. The selection includes cheeseburgers, ham and cheese soufflé, tacos, spaghetti with meat sauce, and gingerbread by the glass.

Clients with amyotrophic lateral sclerosis and others with swallowing difficulties often find that frozen slush is easier to swallow than liquid (Figure 4-13). A slush mug is kept in the freezer. When ready to use, juice or another beverage is poured in and thickens into an icy slush in minutes. Non-toxic, dishwasher safe. Cost is about $8 each. **Manufacturer:** 224. **Source:** 325.

Designed to meet needs of clients with dysphagia, a swallowing instruction set includes a six-page manual plus five color-coded pads of sheets, each with a different level of swallowing ability, and four sheets (144) of stickers with specific instructions, i.e., take small bites, sips (Figure 4-14). **Source:** 522.

A feeding precaution poster kit alerts health care providers to swallowing and feeding disorders of dysphagic patients. It reduces the risks of aspiration and increases overall swallowing function. Kit includes four posters and grease pencil. Cost is about $10 from source 461.

The client with dementia often eats better when given finger foods (Figure 4-15). These allow control over a basic activity even when social rules have been forgotten. Bite-sized pieces of food eaten independently also reduce the frustration and anger aimed at a caregiver who is attempting to feed a confused individual. See Resources for helpful brochure.

The Geri-Feeder (Figure 4-16) facilitates feeding for persons unable to self-feed. The clear plastic container allows the caregiver to see how much food has been taken. A similar unit is designed for starting infants on semi-solid foods. Unit minimizes amount of air swallowed with food. Dishwasher safe. **Source:** 465.

RESOURCES

Addresses for publishers, periodicals, and organizations are given in Section Four.

PUBLICATIONS

About Anorexia Nervosa. (1986). South Deerfield, MA: Channing L. Bete. Illustrated booklet describes symptoms, possible causes, need for treatment, gives resources. $1.25 per copy.

Caring for the Person with Dementia: Finger Foods Make Mealtimes Easier. Free public service brochure from the Hebrew Home for the Aged at Riverdale. Tips and recipes.

Cherney, L. R. (Ed.). (1993). *Clinical Management of*

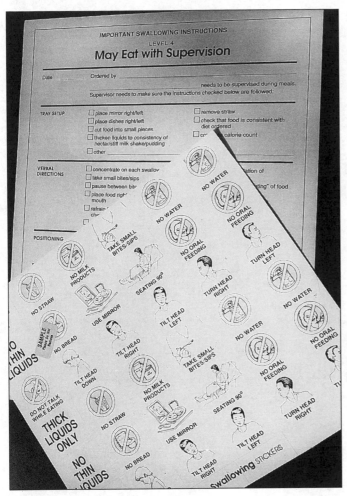

Figure 4-14. This swallowing instruction set is designed to meet needs of clients with dysphagia. (From *Swallowing Instruction Sheets and Stickers,* copyright 1992, Therapy Skill Builders, San Antonio, TX. Reprinted with permission.)

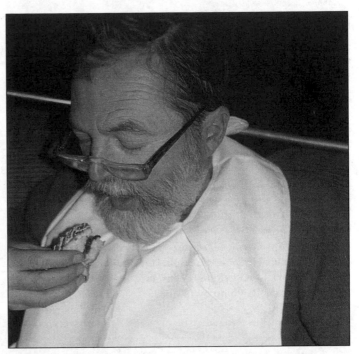

Figure 4-15. The client with dementia often eats better when given finger foods. (Photo by J.K.)

Dysphagia in Adults and Children (2nd ed.). Rehabilitation Institute of Chicago Publication Series. Frederick, MD: Aspen. $64. Evaluation, diagnostic procedures, treatment procedures, quality assurance monitors.

Dickey, M. K., & Wilkinson, S. C. (1992). Swallowing Instruction Sheets and Stickers. San Antonio, TX: Therapy Skill Builders. $34.95. **Source:** 522.

Eating Disorders. Free brochure on anorexia and bulimia from the U.S. Consumer Information Center.

Feeding/Dysphagia: Resource Guide. Bethesda, MD: American Occupational Therapy Association. #4250, $10 AOTA members, $20 non-members. Bibliographies, audiovisuals, resource personnel.

Logemann, J. *Swallowing Problems: How Can They Be Identified, Evaluated and Treated?: A Caregiver's Manual.* Brochure available free from Menu Magic. **Source:** 356.

National Association of Anorexia Nervosa and Associated Disorders. Free information packet.

Piran, N., & Kaplan, A. S. (1990). *A Day Hospital Group Treatment Program for Anorexia Nervosa and Bulimia Nervosa.* New York: Brunner/Mazel. Eating Disorders Manual No. 3.

Posner, T. E., & Eckford, C. (1991). *Dysphagia Resource*

Manual. Bethesda, MD: American Occupational Therapy Association. #4250A, $18 AOTA members, $25 non-members. Manual for instructing dining room personnel and family/care-givers in management of problems associated with dysphagia. Oral/motor exercises, adaptive equipment, charting progress. Includes *Feeding/Dysphagia Resource Guide.*

Rader, T., & Rende, B. (1992). *Swallowing Disorders: What Families Should Know.* San Antonio, TX: Therapy Skill Builders. 13-page booklet for adult clients, $10 for set of 10. **Source:** 522.

Rudolph, M. (1990). OTs prove instrumental in finding solutions for people who can't eat normally. *Advance for Occupational Therapists.*

Sonies, B. C. (1996). *Dysphagia: A Continuum of Care.* Frederick, MD: Aspen. $49. Clinical considerations, dysphagia and respiratory/pulmonary function, models for centers of care, education and training, legal and ethical concerns, effects of changes in health care delivery.

Speech Problems and Swallowing Problems in Parkinson's Disease. (1989). New York: The American Parkinson Disease Association.

Swigert, N. B. (1996). *The Source for Dysphagia.* East Moline, IL: LinguiSystems. $37.95. Questions to ask during medical history interviews, swallowing assessment, patient criteria, family decision making, goals, treatment planning techniques. **Source:** 329.

Wilson, J. R. (1985). *Non-Chew Cookbook.* Glenwood Springs, CO: Wilson Publishing. $17.45. Recipes developed for attractiveness and palatability as well as nutritional needs. For patients on liquid or soft diet. **Source:** 579.

AUDIOVISUALS

Please see Chapter 2.

Logemann, J. *Precautions for Feeding Dysphagic Patients: An Inservice Training Program for Feeding Staff.* Gaylord, MI:

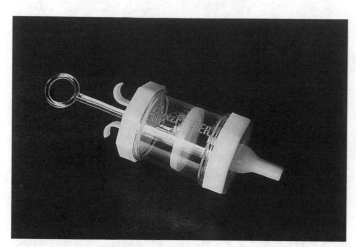

Figure 4-16. The Geri-feeder assists an attendant in feeding a client who is unable to feed himself. It is designed for semi-solid foods. (Manufactured by Infa Feeder, Inc., a division of Sassy®, Inc., Northbrook IL. Photo by J.K.)

Northern Speech Services Inc. Video, 50 inservice manuals and 50 individualized feeding plan forms. Cost is $235 for ¾-inch videotape, $225 for ½-inch VHS. Role of positioning on safety of swallowing, controlling food consistency, amount per swallow, time between swallows, warning signs of difficulty. Documenting feeding controls and instructions. Additional video/manual programs from Northern Speech Services, Inc., include *Assessment of Swallowing Physiology* and *The Diagnosis and Treatment of Dysphagia*. **Source:** 384.

5

The Client Who is Receiving Hospice Care

The concept of hospice is that when the quantity of life cannot be increased, the quality of life can be attended to.

Tailoring time to the needs of the hospice patient is our primary goal. This is true whether the cause is cancer, AIDS, amyotrophic lateral sclerosis, or another disease. As health care workers, we can bring suggestions for better nutrition as well as enhance recall of memories and add joy to each day.

The therapist helps promote continued independence by adapting the physical environment and assists both the client and caregivers in adapting to constantly changing circumstances. Referrals for occupational and physical therapists may include assessment of the environment from bed positioning and static splints or skin protectors for feet and elbows, to handling remote controls for television, bed positioning, lights, intercoms and other communication aids, reachers, overbed tables or trays, commodes or bathroom modifications, and transfer aids. Adapted eating aids and clothing can increase comfort. Assessment of psychosocial needs should address depression, loss of role and self-esteem, boredom, anger, and inability to engage in former activities. Energy conservation may allow the continuation of favorite pursuits. New leisure skills, which add excitement and reduce focus on pain, may be incorporated into therapy sessions from sorting photographs to recording memories, messages, favorite family stories, crafts, and recipes. Personal wishes that the health care professional may communicate include favorite music and foods, which the patient can sometimes help make or have friends and family provide. Small projects, such as a quick-stitch pillow for a young grandchild, planted bulbs, a simple wreath, or even Christmas cookies made in bed, become "memories of art" for the family.

Many hospice clients wish to remain at home in familiar surroundings and with loved ones. Not all are bedbound. Most actively assume family roles whether up and around or not. If your client is able to prepare meals, finding ways to extend energy is important. Arranging for help within the home on a daily or respite basis allows the family to more normally continue regular activities.

Senior companion assistance provides friendship and security to the patient alone at home (Figure 5-1). It also allows the family to pursue normal activities.

Maintaining good nutrition is paramount. The side effects of treatment often affect appetite. You may be called upon to find ways to make eating palatable. Several cookbooks are available for those undergoing chemotherapy, radiation, or other routines. See Chapter 23.

Adapted eating aids help the patient with limited mobility continue self-feeding. Also see Chapter 22 in *Mealtime Manual*, as well as Chapter 4 in this guide.

Soft cutlery is designed for people who need help with feeding (Figure 5-2). The soft rounded edges of the utensils feel comfortable in the mouth and are shaped so that it is easy to give food to a person who cannot open his or her mouth very wide. The long handles allow the person being fed to hold onto the utensils along with the caregiver. The large diameter handle affords the feeder a comfortable grip and good balance. **Source:** 191.

The extended curved lip of a dose cup lets a person drink without leaning his or her head back (Figure 5-3). The design allows good contact with the lips and is graduated with a 1 dl mark. **Source:** 191.

For the person who has difficulty swallowing a pill, an Ezy-Dose® drink-a-pill glass eliminates the gagging reflex when consuming solid medication (Figure 5-4). A small shelf inside the lip of the glass holds a pill up to one-inch long and 3/8-inch in diameter. The glass is filled to a marked line with water and designed so that the pill goes down with a swallow. Cost is about $2 from pharmacies and hospital supply firms. **Manufacturer**: 53B.

Note: Many coated pills should not be crushed prior to administration, because protective coatings affect slow release or bitter taste. If a client cannot swallow whole pills, discuss the problem with his or her physician.

Preparing nutritious, easy-to-swallow snacks becomes streamlined with an electric hand blender (Figure 5-5). It whips up fruit and yogurt drinks or double-milk milkshakes right in the drinking container and purees foods for easier swallowing. Cost is about

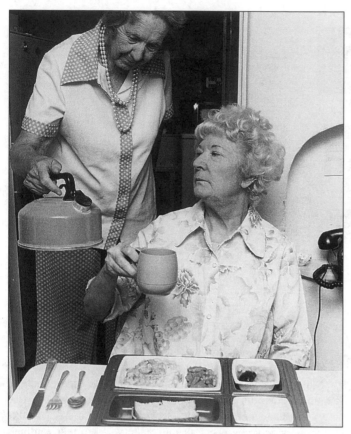

Figure 5-1. Senior companion assistance aids the patient alone at home. (Photo courtesy of ACTION®, Washington, DC.)

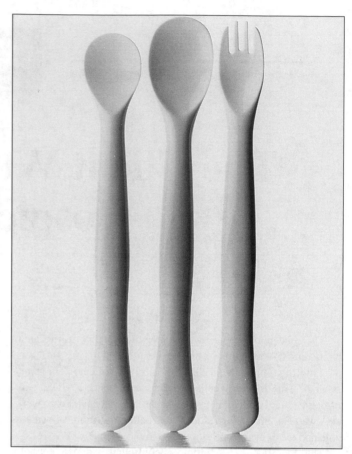

Figure 5-2. This soft cutlery is designed for people who need help with feeding. (Cutlery by RSFU Basic. Photo courtesy of Etac USA, Inc., Waukesha, WI.)

$20 and up from housewares stores. **Manufacturers** include Braun, 92; Rival, 446; and Toastmaster, 530.

Communicating with the hospice patient may be difficult if the person has diminished voice volume or is unable to speak. The use of electronic aids or a communication board increases independence and reduces frustration or stress. A small microphone with a headset increases voice volume so staff, family, and friends can hear requests. An occupational or speech therapist can set up a unit and teach the patient how to use it. **Sources** include 337, 418. See environmental controls in Chapter 6.

The "silent speaker" gives "freedom of speech" to a patient who is prevented from voicing needs but can point with a finger or circle words with a pen (Figure 5-6). A concise list of key words and phrases with two views of a human figure help localize areas of concern. These are supplemented by an alphabet and numbers. It was designed by two nurses, Joan Downey and Margaret Freidin, who saw a need on the wards, tested the words, then put them in an organized form on a laminated sheet. Cost is about $7.50 for a two-sided, bilingual English/Spanish sheet with an attached pen. For information and pricing on other lists, including one for aides, write **source** 533.

Younger family members should have the option of sharing in the care of the ill person. This increases their feeling of belonging and of not being neglected, and reduces feelings of helplessness. Helping a parent prepare food, giving a hand with therapy exercises, playing a board game together, and taking on special jobs that may require a little stretching all help a child adjust. See Chapter 23 and Chapter 6.

Health care professionals may receive training in bereavement and hospice work through seminars as well as several videos and publications. The AARP offers a complete seminar/program. See Resources.

The role of the nurse, therapist, and other caregivers in hospice demands flexibility, creativity, an acceptance of the inevitable, the ability to reach out, love, and bring beauty, however small, to a patient whose world may be as tiny as a serving of homemade mousse, a special flower, a brilliant autumn leaf, or a bright poster of the world outside—in sum, to share and bring fullness and joy to remaining time.

ORGANIZATIONS

Many local groups exist to assist the family through the grieving process. Some counsel and support the family before the death of a member. This is especially important for helping children understand and accept what is happening. Check with local hospitals, churches, senior centers, and organizations that deal with the disease from which the individual suffers, like the American Cancer Society or the Amyotrophic Lateral Sclerosis Association. These are a few nationwide groups. Addresses are in Appendix C or contact local chapters:

- The Compassionate Friends: helps parents who have lost a child.

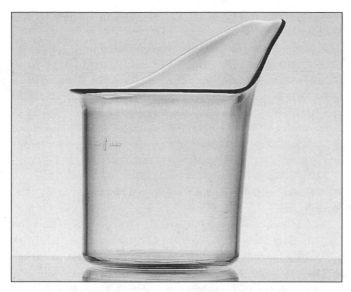

Figure 5-3. The extended, curved lip of this dose cup lets a person drink without leaning his or her head back. (Dose cup by RSFU Basic. Photo courtesy of Etac USA, Inc., Waukesha, WI.)

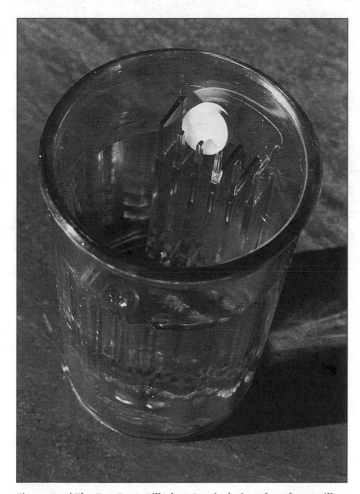

Figure 5-4/ The Ezy-Dose Pilltaker Cup is designed so that a pill may be placed on a small shelf. When the patient swallows it with water, the tablet goes over the back of the tongue and down. (Manufactured by Apothecary Products, Inc., Burnsville, MN. Photo by J.K.)

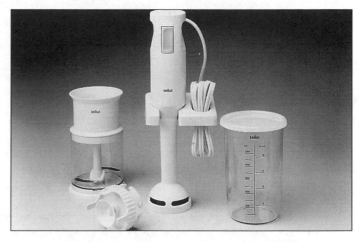

Figure 5-5. Preparing nutritious, easy-to-swallow snacks becomes streamlined with an electric hand blender. (Photo courtesy of Braun Inc., Lynnfield, MA.)

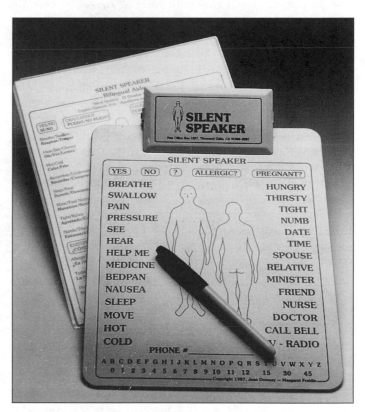

Figure 5-6. The "silent speaker" gives "freedom of speech" to a patient. (Photo courtesy of Trademark Medical, Inc., Fenton, MD.)

- Grant-A-Wish Foundation: grants wishes of terminally ill children.
- Make-A-Wish Foundation of America: grants wishes of terminally ill children.
- National Hospice Organization.
- Theos Foundation: for the widowed and their families.
- Widowed Persons: for widows and widowers, peer support. Also see Chapter 2 and Chapter 23.

RESOURCES

Addresses for publishers, periodicals, and organizations are given in Section Four.

PUBLICATIONS

Aronheim, J., & Weber, D. *Final Passages: Positive Choices for the Dying and Their Loved Ones*. New York: Simon & Schuster. $18.

Bratman, F. (1995). *Everything You Need to Know When a Parent Dies* (rev. ed.). New York: Rosen. $15.95. Tells teenagers where to go for information when they suffer this loss and how others have dealt with it.

Brown, J. (1995). *The Choice: Seasons of Loss and Renewal After a Father's Decision to Die*. Berkeley, CA: Conari. Traces a path to renewal that includes considerations of the meaning and process of death and the nature of choice in our lives. Begins after the death of the author's father.

Buckman, R. (1992) *How to Break Bad News: A Guide for Health Care Professionals*. Buffalo, NY: University of Toronto Press. $17.95.

Buckman, R. (1992). *I Don't Know What to Say: How to Help and Support Someone Who Is Dying*. New York: Random House. $13. Also Key Porter, Toronto. Talking and listening, transitions, practicalities, communicating with health professionals, supporting organizations.

Buckinghan, R., & Huggard, S. (1993). *Coping With Grief* (rev. ed.). New York: Rosen. $15.95. Explains the specific stages of grieving to guide teens through their losses.

Carroll, D. (1991). *Living with Dying: A Loving Guide for Family and Close Friends* (rev. ed.). New York: Paragon House. $19.95.

The Channing Bete Company publishes materials related to hospice care. The booklets include *Preparing Your Advance Medical Directives* and *About Patient Rights*, $1.25 each, and there is also an 18-minute VHS video for patients and families called *Advance Directives: The Decision is Yours*. Produced by Medcom®, 1992, $75. **Source:** 114.

Draimin, B. H. (1994). *Everything You Need to Know When a Parent Has AIDS*, and *Coping When a Parent Has AIDS*. Both from New York: Rosen. $15.95 each. Teens can learn where to turn for help through stories of teens in the same situation.

Final Details: A Guide for Survivors When Death Occurs: Planning for Difficult Times. Distributed by the American Association of Retired Persons. Free.

Fumia, M. (1992). *Safe Passage: Words to Help the Grieving Hold Fast and Let Go*. Berkeley, CA: Conari. $10.95. Book of meditations on grieving written by a woman who lost her son.

Gordon, B. S. (1986). *The First Year Alone*. Dublin, NH: William L. Bauhan. $7.95. **Source:** 77.

Guidelines for Occupational Therapy Services in Hospice,. Bethesda, MD: American Occupational Therapy Association, Inc.

Hospice Benefits/Medicare: A Special Way of Caring for the Terminally Ill. Free brochure from the Health Care Financing Administration.

Kilburn, L. H. (1988). *The Hospice Operations Manual*, Arlington, VA: National Hospice Organization.

Kubler-Ross, E. (1993). *AIDS: The Ultimate Challenge*. New York: Macmillan. $10.

Kushner, Rabbi H. S. (1986). *When Bad Things Happen to Good People*. New York: Avon. $6.95.

LeShan, E. (1976). *Learning to Say Good-Bye: When a Parent Dies*. New York: Macmillan. $12.95. Written to help teenagers understand, it is also good for other members of the family.

Lustbader, W. (1991). *Counting on Kindness: The Dilemmas of Dependency*. New York: Free Press, Macmillan. $17.95. Journey into world of dependency, soothingly discussed from both sides.

Marcil, W., & Tigges, K. (1992). *The Person with AIDS: A Professional and Personal Perspective*. Thorofare, NJ: SLACK Inc. $26.

McClelland, S., & Prescott, S. (1990). *"If There's Anything I Can Do:" An Easy Guide to Showing You Care*. Gainesville, MD: Triad. $8.95. How families and friends can help during a personal crisis.

Menton, T. (1991). *Gentle Closings: How to Say Good-Bye to Someone You Love*. Philadelphia: Running Press Book. $12.95.

Menton, T. (1994). *After Good-Bye—How to Begin Again After the Death of Someone You Love*. Philadelphia: Running Press Book.

Mills, J. C. (1993). *Gentle Willow: A Story for Children About Dying*. New York: Magination Press, Brunner/Mazel. $11.95. Written for children who may not survive their illness as well as for others dealing with death of friends and family.

Moffat, B. C. (1987). *When Someone You Love Has AIDS: A Book of Hope for Family and Friends*. New York: NAL Dutton, Penguin. $8.95.

Sankar, A. (1991). *Dying at Home: A Family Guide for Caregiving*. Baltimore: Johns Hopkins University Press. $22.95. Caregiver's role, use of formal support, social support, tasks of caregiving, nutrition, personal accounts, resources.

Shapiro, E. R. (1994). *Grief as A Family Process: A Developmental Approach to Clinical Practice*. New York: Guilford. $31.50. How to help families transform their attachment to the deceased family member to enhance family development. Examples from a wide variety of cultural traditions.

Siegel, B. S. (1986). *Love, Medicine and Miracles: Lessons Learned about Self-Healing from a Surgeon's Experience with Exceptional Patients*. New York: HarperCollins. $15.95.

Tatelbaum, J. (1980). *The Courage to Grieve: Creative Living, Recovery, & Growth Through Grief*. New York: HarperCollins. $9.95. Written for those grieving as well as the counseling professional.

Tigges, K. N., & Marcil, W. M. (1988). *Terminal and Life-Threatening Illness: An Occupational Behavior Perspective*. Thorofare, NJ: SLACK Inc. $20.

Tigges, K. N., & Sherman, L. M. (1983, April). The treatment of the hospice patient: From occupational history to occupational role. *American Journal of Occupational Therapy*, 37(4), 235-238.

Van den Berg, M. (1994). *The Three Birds: A Story for Children About the Loss of a Loved One*. New York: Magination Press, Brunner/Mazel. $8.95. For young children facing the death of a parent.

AUDIOVISUALS

Living fully until death. From the series *The Doctor is In*. Dartmouth Medical Center. No. CM-195, 28-minute video, $149. Three patients, each with a terminal illness, discuss paths they have found toward coming to terms, taking control of the rest of their lives, and confronting the unknown. And Mednick, J. *The Way We Die*. No. CM-154, 25-minute VHS video, $195. Interviews with medical personnel, terminally ill patients and their families; encourages health care professionals to work with their patients to devise treatment programs in accordance with their needs and values. Also Johnson, J. *Inner Views of Grief*. No. CM-161, 30-minute video, $195. Five young adults discuss reactions to how they coped with death of a close one. And Kara. *Encounters with Grief*. No. CM- 091, 13-minute VHS video, $145. All from Clinician's View; **Source:** 124.

Spousal Bereavement and Primary Health Care. (1991). Washington, DC: American Association of Retired Persons. For health care professionals. Seminar kit includes 14-minute VHS video about effective treatment for the newly widowed and a Leader's Guide plus participant's materials: "Spousal Bereavement and Primary Health Care" brochure from AARP's Widowed Persons Service, "Knowing the Facts About Medication and Bereavement" brochure, "Possible Distinctions Between Depressive Grief and Clinical Depression" a check list, "Widowed Persons Service" a brochure, and "On Being Alone" booklet for the newly widowed. Available for free short-term loan to AARP chapters, RTA units, WPS units, and other non-profit organizations serving the interests of older people from AARP A/V Programs, Dept. ES, Program Scheduling Office.

To purchase kit with leader's guide, sample hand-outs, and video, the cost is $20 from AARP A/V Programs.

Ufema, J. *Dealing with Death and Dying*. Springhouse, PA: Springhouse Publishing. Guidance for health care professionals on how to give a patient greater control over his or her situation, work through fears and repressed anger, create positive communication between patient and family, encourage discussion of concerns, understand client who says he or she wants to die, help maximize final days, deal with physician who refuses to reveal bad news. 45-minute color VHS, $39.95. **Source:** 492.

The Caregiver and the Family

Caring for an older or disabled family member is a situation more and more people are facing. As medical costs escalate, hospitals discharge patients earlier, laws change releasing individuals from state institutions, and the longevity and prevalence of diseases such as AIDS and Alzheimer's increase, people cared for at home require additional services. The average length of caregiving time for those older than 70 years of age, according to the American Association of Retired Persons, is between five and seven years.

Even in the most loving situations, caregiving is a stressful, often depressing, sometimes guilt-ridden, angering, or exhausting experience. Caregivers are caught in the middle, bearing the burden of both their own problems and those of the person(s) for whom they are responsible. Ninety percent of this care falls on women, many of whom are in the work force. As health care professionals, we must be prepared to offer help, suggestions, and alternatives in handling multi-faceted situations. Also, we need to be alert for any evidence of elder abuse. Referring family members and patients to support and self-help groups allows communication, which reduces frustration and releases some of the stresses through sharing.

Many organizations offer help. The Visiting Nurse Association of America has more than 500 chapters nationwide that provide medical and household assistance. The National Association for Home Care has a hotline for referrals to local home health agencies. Family Service America, a non-profit organization that helps families solve complex problems of elder care through counseling, support groups, and specialized services, has 290 member agencies and will refer you to the nearest one. The National Family Caregivers Association and the Family Caregiver Alliance can direct one to long-term care resources. The Alzheimer's Disease and Related Disorders Association has 1500 support groups throughout the country and a free, 24-hour information line; each chapter provides free service referrals. Children of Aging Parents, a non-profit organization, provides help in setting up support groups, gives peer counseling in person and by telephone, publishes a newsletter (*The CAPsule*), and has a variety of publications

(some in Spanish) for caregivers. The Well Spouse Foundation provides help for the caregiving partner through support groups and publications. Also see organizations listed under separate chapters, such as Chapter 11, i.e., Parkinson's Disease Foundation, National Multiple Sclerosis Society, United Cerebral Palsy Associations, and the National Association of Area Agencies on Aging. Addresses are in Appendix C.

There are four types of respite programs to provide short-term relief for the caregiver. The first may be a health care worker or volunteer, as with hospice programs, who comes in for a few hours on a regular basis. This allows the caregiver to plan shopping, children's activities, exercise, and social and other breaks. Occasionally, these breaks can be planned by coordinating services from a home care agency so that treatments and visits by the professionals are scheduled back-to-back.

The second type brings an alternate caregiver into the home for a specified length of time, permitting the major caregiver and other members of the family a longer break, even overnight or for several days.

The third program transfers the patient for a short period of time to an in-patient facility, again giving the caregivers a chance to re-group.

A fourth alternative is a day care program that allows the client who is well enough to travel a chance to socialize and learn with others while the family or other caregivers attend to other responsibilities. See Resources.

TRANSFERS

Along with the routines and emotional stress of caregiving are physical demands, especially getting the client out of bed for eating, bathing, toileting, exercises, and socialization. Back injuries are an all too common disability among caregivers. The physical or occupational therapist should train the caregiver in proper methods of transferring and lifting. The list of ways to save your back from Chapter 14 (reproducible page in Appendix G) may be given to the caregiver as a reminder. Also see Resources for com-

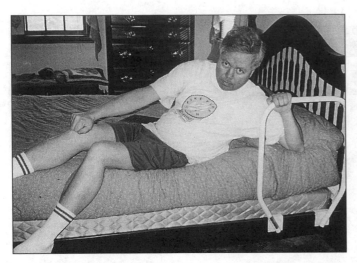

Figure 6-1. A transfer handle attached to a bed provides stability for the client who needs assistance rising. (Photo of Bed-Bar® courtesy of Brown Engineering Corp., Westhampton, MA.)

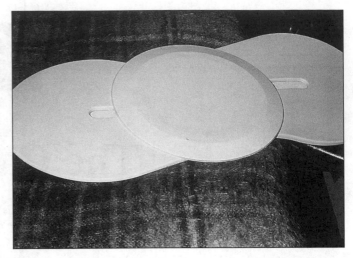

Figure 6-2. The BeasyTrans™ system uses a lateral sliding technique like regular transfer boards, but with a marked difference. A rotating seat slides across the frictionless base, allowing the caregiver to more easily transfer a patient. (BeasyTrans™ system from Beatrice M. Brandtman, Inc., Lake Forest, IL. Photo by J.K.)

panies offering reproducible materials on transferring and lifting.

Equipment may reduce the stress of transferring and positioning a patient. Bed ladders and hand-blocks or push-up bars save a caregiver's back by allowing the patient more mobility in and around the bed. The blocks or bar frame keep the client's hands from sinking into the bedding so that moving to the side of the bed is easier. The patient must have adequate power in his or her upper limbs, but even when using one hand a single block helps a caregiver move the patient more easily. Cost of blocks is about $29 per pair from hospital supply firms.

A transfer handle attached to the bed provides stability for the client who needs assistance rising (Figure 6-1). It may be used to come to an upright position for ambulating or to give support while transferring to a wheelchair. Units are designed for home or hospital beds. Patients who may find a transfer handle helpful include people with Parkinson's, multiple sclerosis, hemiplegia, and general weakness. As with other transfer techniques and aids, training by a therapist in the correct technique is needed to ensure suitability for the client's level of function and to increase safety and ease for both the caregiver and the client. Cost is about $50 and up, depending on model. **Manufacturers:** 97, 366. **Sources:** 97, 366, 383.

If the patient cannot rise when transferring, other equipment may be required. The aid may be as simple as a transfer board or as complicated as a lift. Both aids require training of the patient and caregiver for efficient and safe use. Transfer boards and lifts are carried by hospital supply firms. Boards cost about $28 and up, depending on size, material, and style. **Sources:** 8, 11, 140, 198, 383, 461, 483, 503, 518.

The BeasyTrans™ system uses a lateral sliding technique like regular transfer boards but with a marked difference (Figure 6-2). A rotating seat slides across the frictionless base, allowing the caregiver to more easily transfer a patient up to 400 pounds from bed to chair, without pulling and back strain. The BeasyTrans™ system comes in two lengths: 27.5 and 40 inches. Free video is available from **Manufacturer/Source:** 81.

A transfer disk has a rotating top with a solid base (Figure 6-3). When placed under the client's feet, it allows one person to trans-

fer a patient who can stand but cannot move his or her feet from the bed to a wheelchair or other chair. Feet are first placed on the disk; the patient then stands with the support of a caregiver and is slowly turned so that his or her back faces the seat or bed to which he or she is being transferred. It is especially helpful when an individual is stiff because of a neurological disability like Parkinson's disease or cerebral palsy. Cost is about $59 and up, depending on size, from hospital supply firms. **Sources:** 33, 81.

If a client is severely involved, a lift may need to be considered. Basic lifts may be rented from home health supply firms, the cost of which is usually covered by insurance. **Manufacturers** of lifts include Access Unlimited (multi-lift which may be used for bed, car, bath), 10; Barrier-Free Lifts (attached to ceiling) 75; Columbia McKinnon (electric, battery-operated) 131; Rand Scott (manual) 431B; Sears Roebuck (manual and pneumatic) 468; Sunrise Medical (manual and pneumatic) 499; Wy'East (lift transfers patient in prone position then concerts to chair) 587. Non-profit organizations that provide support services for a specified disease will sometimes loan or fund purchase of a lift. The family and aides should receive instruction in the use of a lift by a trained professional. This will teach them how to protect and reassure patient, and will determine the correct positioning, and right selection of a sling. Some patients with marked weakness or spasticity require slings with head support.

The Pivot Pole® improves functional mobility, allowing a client to get up for meals and join family and friends more easily (Figure 6-4). It holds the weight of the person being transferred, rather than the caregiver, and may allow the client to transfer almost independently with training. The individual must have adequate upper extremity strength and trunk and neck control to maintain a sitting posture with support. Two models include a T-bar model for people with adequate strength in the upper extremities to grasp and hold for standing pivot transfers (paraplegics, amputees, obesity) and a forearm model for those with less function and grasp in the upper extremities. The Pivot Pole® may be rolled from room to

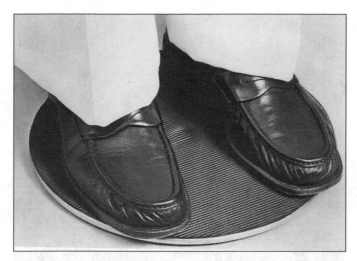

Figure 6-3. A transfer disk allows one person to transfer a patient who can stand but cannot move his or her feet from the bed to a wheelchair or other chair. (Photo courtesy of AliMed®, Inc., Dedham, MA.)

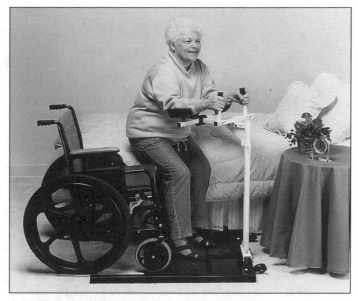

Figure 6-4. The Pivot Pole® improves functional mobility, allowing a client to get up for meals and join family and friends more easily. (Photo courtesy of North Coast Medical, Inc., San Jose, CA.)

room when tipped back on casters and fits through any wheelchair-accessible doorway. Information and a free video is available from: 383. Cost is $625 for the T-bar model and $695 for the forearm model. **Sources:** 1, 383.

Keeping track of a patient who is apt to wander causes extra worry for a caregiver. This is a common problem for people with Alzheimer's disease. Gates work in some cases, but an alarm unit gives an immediate warning.

The Bed-Check and Chair-Check are portable, battery-operated devices that monitor the individual and immediately alert a caregiver if the patient tries to get up. The aid helps prevent falls and also allows the caregiver to sleep at night without fearing that a person with Alzheimer's disease or other problem will walk and fall downstairs or wander out of the house. **Source:** 83.

The client with severe, chronic disability or weakness due to progressive disease may still control a number of functions from bed, wheelchair, or chair with the use of an environmental control unit (Figure 6-5). The feasibility and assessment for use must be done with an occupational therapist or rehabilitation engineer. Units may be operated by various methods, i.e., buttons, microswitches, and voice commands. **Manufacturers** and distributors of environmental control units include 139, 418, 428, 506, 512.

See Resources on assistive technology at the end of this chapter and also in Appendix F. The American Occupational Therapy Association offers continuing education programs in assistive technology. *Team Rehab* magazine has monthly articles on the application of assistive technology.

TOILETING AND PERSONAL HYGIENE

Toileting and handling personal hygiene is a major daily activity and requirement of caregiving. As with other activities, caregivers must be taught to wear protective clothing, including gloves, while toileting and bathing a client.

Assessment of the bathroom includes ability of the client to get to and from the bathroom (during the day as well as at night); location of bathroom and whether there is a unit on the floor where the major portion of each day is spent; space to maneuver within bathroom; width of the door (adequate clearance for wheelchair or glider chair); physical ability of the client to handle personal cleaning; and design, usability, and modifications needed for safety and comfort with a tub or shower. The health care professional can ease the burden on the family and caregiver through training of the client and recommendations of equipment that increase safety and reduce physical as well as emotional strain.

Equipment may include a commode for use during the day or just at night to avoid trips to the bathroom when the client is unstable and not fully awake. The cost of a bedside commode is covered by Medicare and most insurance companies. Rails over the toilet seat and a raised seat are not covered, but if the right commode is ordered, this can be shifted to the bathroom as the client's strength and mobility increase. Bedside commode **manufacturers** include 18, 258, 336, 405, 454, 468, 499, 580.

When a client has progressive weakness or limited upper extremity function, handling personal hygiene after toileting is often difficult or impossible. Toilet tongs may assist a few clients. However, the best answer for preserving dignity and reducing strain on caregivers, although initially more expensive, is an electric bidet unit.

The Lubidet® personal hygiene system includes a bidet attachment and outlet (Figure 6-6). It is UL and UPC listed. The warm water and air help prevent urinary tract infections, vaginal yeast infections, and reduce hemorrhoidal discomfort or constipation by softening anal sphincter muscles. Cost is about $450 through rehabilitation supply firms. **Manufacturer:** 335. **Sources:** 383, 461. Similar unit: 324. Bidet attachment units are also **manufactured** by American Bidet, 38; Sanlex, 462. Note: send for brochures and check measurements before ordering, because models vary in the amount of side space required for controls.

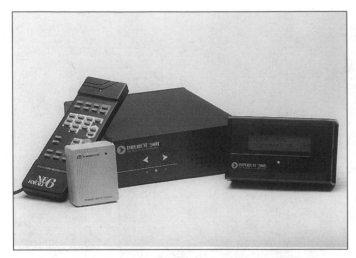

Figure 6-5. The client may still control a number of functions from bed, wheelchair, or chair with the use of an environmental control unit. (Photo courtesy of Teledyne Brown Engineering, Huntsville, AL.)

Incontinence affects more than 15 to 20 million people in the United States and Canada. Ninety percent of these individuals live at home, and not all of them are elderly. It is a problem for both the client and caregivers. It creates insecurity, a lowered sense of control over one's life, and is one of the most common reasons that a client shuts himself or herself away from socialization with friends and even family. Finding ways to handle incontinence increases dignity for the client and allows more activities away from home.

Incontinence aids for children and adults are available through local and mail-order firms. The nurse and physician should discuss the causes as well as equipment and bladder/bowel training with the client and family. Scheduling of meals and diet must be included. The client may be reducing fluid intake to a level that affects his or her health. The therapist can teach exercises to strengthen bladder muscles and can recommend side-opening underwear for clients who use wheelchairs, wear leg braces, or have limited upper extremity function. **Source:** 107. Several organizations provide literature and audiovisuals for professionals and for people with incontinence.

Some of these include the American Medical Directors Association, the Bladder Health Council, the National Association for Continence, and the Simon Foundation. Addresses are in Appendix C. Also see Resources in this chapter.

COMMUNICATION WITH THE CLIENT

Communication within a house may be eased and steps reduced with an intercom system or personal pager. Cost of an intercom may be as low as about $30. A battery-powered pager that beeps when a button is pressed to summon help from up to 100 feet away is about $50; a unit that vibrates rather than beeps is about $90. No installation is required. **Sources:** 229, 383.

When a client's language or involvement caused by a disability disturbs normal talking, finding a method to communicate allows the patient to maintain more control and dignity and also reduces

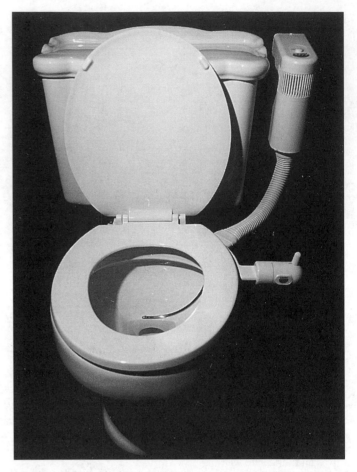

Figure 6-6. The Lubidet® personal hygiene system includes a bidet attachment and outlet. The warm water and air help prevent urinary tract infections, vaginal yeast infections, and reduce hemorrhoidal discomfort or constipation by softening anal sphincter muscles. (Photo courtesy of Lubidet USA, Inc., Denver, CO.)

stress on the family and caregivers. A speech or occupational therapist should assess the situation for the most appropriate solutions. If the onset of inability to speak is gradual, as in amyotrophic lateral sclerosis, selection of alternative communication and training in its use may be provided. Some suggestions are given in Chapter 5. These include a board for pointing and a microphone for amplifying volume. Additional methods include a computer with a voice synthesizer, which is sometimes available on a loan basis through a local hospice organization, or a hand-held talking device that spells out words on a digital read-out or tape. Some units store up to 20 messages that may be retrieved by the client using visual or tactile symbols. Cost is about $225 and up. **Sources** for alternative communication units include 154, 226, 418.

Aids to keep a patient oriented include a large calendar that may be marked off daily. A Reality Orientation Chart that gives the single day, month, year, and weather may be helpful for the individual with cognitive loss or dementia. **Source:** 434.

RESOURCES

Addresses for publishers, periodicals, and organizations are given in Section Four.

PUBLICATIONS

The American Association of Retired Persons provides several publications on caregiving and long-term care. These include D12895—*A Checklist of Concerns/Resources for Caregivers*, 50 for $4; D955—*A Handbook About Care in the Home*, 50 for $12; D12957—*A Path for Caregivers*, 50 for $6; D12748—*Miles Away and Still Caring: A Guide for Long Distance Caregivers*, 50 for $10; *Coping and Caring: Living with Alzheimer's Disease*, 50 for $12.50; D13803—*Care Management: Arranging for Long Term Care*, 50 for $7.50.

American Red Cross. (1993). *A Guide to Home Care for the Person Living with AIDS*. Washington, DC: Author.

Bass, D. S. (1990). *Caring Families: Supports and Interventions*. Silver Spring, MD: National Association of Social Workers. $21.95.

Bauch, E. (1989). *Extended Health Care at Home*. Berkeley, CA: Ten Speed Press. $9.95. Practical and emotional aspects of home care, whether recuperating from trauma or facing chronic or life-threatening illness. Choice of physician, facilities, working with pharmacist, finding health professionals, preparing the home, supplies, medications, special needs of patients with cancer, Alzheimer's, AIDS, and other conditions.

Bedell, G. (1994). *HIV/AIDS: A Consumer Guide for Daily Living*. Bethesda, MD: American Occupational Therapy Association. $4.50 AOTA members; $5.50 non-members. Designed for use by people with HIV/AIDS and their caregivers in collaboration with their occupational therapists. Reviews general HIV/AIDS-related problems in self-care, home living, work, and leisure time.

Biegel, D. E., Sales, E., & Schul, R. (1990). *Family Caregiving in a Chronic Illness*. Thousand Oaks, CA: Sage. $45.

Caring Magazine. Focuses on the needs of health care professionals and caregivers. In-depth, interdisciplinary articles.

Carlin, V. F., & Greenberg, V. E. (1992). *Should Mom Live With Us? And Is Happiness Possible If She Does?* Lexington, KY: Free Press.

Carter, R., with Golant, S. K. (1994). *Helping Yourself Help Others: A Book for Caregivers*. New York: Times Books, Random House. $20.

Children of Aging Parents distributes materials to assist caregivers: Starter Packet for Self-Help Groups (*Manual* and *Instant Aging: Sensitivity Manual*), $25; *Care Giving Directory—Geriatric Care Managers, Caregiver Support Groups and Health Related Services*, $20 (list of care managers from one state, $2; for support groups and resources from one state, $2); Tips for Caregivers Packet (leaflets on home care, nursing homes, housing options, "red tape," understanding the elderly, etc., $5; Selected bibliography of manuals and books, $2; *I Was My Father's Parent*, $2; *Caring for the Alzheimer's Patient*, $2; *As Your Parent Grows Old*, $1.50; *Do's If Your Parent Lives with You*, $.50; *The Caregiver: Taking Care of One's Self*, $1; *Special Products for the Elderly and Handicapped*, $21.

Cohen, D., & Eisdorfer, C. (1995). *Seven Steps to Effective Parent Care: A Planning and Action Guide for Adult Children with Aging Parents*. New York: Putnam Berkley.

Committee on Handicaps Group for the Advancement of

Psychiatry. (1993). *Caring for People with Physical Impairments: The Journey Back* (Report #135). Washington, DC: American Psychiatric Press.

Davidson, F. G. (1994). *The Alzheimer's Sourcebook for Caregivers*. Los Angeles: Lowell House.

Deily, J. *Experiencing Sensory Loss: A Manual for Caregivers*. Jefferson Area Board for Aging. Covers losses in vision and hearing in detail; an occupational therapist suggests solutions for increasing communication.

Dickey, R. (1996, July). Assessment for selection of environmental control. *Team Rehab*, 23-26.

Dippel, R. L., & Hutton, J. T. (1991). *Caring for the Alzheimer's Patient*. Anherst, MA: Prometheus.

Evans, J. *Caring for the Caregiver: Body, Mind and Spirit*. American Parkinson's Disease Association Educational Supplement No. 4. Free reprint of article by medical social worker from the Association.

Family Concerns: Caring for an Older Relative. (1990). San Antonio, TX: The USAA Foundation. Free. Determining level of care needed, resources for independent and dependent seniors, nursing home checklist.

Gartley, C. (Ed.). *Managing Incontinence: A Guide to Living with Loss of Bladder Control*. The Simon Foundation, $12.95. Incontinence is not limited to the very young or old. Book offers ways for people with incontinence to live normal, happy lives. Gives medical information, practical help, and product information. Sharing this with your clients and their families may help them find solutions to one problem.

Giblin, N., & Bales, B. (1995). *Finding Help: A Reference Guide for Personal Concerns*. Springfield, IL: Charles Thomas. $29.95.

Guide to Running a Respite Care Program in the 1990's. New York State Office for the Aging. $4 from the Long Term Care National Resource Center at UCLA/USC.

Harbaugh, G. L. (1992). *Caring for the Caregiver*. Washington, DC: The Alban Institute. **Source:** 31.

Heath, A. (1993). *Long Distance Caregiving*. San Luis Obispo, CA: American Source, Impact.

Horne, J., & Thomas, J. R. (Eds.). (1991). *A Survival Guide for Family Caregivers: Strength, Support, and Sources of Help for All Those Caring for Aging or Impaired Family Members*. Minneapolis: CompCare.

How to Help a Family Member Who Has a Bladder Control Problem. Free from Caring Products International, Inc. **Source:** 111.

Ideabook on Caregiver Support Groups, #2010. Washington, DC: National Council on the Aging. $7. Report on mutual help groups for families of frail and dependent older people. Includes state-by-state directory of nearly 800 support groups.

Incontinence. #1240, Krames Communications. 16-page, illustrated booklet for patients, promotes doctor-patient teamwork, includes assessment diary. **Source:** 308.

Jevne, R. F. (1991). *It All Begins with Hope: Patients, Caregivers & the Bereaved Speak Out*. San Deigo: Lura Media. $13.50. First-person accounts, photographs, and reflective insights. Reveals resilience of the human spirit. Becoming hopeful instead of hopeless. **Source:** 339.

Kievman, B., with Blackmun, S. (1989). *For Better or Worse:*

A Couple's Guide to Dealing with Chronic Illness. Chicago: Contemporary Books.

Lange, M. (1996, October). Selecting an ECU. *Team Rehab,* 57-59. At-a-glance Environmental Control Unit comparison chart.

Levin, N. J. (1997). *How to Care for Your Parents: A Handbook for Adult Children.* New York: Norton. $22.

Lifting and Moving Patients Safely. South Deerfield, MA: Channing L. Bete. Illustrated booklet explains basics of body mechanics, highlights proper techniques, suggests when assistance is warranted. $1.25 per copy.

Ludlum, C. D. (*Getting From Here to There: A Manual on Personal Assistance.* Storrs, CT: A.J. Papannikou Center on Special Education and Rehabilitation, University of Connecticut. Author's guide with tips used when she moved to her own home, including job descriptions, hiring techniques, reproducible forms, and resources.

Lustbader, W., & Hoogman, N. (1994). *Taking Care of Aging Family Members: A Practical Guide.* New York: Free Press, Simon & Schuster.

MacNamara, R. D. (1991). *Creating Abuse-Free Caregiving Environments for Children, the Disabled and the Elderly: Preparing, Supervising and Managing Caregivers for the Emotional Impact of Their Responsibilities.* Springfield, IL: Charles C. Thomas. $43.75.

Martelli, L. J. (1993). *When Someone You Know Has AIDS: A Practical Guide* (rev. ed.). New York: Crown.

Moe, B. (1992). *Coping with Chronic Illness.* New York: Rosen. $15.95. Through stories of young people, teenagers learn about dealing with a permanent illness and adjusting to one's limitations by having a healthy attitude and positive outlook.

Nelson-Morrill, C. (Ed.). (1993). *Florida Caregivers Handbook,* Revised Second Edition. Tallahassee, FL: HealthTrac.

Oregon State University Pacific Northwest Extension Service has several helpful publications by Schmall, V. L., et al., for caregivers and families, including *Aging Parents: Helping When Health Fails,* PNW246, $.50; *Coping with Caregiving: How to Manage Stress When Caring for Elderly Relatives,* PNW315, $1; *Families and Aging: A Guide to Legal Concerns,* EC1221, $1.25; *Helping Your Older Family Member Handle Finances,* PNW344, $.50. **Source:** 393B.

Ossman, N. H., & Campbell, M. (1990). *Adult Positions, Transitions, and Transfers: Reproducible Cards for Caregivers.* San Antonio, TX: Therapy Skill Builders. $35. OT and PT cover 28 situations for adult and geriatric clients. Shows caregiver how to help patients develop good habits, ensure safety, and encourage active patient participation. Kit comes with *Therapist Guide* and *Caregiver Guide.* **Source:** 522.

Ostuni, E., & Santo Pietro, M. J. (1991). *Getting Through: When Someone You Love Has Alzheimer's Disease.* Vero Beach, FL: The Speech Bin. **Source:** 488.

Peterkin, A. (1992). *What About Me? When Brothers and Sisters Get Sick.* New York: Magination Press, Div. of Brunner/Mazel. $8.95. For ages four to eight, to be read with parents to help the isolated healthy child.

Ratto, L. L. (1992). *Coping with a Physically Challenged Brother or Sister.* New York: Rosen. $15.95. Step-by-step methods of coping, written for teenagers.

Reference Guide to Incontinence. Silver Spring, MD: Agency for Health Care Policy and Research, Columbia, MD: American Medical Directors Association.

Rob, C., with Reynolds, J. (1992). *The Caregiver's Guide: Helping Elderly Relatives Cope with Health and Safety Concerns.* Boston: Houghton Mifflin. $22.45. Recognizing physical and mental problems, increasing independence for longer, locating social services, resources.

Silverstone, B., & Hyman, H. K. (1990). *You and Your Aging Parent: The Modern Family's Guide to Emotional, Physical, and Financial Problems.* New York: Pantheon, Random House.

Susik, D. H. (1995). *Hiring Home Caregivers: The Family Guide to In-home Eldercare.* San Luis Obispo, CA: American Source Books.

Urinary Incontinence in Adults: Acute and Chronic Management Update. Agency for Health Care Policy and Research. Guide designed for use by caregivers to improve quality of life for their charges and to allow them to stay at home longer. Guidelines may be accessed through AHCPR's home page on the Internet at http://www.ahcpr.gov/guide/. A quick reference guide *Managing Acute and Chronic Urinary Incontinence* and a consumer guide *Understanding Incontinence* (in English or Spanish) is free from the AHCPR Publications Clearinghouse.

Well Spouse Foundation. Four pamphlets: *Anger, Guilt, Isolation,* and *Looking Ahead.* $1.50 each. Bimonthly members' newsletter, *Mainstay.* Individual membership $20 per year.

Wheeler, E., & Dace-Lombard, J. (1990). *Living Creatively with Chronic Illness: Developing Skills for Transcending the Loss, Pain and Frustration.* San Bernadino, CA: Borgo. $29.

AUDIOVISUALS

Bosch, J. V. *Elder Abuse: Five Case Studies.* 40-minute video, $245; Davis, D. *The Golden Years?* KCTS Television, 60-minute VHS video, $99; and Feinberg, J. *A Safer Place.* Illinois Department of Aging, 20-minute VHS video, $89. Three videos on elder abuse available through Fanlight Productions. Descriptive brochure. **Source:** 200.

Hope, L. *Another Home for Mom,* KGW-TV, 30-minute video, $195; Bosch, J. V. *My Mother..My Father,* 33-minute video, $295, and *My Mother, My Father...Seven Years Later,* 42-minute video, $295, with Kaufman, N. J. in association with Consumers Union. *Study Guide; To Care: A Portrait of Three Older Caregivers,* 28-minute VHS video, $195; and Feinberg, J. *Respite: Taking Care,* Kellogg Respite Care Project, 22-minute video, $145. Five videos on caregiving, all available through Y13 Productions. Descriptive brochure. **Source:** 588.

Family Seminars for Caregiving: Helping Families Help. Facilitator's Manual. (1985). University of Washington Press. Looseleaf binder, $50. Including "It's the Little Things," 69 35-mm slides in carousel and 20-minute audiocassette, $135. **Source:** 550.

Kirn, H. *Caring....Sharing: The Alzheimer's Caregiver,* 38-minute VHS video, $195; Fabares, S. *Someone I Love Has Alzheimer's Disease,* Lifestyle Productions, 17-minute VHS video with curriculum guide, $145; Stauffacher, C. *Something Should Be Done About Grandma Ruthie,* 54-minute VHS video, $195. Three videos on Alzheimer's and caregiving, all available from Fanlight Productions. Descriptive brochure. **Source:** 200.

Neef, N. A., et al. (Producers). *Caring for Persons with Developmental Disabilities: A Training Program for Respite Care Providers*. Champaign, IL: Research Press. Video training program teaches skills needed to care for individuals with a wide range of developmental disabilities. Six tapes cover preparation (dressing safely for job, key information from parents, manual communication signs), daily routines (mealtime, feeding patients with oral-motor problems, toileting, bedtime, using routine activities to strengthen existing skills), physical medical management (transfers, lifting, hyperextension, medication), behavior management (preventing misbehavior, management strategies), emergencies (cessation of breathing, poisoning, bleeding, choking, seizures), and parent return (positive behavior, departures from routine, medical problems, behavior problems). Leader's guide and pre- and post-assessment forms, $495 plus $4 shopping. One-day preview available; call or write for next available date. **Source:** 441.

Tigges, K. N., & Marcil, W. M. *Home Care Needs and Techniques*, 50-minute VHS video and companion book, *Caring for Someone in Your Home*, $15.95. Also Tigges, K. N. *Home Care Needs in the Bathroom*, 30-minute VHS video. Wide ranging approach to adapting the bathroom from easy-to-find aids to specialized equipment. Covers tub safety, showering, grab bars, commode assists, and general safety. And Davis, V. *Personal Home Care Issues: Mastectomy, Circulation, Incontinence*, 35-minute VHS video. Demonstrates various products and resources available to allow effective management of personal problems. Cost of videos is $49.95 each, distributed by Clinician's View. **Source:** 124.

Transfer Skills. Y13 Productions. 19 minutes, VHS video. Physical therapist shows nurse how to employ correct body mechanics during patient transfers, including bed to chair, chair to toilet, and floor to chair. $99 plus $6 handling and shipping. **Source:** 588.

Stress-Reduction Techniques

Everyone is under stress, including caregivers, other family members, and health professionals. Good or positive stress helps us accomplish goals in a realistic manner and length of time. Bad or negative stress incapacitates and creates barriers to good health and enjoying the processes of life. By learning how to relax, solve problems, and communicate more effectively, a person can minimize stress and use positive stress to achieve increased independence and success. Relaxation has also been shown to help speed healing and to slow the pace of immune diseases, such as HIV/AIDS.

If the stress is making it impossible for a patient, caregiver, or family to function, ways to help reduce stress should be incorporated into the home management program. It is often while doing routine tasks that people talk about problems and seek, as well as accept, solutions. Along with good nutrition and physical skills, methods of relaxation and problem solving may be dispensed.

This guide looks mainly at physical and cognitive disabilities. Many individuals, however, have mental or emotional problems that go beyond its intended scope. Health professionals, including psychiatric nurses and occupational therapists, combine skills to work with both aspects of an individual's needs. Other professionals include pastoral counselors, social workers, psychiatrists, and psychologists. Some of the stress-reducing techniques discussed here may be applied.

Building a therapeutic relationship takes time. Just as the person with low energy must set priorities, the individual who feels overstressed needs time to set down or formulate problems and then must take small steps to find solutions. Understanding how your client or a caregiver reacts to stress is a base on which to build. This includes physiological, cognitive, and behavioral responses. Some of the books in the Resources may be recommended to the caregiver.

Long-term physical reactions to stress increase the risk of heart disease, depression, and other physical and emotional disorders. The individual should be taught to recognize stress-related symptoms. The first is usually increased muscle tension and tightness, especially in the face, neck, and back. This may lead to

headaches. Second is dysfunction of the gastrointestinal tract and stomach leading to heartburn, diarrhea, or constipation. Third is rapid pulse and elevated blood pressure, which can lead to hypertension and other cardiovascular diseases. Constricted blood vessels result in cold hands or migraine headaches. Troubling thoughts and feelings increase worry, anxiety, and poor self-image. Sleep is disrupted, reducing energy. The person may feel depressed and experience loss of appetite or compulsive eating, irritability, and mood swings.

Teaching a patient about the physical strains created by stress helps pinpoint that there are problems, but not what they are. This requires a second phase. The "stressors" should be listed, with sliding scale values given to those considered major life crises or events down to minor hassles.

For the older client, stresses may include moving to a new location and losing one's former support group, a change in role, loss of spouse and friends, limited income, changes in appearance, and declining physical abilities. As we grow older, it takes longer for the body to recover from the physiological changes caused by stress.

For the younger person, guilt over poor health and dependency on others plus the upheaval in one's vision of future plans contribute to the stress. By writing down the stress-causing factors, the individual can isolate and tackle them more effectively.

Conquering stress involves many factors:
- Effective time management.
- Setting of priorities.
- Having adequate rest or sleep.
- Cognitive relaxation or meditation.
- Counseling.
- Delegating jobs.
- Finding new or positive outlets and channels for tensions, anger, and frustration.
- Finding support networks or respites.

See Appendix G for a reproducible list of "Rules to Reduce Stress." Post these rules so your client can review them daily.

Within the home care setting, cognitive relaxation may be taught as a beginning or ending to a treatment session. Learning the patient's likes allows the therapist to use images that increase relaxation. For the patient with chronic obstructive pulmonary disease or asthma, sitting and visualizing a balloon floating freely in light air and following it over gentle fields and hills leads to a relaxing of the body. As the patient learns to concentrate on such images, the level of relaxation increases. Making a menu of pleasurable experiences for visualizing on one's own lets the patient choose an image according to his or her mood or needs. Meditation done on a daily or twice-daily basis for 20 minutes can reduce stress and has been proven to reduce blood pressure (study reported in *Hypertension*). Your client, the caregiver, or you should sit quietly in any comfortable position with eyes closed. If worrisome thoughts intrude, continue sitting quietly. To help focus, you may suggest that your client find a short mantra to repeat. Materials on meditation are listed in the Resources.

Walking is another way for a patient to reduce stress. All homemaking training does not have to be done around the kitchen table. The steady, rhythmic action of walking helps both conscious and unconscious thinking. Identifying a problem before the walk begins, then quietly thinking about it while one is walking may lead to new insights. Walks may be started in therapy as part of a full day's program, then independently carried on by the patient.

Nutrition affects stress levels. Stimulants including those with caffeine should be avoided; at least eight glasses a day of herbal teas and water are recommended. When working on meal planning, your client may want to consider eating six small meals a day to avoid the dips that longer waits and larger meals create. Protein seems to stimulate norepinephrine, a natural antidote to mental fatigue. Complex carbohydrates like pasta, bread, and beans boost the levels of the amino acid tryptophan, which raises levels of "feel good" serotonin in the brain. An afternoon snack might combine high-in-protein low-fat cheese and whole wheat bread.

Other techniques to consider include teaching your client to take short periods of time to breath effectively (with long, slow, deep breaths from the diaphragm) and keeping a stress diary. Writing down thoughts actually helps to dispel them or to work out solutions.

Some patients may actually need to increase their stress level to achieve a balanced lifestyle. The newly retired individual, for example, with too much time on his or her hands might benefit from a volunteer job that re-invests energy in a new responsibility or leisure skill.

Learning to cope with stress in a positive way helps an individual handle pain and chronic disease. Chapter 14 has several references for relaxation tapes and materials.

RESOURCES

Addresses for publishers, periodicals, and organizations are given in Section Four.

PUBLICATIONS

Bell, L., & Seyfer, E. (1987). *Gentle Yoga: Yoga for People with Arthritis, Stroke Damage, Multiple Sclerosis, in Wheelchairs, or Anyone Who Needs a Guide to Gentle Exercise*. Berkeley, CA: Celestial Arts, Ten Speed. $7.95.

Benson, H. (1975). *The Relaxation Response*. New York: Avon. $3.99.

Benson, H. (1996). *Timeless Healing: The Power and Biology of Belief*. New York: Scribners. $24. Explores connection between science and power of the human spirit; relaxation response and resources included.

Blumenfeld, L. (1993). *The Big Book of Relaxation*. Roslyn, NY: The Relaxation Co. $14.95. Simple techniques to control stress in one's life.

Coleman, D., & Gurin, J. (1993). *Mind/Body Medicine: How to Use Your Mind for Better Health*. Yonkers, NY: Consumer Reports® Books. $24.95.

Coping with Stress. Free booklet, in large print, from the National Multiple Sclerosis Society. Outlines causes, mechanisms for coping, and relaxation techniques your client can practice independently.

Cotton, D. H. G. (1990). *Stress Management: An Integrated Approach to Therapy*. New York: Brunner/Mazel. $30. Conceptual framework to help therapist and client understand and control both positive and negative stress. Steps to build therapeutic relationship, identify and delineate stress-related problems, formulate individualized treatment plan, organize treatment strategies, and help client apply new stress-management skills.

Davis, M., et al. (1995). *The Relaxation and Stress Reduction Workbook*. Oakland, CA: New Harbinger. $14.95. Interactive guide with self-assessment questionnaires, suggested exercises, symptom effectiveness chart with recommendations for techniques that are most effective for specific symptoms, checklists, and fill-in-the-blank pages. A separate publication is available for individuals interested in conducting group programs, *Leader's Guide to The Relaxation and Stress Workbook*, also by M. Davis. **Source:** 376B.

A Guide to Managing Stress. San Bruno, CA: Krames Communications. Patient education aid. 16-page booklet, 40 color illustrations, shows how to recognize positive and negative stress feelings. Step-by-step instructions on various relaxation techniques and tips for reducing stress. **Source:** 308.

Hansen, M., et al. (1990). *Understanding Stress: Strategies for a Healthier Mind and Body*. Bethesda, MD: American Occupational Therapy Association. #1670, $4.50 AOTA members, $6 non-members, plus handling. Illustrated booklet identifies common causes of stress, suggests positive responses to situations, presents real-life case scenarios, and offers constructive solutions.

Hanson, P. (1987). *The Joy of Stress*. Kansas City, MO: Andrews and McMeel. $8.95. Discusses relief of tensions by involving different circuits of the brain and body that are used in daily occupations.

Horowitz, K. E., & Lanes, D. M. (1992). *Witness to Illness: Strategies for Caregiving and Coping*. Reading, MA: Addison-Wesley.

Karr, K. L. (1992). *Taking Time for Me: How Caregivers Can Effectively Deal with Stress*. Buffalo, NY: Prometheus.

Le Shan, L. (1987). *How to Meditate: A Guide to Self Discovery*. New York: Bantam Doubleday Dell. $5.50.

Mason, L. J. (1985). *Guide to Stress Reduction*. Berkeley, CA: Celestial Arts, Ten Speed. $9.95. Exercises to reduce stress; may be used with client, caregiver, or by professional. Includes visualization and imagery exercises.

Navarra, T. (1995). *Wisdom for Caregivers*. Thorofare, NJ: SLACK Inc. $12. Collection of ideas, observations, and thoughts to reduce stress and offer support with a dose of appreciation to health care professionals and other caregivers.

Norton, S. (1977). *Yoga for People Over 50: Exercise Without Exhaustion*. Santa Cruz, CA: Devin. Check your local library.

Ornstein, R., & Sobel, D. (1989). *Healthy Pleasures*. Reading, MA: Addison-Wesley. $16.95.

Ornstein, R., & Sobel, D. (1986). *The Healing Brain*. New York: Touchstone, Simon & Schuster. $8.95.

Rosenfeld, M. S. (1993). *Wellness and Lifestyle Renewal: A Manual for Personal Change*. Bethesda, MD: American Occupational Therapy Association. #1978, $20 AOTA members, $28 non-members. Manual/workbook helps clients reassess current lifestyle due to illness or injury. Exercises are designed to be done by a group or by the therapist and a client.

Sobel, D. S., & Ornstein R. *The Healthy Mind, Healthy Body Handbook*. Institute for the Improvement of Human Knowledge. Order from ISHK Book Service, $14.95. Self-help strategies for coping with anxiety, depression, anger, trauma, insomnia, chronic illness, and pain. Relaxation to communication skills, using imagery techniques, humor, and healing. **Source:** 283.

Stress Techniques. Atlanta, GA: Arthritis Foundation. Free 16-page brochure on ways to manage stress. Ask local chapter or call the National Office.

PERIODICALS

See Appendix D for addresses and rates.

CardiSense. Free newsletter for health care professionals and people taking heart medications. Often has articles on life management skills and reducing stress.

Mental Medicine Update: The Mind/Body Health Newsletter. The Center for Health Sciences, the Institute for the Study of Human Knowledge. Articles and book reviews on handling stress, pain, anger, and communicating with health care practitioners.

AUDIOVISUALS

Time-Life Medical Series: Stress and Anxiety. With C. Everett Koop. Omaha, NE: Infovision. $25. Four parts: Understanding the diagnosis; what happens next; treatment and management; and issues and answers. Program comes with and refers to a personal workbook. **Source:** 280.

8

The Client Who Uses One Hand or Has Had a Stroke

Most patients limited to use of only one hand are hemiplegic individuals who have suffered a cerebral vascular accident or stroke. In the United States, there are now more than 500,000 people who have had strokes. Each year, 25,000 Americans younger than 25 are diagnosed with strokes.

Other clients may be functioning with one hand because of a temporary problem such as a fracture, or a permanent injury such as disability from birth, a brachial plexus, or other neurological paralysis or amputation. Our discussion here focuses on the post-stroke client, but the one-handed techniques are applicable to anyone.

Assessment of the hemiplegic or post-stroke patient includes physical status of the arm and leg, trunk balance and ambulation skills, perceptual/cognitive limitations, visual status, oral and written abilities, and goals of the patient, i.e., role at home and/or work. The individual usually has the inability to use one hand and arm and has a poor gait. He or she still may be confined to a wheelchair or have general poor balance when using a cane with the good hand. Receptive and/or expressive aphasia may be present if hemiplegia is on the dominant side. Perceptual losses, which reduce awareness of safety factors, are more frequent when hemiplegia is on the non-dominant side. A visual loss of field on the affected side (hemianopsia) is common. If there is loss of sensation in the affected arm, denial or non-recognition of that side may also be present.

A difference in goals is often defined by the age of the person. Older clients frequently depend on their children or spouses for support. An increasing number of younger stroke patients, on the other hand, must return to full family and work responsibilities, including bringing up children.

Any treatment plan for the person who has survived a stroke and has perceptual, cognitive, and physical limitations must be carefully coordinated with all therapeutic disciplines. Within the institution, the client will still be recovering physically and will be just beginning to assess his or her status and needs. Strength and ability to concentrate on a task may be poor. Progress differs widely. At home, depending on the speed of discharge from the hospital, the patient may be ready to accept a full program, a return to former routines, or may still be physically and emotionally fragile.

Homemaking rehabilitation for the client who has had a stroke often requires cognitive as well as physical retraining (Figure 8-1). The occupational therapist evaluates the patient in terms of safety, memory, coordination, visual limitations, and perceptual deficits. Familiar activities not only permit realistic evaluation but help increase patient's confidence.

Teaching one-handed techniques with the non-affected arm is an immediate need. Even before the hemiplegic develops function in the affected arm, using it as an assist is important and helps overcome denial of that side. Tasks such as mixing and opening packages call both hands into use, letting the weight of the affected arm stabilize.

Tasks that require training may include the following:
- Food preparation: handling knife; peeling and slicing; measuring; stirring or mixing in bowls and pans; draining hot pots; breaking eggs; opening cans, jars, and other containers; beating with rotary mixer; carrying water or pans; lighting or setting range top and oven; using appliances; and retrieving items from cabinets.
- Serving: setting and clearing table; getting out flatware and dishes; transporting casseroles and hot foods; and carrying liquids.
- Cleaning up: scrubbing pans; loading dishwasher; putting clean items away; cleaning counters and stove top; wiping up spills; mopping or sweeping; and handling vacuum cleaner.
- Shopping: planning meals; making shopping list; and doing actual marketing or delegating it to someone else.

Specific suggestions for techniques and aids for these areas are given in *Mealtime Manual*, Chapter 1.

Homemaking areas outside of meal preparation include laundry, sewing, child care, and housecleaning.

Meal preparation and homemaking training are not limited to relearning skills. There is the necessity to change old habits due to new health and diet concerns. There is a redefining of role. Memory and cognitive abilities may be affected. Additional

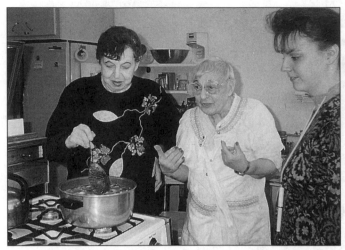

Figure 8-1. Homemaking rehabilitation for the client who has had a stroke often requires cognitive as well as physical retraining. (Photo courtesy of the O.T. Dept., Howard A. Rusk Institute of Rehabilitation Medicine.)

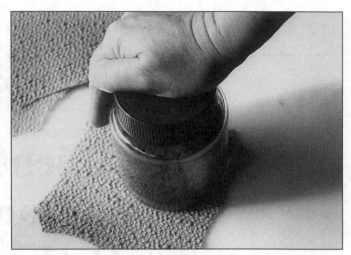

Figure 8-2. A gripper pad secures objects to the counter. (Gripper pads by Compac Industries, Atlanta, GA. Photo by J.K.)

stresses include doctors' bills, therapists, and how to cut back on, or if to cut back on, activities.

If aphasia is part of the picture, communication is difficult. Memory and cognitive function may also be impaired, requiring additional perceptual and safety training. One patient commented that between her mild aphasia and her husband's increasing word-finding difficulty, "It takes two of us to get a good sentence out."

The post-stroke patient often feels the future is uncertain. Depression is a prevalent reaction. Mood swings are common. Anxiety about a second stroke affects behavior and mental status.

The last stage of rehabilitation from a stroke is reorganization. This is when the person becomes aware of emotional and social isolation. Joining a stroke support group lets a client share feelings and develop coping mechanisms. Daily phone calls between post-stroke patients motivate and develop increased independence. To find a group, check with the nearest chapter of the American Heart Association, local hospitals, or visiting nurses' associations. Referral is easier if you accompany the patient and spouse or caregiver to the initial session. For health professionals wishing to start a support group, information is available from the American Heart Association, the National Stroke Association, and the Courage Center. Addresses are in Appendix C.

If your client has aphasia, reading recipes and other materials may not be possible. Using familiar simple recipes, ones known by heart, is a first step. Cookbooks designed for the developmentally delayed allow cooking by picture. See Chapter 21. A photo phone book or a memory-dial phone allows the patient to reach frequently called numbers. The family may design one with the numbers for the spouse's workplace, children, visiting nurses, doctors' office, emergency 911, fire department, and others. Make the numbers large, and draw or use photos of each person. See Chapter 3 for an adapted phone dialer. Organizations that offer information for the individual with aphasia are the Academy of Aphasia, the American Speech,

Language and Hearing Association, and the National Aphasia Association. Addresses are in Appendix C.

To stabilize objects while working, the client may put a damp paper towel or friction-type material under the bowl or pan.

A gripper pad secures a bowl, plate, jar, or other object to the counter (Figure 8-2). The textured pad shown, called the Mighty Gripper, also increases grip when opening a jar. **Manufacturer:** 133. Cost is about $1.60 for a package of four from housewares and grocery stores. A similar material, MediGrip® is made by 554.

For other non-slip materials, see Chapter 4 and Chapter 11. Other stabilizing techniques and devices for the person working with one hand are discussed and illustrated in *Mealtime Manual*, Chapter 1. Some of the aids for the individual using one hand may be simply adapted or constructed.

A suction-based brush may be purchased ready-made or adapted with Poly Lock® hook and loop closure (Figures 8-3A, B). Suction-based brushes for use with vegetables, kitchen clean-up, fingernails, and dentures are available through rehabilitation and self-help firms. **Sources:** 33, 140, 319, 383, 461.

An adapted cutting board with two nails to secure items being cut is a basic kitchen aid. See *Mealtime Manual*. A paddle-shaped board with a handle is easier to pick up with one hand than a rectangular board. **Manufacturers** of paddle boards include 20, 193, 210.

A wooden pan handle holder stabilizes the pot while the patient stirs with one hand (Figure 8-4). Suction cups or strong magnets secure it to the top or side of a small range. Dampen suction cups before securing holder; release if necessary by slipping point of table knife under edge. This prevents weakening attachments to the wood. Idea from *Home Economics Guide: With One Hand*, Cooperative Extension Center, University of Missouri-Columbia, 1981, out of print.

A pull-out bread board becomes a bowl holder when a circle slightly smaller than the bowl is cut out of one side (Figure 8-5). The inner surface may be lined with rubber, or a damp sponge cloth may be used to stabilize the bowl.

Teaching your client to sit while working not only increases safety but lets the knees and lap become a holding aid (Figure 8-

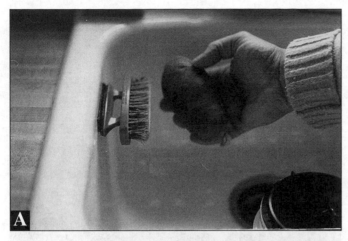

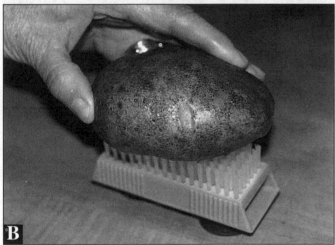

Figure 8-3A,B. A suction-based brush may be purchased ready-made or adapted with Poly Lock® hook and loop closure. (Figure 8-3A: Photo courtesy of Consumer Care Products, Sheboygan, WI. Figure 8-3B: Photo by J.K.)

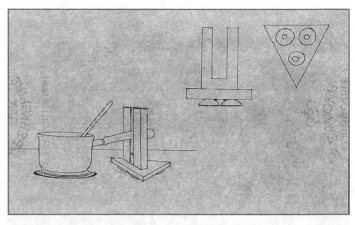

Figure 8-4. A wooden pan handle holder stabilizes the pot while the patient stirs with one hand. (Illustration by G.K.)

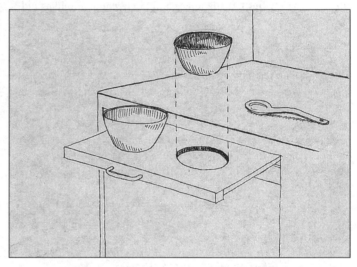

Figure 8-5. A pull-out bread board becomes a bowl holder when a circle slightly smaller than the bowl is cut out of one side. (Illustration by G.K.)

6). Tongs pick up food more securely than a fork and release an item easily when working with one hand (Figure 8-7).

RESOURCES

Addresses for publications, periodicals, and organizations are given in Section Four.

PUBLICATIONS

Also see *Mealtime Manual*, Chapter 1.

The American Heart Association's newsletter for stroke patients and their families, *Stroke Connections*, is produced six times a year and is available by subscription. Sample copy, $.50.

Other publications from the American Heart Association include *Straight Talk About Stroke*, H51-1093, $5. Twenty-two reproducible, two-sided fact sheets. Topics include aphasia, high blood pressure, and rehabilitation. For stroke survivors and family members. *AHA Family Guide to Stroke*, H67-0056, $23. For family members and stroke survivors, in-depth information about warning signs and cases, diagnosis, medical treatment, rehabilita-

tion, and living with a stroke. Gives tips on adapting one's home and habits, tells what will happen as recovery continues. Booklets include *How Stroke Affects Behavior*, H50-1123, 50 for $6.50; *Brain Attack: The Family's Role in Caregiving*, H50-1072, 25 for $5.50; *Recovering from Stroke*, H50-1124, 25 for $12. Large-format, large-print book for stroke survivors shows how to do familiar tasks in new ways, discusses perception, coordination, personal care, exercise, medications, and mental and emotional factors. *Caring for a Person with Aphasia*, H55-1127, 25 for $8.50. *The One-Handed Way*, H50-1120, $2.50 per copy. Nearly 300 day-to-day challenges with methods for handling them with one hand. *The Language of Stroke*, H50-1125, $4 per copy. Stroke-related vocabulary of medical and biological terminology, H50-1125, $4 per copy. Also see AHA cookbooks in Resources, Chapter 29.

Burns, M. S., et al. (1996). *Clinical Management of Right Hemisphere Dysfunction* (2nd ed.). Frederick, MD: Rehabilitation Institute of Chicago Publication, Aspen. $56.

Courage Stroke Network, c/o Courage Center, provides information on coping with stroke and referral to stroke groups.

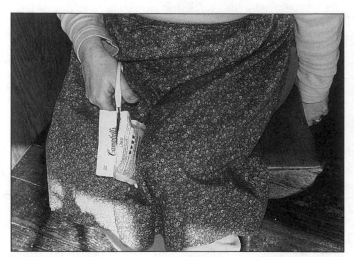

Figure 8-6. Teaching your client to sit while working not only increases safety but lets the knees and lap become a holding aid. (Photo by J.K.)

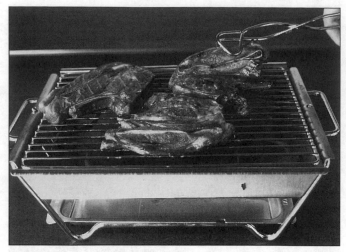

Figure 8-7. Tongs pick up food more securely than a fork and release an item easily when working with one hand. (Photo by J.K.)

CVA (Stroke): Resource Guide. Bethesda, MD: American Occupational Therapy Association, #4220, $10 AOTA members, $20 non-members. Bibliographies and list of audiovisuals and resource personnel.

Fishman, S. (1988). *A Bomb in the Brain.* New York: Avon. $8.95. Author's story of stroke and rehabilitation.

Foley, C., & Pizer, H. F. *The Stroke Fact Book—Everything You Want and Need to Know About Stroke—From Prevention to Rehabilitation.* Courage Center. $12.95.

Garee, B. (1987 reprint). *Single-Handed: Devices and Aids for One-handers and Sources of These Devices.* Bloomington, IL: Accent, Cheever. $3.50.

Jay, P. (1991). *Help Yourselves: A Handbook for Hemiplegics and Their Families.* Studio City, CA: Empire.

Johnstone, M. (1991). *Therapy for Stroke: Building on Experience.* New York: Churchill Livingstone. $25.

Learning to Live with Angina and *Learning to Live with Hypertension.* Both from the Patient Information Series, $3 each from Medicine in the Public Interest. **Source:** 355.

The National Stroke Association has a variety of materials available for use with post-stroke patients. *Be Stroke Smart* is their quarterly newsletter with both scientific articles and practical advice for patients. The book *The Road Ahead: A Stroke Recovery Guide* by Karin Schumacher and Cindy Hanna deals with what to expect. $16.95 per copy. *Adaptive Resources: A Guide to Products and Manufacturers,* free. Other materials include five mini-packets: *Prevention and Warning Signs* 3 articles, $1; *Communication Difficulties* 3 articles, $2; *Rehabilitation Guidelines and Resources* 10 articles, $6; *Home and Work Adaptations* 5 articles, $3; *Emotional Aspects* 5 articles, $3. Four *Be Stroke Smart* brochures are $.50 each and include *What Every Family Should Know About Stroke, Suggestions for Communication with an Aphasic Person, Depression—A Natural Reaction to Stroke, The Importance of Proper Diet After Stroke.* Pamphlets are *Stroke—What It Is, What Causes It,* $1; and *Living at Home After a Stroke,* $2. There are also four booklets for distribution to patients: *Home Exercises for Stroke Patients,* 13 pages, $2; *Understanding Speech and Language*

Problems After Stroke, 20 pages, $2; *Stroke: Reducing Your Risk,* 13 pages, $2; *Stroke: Questions and Answers,* 24 pages, $3.

Okema, K. (1993). *Cognition and Perception in the Stroke Patient: A Guide to Functional Outcomes in Occupational Therapy.* Frederick, MD: Rehabilitation Institute of Chicago Publication Series, Aspen. $63. Organized into three parts: cognitive and perceptual evaluation, goal writing and treatment planning, evaluation and treatment.

Paulin, E. *Ted's Stroke: The Caregiver's Story.* Practical personal answers to questions all caregivers have. With two appendices written by physicians. $14.95 from Courage Center.

Post-Stroke Rehabilitation. (1996). Developed by the Center for Health Economics Research with the AHCPR. Frederick MD: Aspen. $19.95. Clinical practice guidelines.

Practice Guidelines for Adults with Stroke. (1996). Bethesda, MD: American Occupational Therapy Association. $20 AOTA members, $25 non-members. Reference tool for health care facility managers, managed care organizations, third-party payers, and OT practitioners. Defines evaluations, frequency, duration of treatment, and gives explanation of billing codes.

Rasmussen, M. (1990). *The Language of Stroke: A Guide to Understanding the Medical Terms of Stroke.* Golden Valley, MN: Courage Press. $4.95. Dictionary of terms used in referring to stroke.

Resource Guide to Stroke. Free from the National Association for Rehabilitation Information Center.

Sarno, M. (1991). *Acquired Aphasia* (2nd ed.). Westminster, CA: Academy Press. $55.

Shirk, E. (1991). *After the Stroke: Coping with America's Third Leading Cause of Death.* Buffalo, NY: Prometheus. $19.95.

Sarton, M. (1988). *After the Stroke.* New York: Norton. $16.95. Journal of author's journey back to health following stroke.

Stroke Rehabilitation: Patient Education Manual. (1995). Frederick, MD: Aspen Reference Group, Aspen. $159. Annual supplements sent on 30-day approval. Hand-outs, guidelines, charts, instructions, and other tools; multidisciplinary approach. Covers medical problems and conditions, as well as physical perceptual/cognitive/language, psychological and social problems and conditions. Major foci on activities of daily living and post-stroke prevention of recurrence.

Youngson, R. M. (1990). *Stroke: A Self Help Manual for Stroke Suffers and Their Relatives*. San Bernardino, CA: Borgo. $24.95.

Zoltan, B. (1996). *Vision, Perception, and Cognition: A Manual for Evaluation and Treatment of the Neurologically Impaired Adult* (3rd ed.). Thorofare, NJ: SLACK Inc. $29. Specific methods for evaluation and treatment with step-by-step testing techniques and guidelines.

Additional organizations involved with stroke include the American Physical Therapy Association, the National Institute of Neurological Disorders and Stroke, and the Rehabilitation Research and Training Center on Enhancing Quality of Life of Stroke Survivors. The NARIC library has more than 1000 documents pertaining to stroke.

PERIODICALS

American Journal of Occupational Therapy. AOTA.
Cognitive Rehabilitation. Neuroscience Publishers.
Hypertension. American Heart Association.
Topics in Stroke Rehabilitation. Aspen.

AUDIOVISUALS

Ewing, S. A., & Pfalzgraf, B. *Pathways: Moving Beyond Stroke and Aphasia*. 28-minute VHS encourages survivors to move through and beyond their illness; six families discuss diverse paths they have taken to work through grief and accept changes in roles and responsibilities. By the same authors and speech pathologists, *What is Aphasia?* is a 28-minute VHS focusing on understanding communication loss due to a stroke and demonstrating strategies used to compensate for losses and learn to communicate effectively. Videos are $49.95 each from Wayne State University Press. An accompanying book called *Pathways: Moving Beyond Stroke and Aphasia* is $34.95 cloth or $17.95 paperbound. **Source: 565.**

Home Care of Stroke Survivors. (1996). Frederick, MD: Aspen Patient Education Video Series, Aspen. Binder includes two full-color videos: *Activities of Daily Living After Left Brain Stroke* (20 minutes); *Activities of Daily Living After Right Brain Stroke*, two companion booklets with photocopy-ready hand-outs to reinforce video training. Set of two, $149. **Source: 61.**

The Homemaker with Use of One Hand: Handicapped Homemaker Film Series, M-2243-X. Howard A. Rusk Institute of Rehabilitation Medicine, New York University Medical Center, under a grant for the Campbell Soup Fund. 28 minutes, 16 mm. Color/sound. Demonstrates the kitchen planning, techniques, and equipment used by a young hemiplegic homemaker. For information, contact Living Media, Inc. **Source: 332.**

Levin, R. *Strok-A-Cize*. VHS, 40 minutes. Strength and flexibility exercises all done in sitting position at a comfortable pace, to be done with family member or caregiver, $50. **Source: 275.**

One Hand Can Do the Work of Two. (1993). VHS, 20 minutes. West Sacramento, CA: A/V Health Services. $32.50. After losing use of dominant hand, woman shows how she taught herself to be independent using one hand. Demonstrates skills in homemaking and activities of daily living. Text recommends viewing supervision by therapist or other professional. Several aids are described but not shown so follow-up by therapist is required to teach patient and to demonstrate appropriate aids. **Sources: 1, 11, 14, 65.**

Stroke Education Videos, 2 sets: #1S *Beginning Stroke Therapy* #2S *Advanced Stroke Therapy*. Y13 Productions. Each set of 3 videos has separate right and left CVA tapes and a transfer techniques video; cost each set, $169. #1S—Setting in hospital includes nurse, physical and occupational therapists, and speech pathologist working with patient; #2S—Prepares patient and family to function at home with specific tasks taught by multidisciplinary team and a home visit by second occupational therapist. Combination five-tape set, including one transfer tape is $269. **Source: 588.**

A Stroke Survivor's Workout Video. VHS, 30 minutes, $20. Led by Nicoli, L., RPT, with flexibility and strengthening exercises. Most exercises done from sturdy chair or wheelchair; some while standing and using a chair for balance, $19.95 from Courage Center. **Source: 150.**

You're Not Alone, H50-1134. Offers encouragement to stroke survivors and their families, helps them to understand physical and emotional lifestyle changes, left- and right-brain effects, role of family and friends, support groups, prevention methods for secondary stroke. *A Gift of Caring*, H50-1135. Role of caregivers, responsibilities, importance of ensuring that caregiver's as well as the patient's needs are met. Two 15-minute VHS videos, $10 each from the American Heart Association.

Exercise videos, designed for people who have sustained a stroke and have one-sided weakness, may help your client continue a daily exercise program when no longer on a rehabilitation program.

CONTINUING EDUCATION

Stroke: Strategies, Treatment, Rehabilitation, Outcomes, Knowledge, and Evaluation. (1996). A self-paced clinical course, Royeen, Charlotte B., Course Editor, #3010. Bethesda, MD: American Occupational Therapy Association. 12 lessons in package, $240 AOTA members, $290 non-members.

9

The Client with Upper Extremity Weakness

Weak upper extremities may be caused by paralysis from spinal cord injury, trauma to the brachial plexus, or the effects of a disease such as multiple sclerosis, poliomyelitis or post-polio syndrome, muscular dystrophy, or amyotrophic lateral sclerosis. Function may also be limited by unwanted motion, as in Parkinson's or cerebral palsy, or by limited range, as in scleraderma, arthrogryposis, cerebral palsy, and arthritis.

The goal is to develop the optimal level of function possible for the individual. Methods include the applications of ergonomics and energy-saving techniques, adapted or built-up equipment, splints or orthoses, gravity-reducing aids, robotics, or an alternate means of providing function.

Independence comes in many forms. The desires of each patient must be taken into consideration. One person with a disease that causes fatigue and weakness opts for assistance in feeding and food preparation. Another individual feels these tasks are the most rewarding of the day and is willing to expend energy and use technological aids to carry out these activities.

AMYOTROPHIC LATERAL SCLEROSIS

Also referred to as Lou Gehrig's disease, amyotrophic lateral sclerosis (ALS) affects between 20,000 and 30,000 people in the United States. There are about 5000 new cases a year, similar to the incidence of multiple sclerosis. Ten percent of these are familial, which suggests a genetic cause, but there is no clinical difference between these and cases with no hereditary ALS.

A progressive neurological disorder caused by degeneration of the large motor neurons of the brain and spinal cord, ALS leads to progressive weakness, poor coordination and wasting of skeletal muscle, paralysis, and death. There is no loss of mental capabilities; in fact, it seems as though the patient is more alert as weakness increases. The onset may be slow with a remission or very rapid. Death occurs within five years, usually sooner.

Every ounce of our energy and knowledge as health care professionals is called into play finding means for the patient with ALS to continue living as fully as possible. Adapted equip-

ment is changed from week to week. Some patients elect to use overhead slings or balanced forearm feeders to maintain function. Others prefer to conserve energy for communication and other activities. Augmentative communication may include use of an amplifying microphone or computer as breathing and talking become difficult. See Chapter 5 and Chapter 6.

Maintaining adequate nutrition is increasingly difficult as swallowing becomes affected. Highly concentrated, nutritionally packed meals that are easy to swallow is one facet of the treatment program. Ice chips and slush are easier to swallow than water. Adapted equipment, such as the dose cup, swivel and narrow spoons, and slush cups make feeding easier. Using a food processor or blender allows sharing of the same meals by the whole family. A few patients may require stomach-tube feeding. See Chapter 4 and Chapter 5.

Agencies that offer support include the Muscular Dystrophy Association for free ALS clinics, equipment funding, and support groups, and the Amyotrophic Lateral Sclerosis Foundation for support groups, information, and possible equipment loans. Other agencies listed in Chapter 5 and Chapter 6 may be helpful.

Research has identified the location of the gene responsible for inherited ALS, and drugs are now available that slow the disease process. Although there is no cure at this time, these are stepping stones to the development of specific diagnostic tests and a cure.

POST-POLIO SYNDROME

In the United States today, there are approximately 641,000 people who had polio during the 1940s and 1950s. Between 25% and 66% of these survivors are experiencing increased problems as they age. These difficulties fall into two groups. The first is increased difficulty in breathing. This manifests itself in fatigue while breathing, headaches, altered swallowing patterns, and sleeping problems that cause one to wake often during the night. The second is pain associated with increasing weakness and overall fatigue. Treatment of the first group should start with a full pulmonary evaluation; treatment of the second should start with a

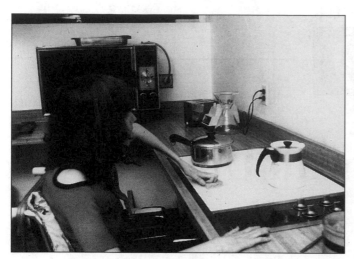

Figure 9-1. This built-in cooktop is flush with the counter, and the large controls turn easily with limited hand function. (Photo courtesy of Barrier-Free Design, O.T. Dept., Howard A. Rusk Institute of Rehabilitation Medicine.)

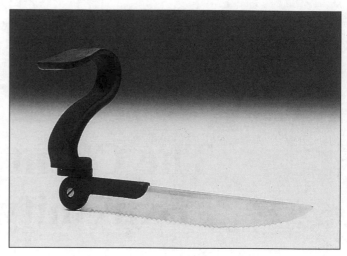

Figure 9-2. This knife with a cuff handle lets the person with loss of grasp safely handle cutting activities. (Photo courtesy of Etac USA, Inc., Waukesha, WI.)

consultation with a physical medicine/rehabilitation specialist. Because this syndrome mimics other diseases, an evaluation to rule out arthritis, diabetes, multiple sclerosis, and anemia is necessary.

The individual with post-polio syndrome must use energy-conservation techniques. Exercise is required only to maintain mobility. Muscle fibers and nerve cells, already damaged by the disease, have been working to capacity, perhaps overcompensating. Resistive exercise will only over-fatigue them. Swimming for exercise is easier on the muscles and joints. Teach the patient to avoid overexertion and to rest as necessary. Weight control and good nutrition are important. Smoking and drinking put extra stress on breathing and sleeping.

"Slowing down" and altering lifestyle are necessary. Conservation is the goal. Use of a cane or crutches, lightweight brace, motorized wheelchair, or scooter may be considered for use both in the house and outside. See Chapter 16. For information on treatment and ongoing research, contact the International Polio Network, the Polio Society, the Post-Polio Program, National Rehabilitation Hospital, Ranchos Los Amigos Hospital, the Roosevelt Warm Springs Institute for Rehabilitation, and the University of California at Los Angeles Post-Polio Clinic. Addresses are in Appendix C.

SPINAL CORD INJURIES

The level and completeness of the lesion affect how much function remains in the shoulders, arms, and hands. Use of environmental controls, easier-to-operate appliances like microwaves, adapted equipment, and careful kitchen planning permit independence in the kitchen for many quadriplegics. People with high-level losses below the fourth cervical vertebrae may participate in food preparation and feed themselves with the use of gravity-reducing orthoses if necessary. Trunk balance should be assessed when a wheelchair is ordered, and lateral support should be provided if required. Loss of sensation requires stringent safety precautions when handling hot pans, using hot water, or carrying

items. If a high-level quad is seen early in rehabilitation in the kitchen, awareness of breathing problems and energy conservation are even more critical.

Work surface height requires careful assessment when working with a client with a high-level spinal cord injury. Both trunk balance and the level of injury determine the optimal height; there will be individual variations. An ideal work surface height allows a quad to stabilize his trunk with his elbows for increased tenodesis function. He or she can work at a wheelchair-height cooktop or with portable appliances without raising the arms above the shoulders. Working efficiently at normal stove height, however, is very difficult and dangerous for an average height quad with a C5,6 lesion, because he or she loses trunk balance when reaching upward. Use of a stove may be possible, though energy consuming, for a C7 quad.

Kitchen planning for the person with quadriplegia or marked weakness in the upper extremities requires a lowered continuous surface on which items may be slid rather than lifted (Figure 9-1). The area under the counter must be open so the homemaker can get close to the work area in her wheelchair.

ADAPTED EQUIPMENT AND ORTHOSES

Specially adapted tools and utensils allow the person with loss of grasp and marked weakness in the upper extremities to perform meal preparation, self-feeding, and other tasks. Tools and aids for people with loss of power in their arms and hands must be designed to use remaining motions. A knife with a cuff allows cutting by moving the shoulder. A quad reacher uses wrist extension to open and is self-closing. It is custom fit for optimum function. **Source:** 191. The universal cuff, shown in *Mealtime Manual*, Chapter 2, has a palmar pocket to hold utensils.

A knife with a cuff handle lets the person with loss of grasp safely handle cutting activities (Figure 9-2). **Source:** 191.

A metal cuff riveted to the handle of a mixing spoon allows a quadriplegic with no grasp in his or her hands to mix and handle foods (Figure 9-3).

Plastic cuffs attached to utensils eliminate the need for active

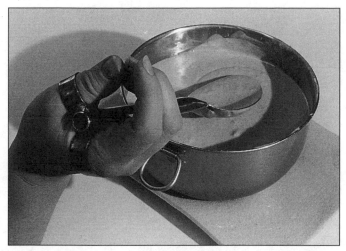

Figure 9-3. A metal cuff riveted to the handle of a mixing spoon allows a quadriplegic with no grasp in his or her hands to mix and handle foods. (Photo courtesy of the O.T. Dept., Howard A. Rusk Institute of Rehabilitation Medicine.)

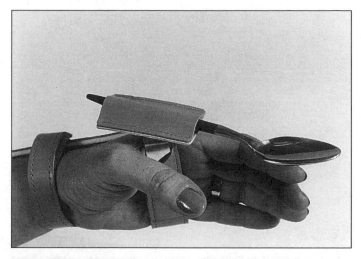

Figure 9-5. An adjustable wrist support stabilizes the hand in a functional position. (Photo courtesy of North Coast Medical, Inc., San Jose, Ca.)

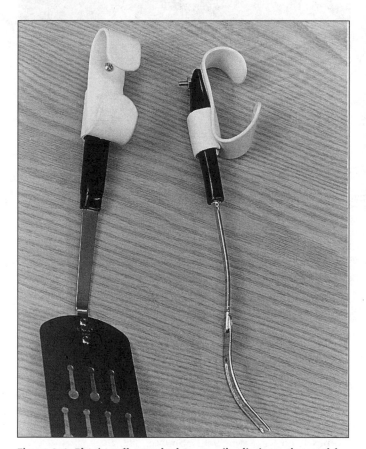

Figure 9-4. Plastic cuffs attached to utensils eliminate the need for active grasp when using a cooktop. (Photo courtesy of the O.T. Dept., Rehabilitation Institute of Chicago.)

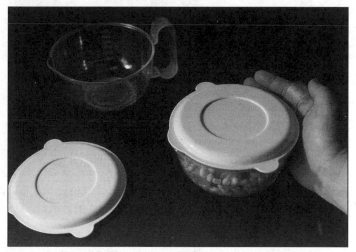

Figure 9-6. Lightweight bowls with closed handles are easier to pick up with weak grasp. (Photo by J.K.)

fit. Cost is about $16 and up from drugstores and home health suppliers. **Manufacturers** include 33, 82, 294B, 303, 354, 481. **Sources** for this and similar supports: 33, 82, 198, 334, 383, 461, 481, 483, 503, 518, 553.

Lightweight bowls with closed handles are easier to pick up with weak grasp (Figure 9-6). The four-cup capacity containers shown may be used in the microwave oven for heating stew, soup, leftovers, casseroles, or to boil water. Bowls may go from freezer to microwave, which allows preparing a one-dish meal ahead of time. Lid has extensions on the lip so it can be removed with light upward pressure. It is top-rack dishwasher safe. Set of two costs about $9 from housewares stores and mail-order firms.

Flexor-hinge, wrist-driven, wrist-hand orthoses allow the quadriplegic to pick up and hold items by using wrist extension and flexion to flex and extend the fingers (Figures 9-7A,B,C,D). With the orthosis, it is possible to lift containers and pans, hold utensils and foods, and operate appliances.

Using a tenodesis orthosis, it is also possible to perform fine

grasp when using a cooktop (Figure 9-4). This allows concentration on the activity rather than maintaining hold on the utensil.

When wrist strength is weak or there is carpal tunnel syndrome or arthritis, an adjustable wrist support stabilizes the hand in a functional position (Figure 9-5). Velcro® closures adjust for a firm

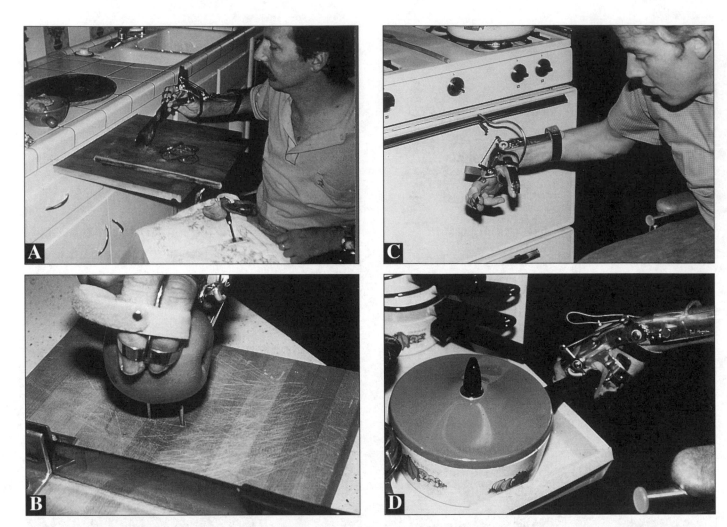

Figure 9-7A,B,C,D. With the orthosis, it is possible to lift containers and pans, hold utensils and foods, and operate appliances. (Photos courtesy of the O.T. Dept., Rancho Los Amigos Medical Center.)

activities, such as writing (Figure 9-8).

When an individual has weakness or limited movement in the arms and shoulders, a sink escalator allows sliding heavier items to and from the sink (Figure 9-9). The aid is made with two boards that are joined with hinges at the middle. Boards should be as light as possible and narrow enough to fit into the sink with room for hands to grasp on either side for removal. Beveling both ends eliminates any lifting. Finish boards with marine waterproof varnish or polyurethane to prevent them from becoming water-logged and warped. Plastic materials may be used, but hinges may not hold up as well over time.

Patients find their own solutions. Lightweight scrubber brushes and sponge mops have soft plastic handles that the user, who has quadriplegia, holds in his or her teeth for washing dishes (Figure 9-10A). This leaves one hand free to hold the dish, and the other free to maintain trunk balance. Cost is about $2 to $3 each from variety stores. **Manufacturer:** 187. Suggestion from IDEA: 273.

Bringing both hands together allows a client with quadriplegia to handle many types of containers (Figure 9-10B). Note arms braced on low surface with table-top appliance.

Ready-made splints and orthoses are available from hospital supply firms. **Sources** include 33, 383, 481, 518. Custom fabrication of

orthoses for patients with weak hands and wrists may be accomplished with a variety of splinting materials by an occupational therapist or orthotist. Several companies offer materials that soften in hot water. Request samples from **manufacturers:** 33, 481, 586.

Overhead slings and balanced forearm orthoses reduce gravity and conserve energy. Both types of aids also build up strength and permit earlier training in self-care and homemaking.

An arm positioner, or balanced forearm orthosis, adjusts forward and backward, up and down to achieve optimum positioning (Figure 9-11). **Manufacturer:** 292. **Sources:** 14, 292, 362, 383.

The ball-bearing feeder with an elevating arm allows self-feeding and other activities when there is severe loss of upper extremity muscle power (Figure 9-12). **Source:** 383.

Adapted controls increase independence and conserve energy for the person with severe loss of upper extremity function. A variety of control interfaces or switches allow the person with severe limitations in mobility to handle many aspects of the environment. This may be as simple as a single rocker or "jelly bean" switch to turn on an appliance (Figure 9-13). **Manufacturer:** 4. **Sources:** 4, 516. At the other end of the scale is an electronic environmental control that operates selected functions, including wheelchair operation, telephone, window opening and closing,

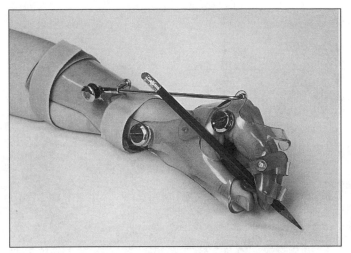

Figure 9-8. Using a tenodesis orthosis, it is also possible to perform fine activities, such as writing. (Photo courtesy of the O.T. Dept., Howard A. Rusk Institute of Rehabilitation Medicine.)

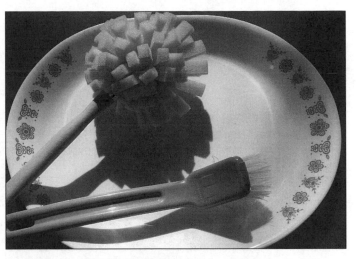

Figure 9-10A. Lightweight scrubber brushes and sponge mops have soft plastic handles that the user, who has quadriplegia, holds in his teeth for washing dishes. (Photo by J.K.)

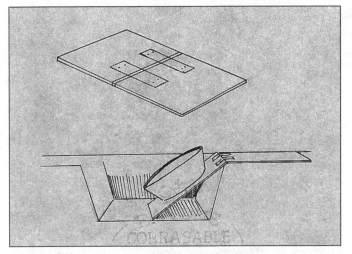

Figure 9-9. A sink escalator allows sliding heavier items to and from the sink. (Illustration by G.K.)

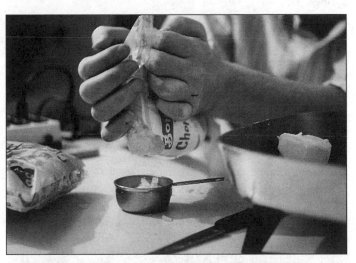

Figure 9-10B. Bringing both hands together allows this client with quadriplegia to handle many types of containers. (Photo by J.K.)

television, radio, fans or air conditioning, door answering, and bed positioning. Types of easy-to-adapt switches include push, rocking, wobble, joystick, pneumatic, and micro. These may be operated by a single motion as limited as sipping or puffing, blowing one cheek against a microswitch, using head control with a mouthstick, or tapping a finger or toe. A full evaluation of the individual's needs, cognitive and physical capabilities, as well as prognosis is taken into account when prescribing a control unit. A rehabilitation engineer and/or occupational therapist carries out the evaluation and program. **Sources** for various types of switches and information include 2, 4, 280B, 294, 418, 506, 532. Also see assistive technology resources in Appendix F.

See other switches in Chapter 2 and Chapter 27.

Beyond orthoses and technology is a third answer that has become familiar to some quadriplegics during the past 15 years. The capuchin monkey has become the arms and legs for quadriplegics (Figure 9-14). The monkey is trained to increase independence by helping the individual eat, drink, read, watch television,

and listen to music. Those who have used the trained monkeys say that they also develop a strong bond and even improve their social lives. Started by Dr. Mary Jane Willard, a behavioral psychologist, to make life better for a friend, the experiment has developed into a non-profit program called "Helping Hands—Simian Aids for the Disabled." Address is in Appendix C.

Dogs have also been trained to help individuals with severe disabilities. See Canine Companions for Independence, Inc., in Chapter 30.

RESOURCES

Addresses for publishers, periodicals, and organizations are given in Section Four.

PUBLICATIONS

Curtis, P. (1982). *Animal Partners: Training Animals to Help People*. Out of print, check with library. New York: Dutton,

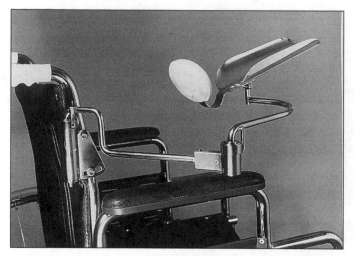

Figure 9-11. This arm positioner, or balanced forearm orthosis, adjusts forward and backward, up and down to achieve optimum positioning. (Photo courtesy of Jaeco Orthopedic Specialties, Hot Springs, AR.)

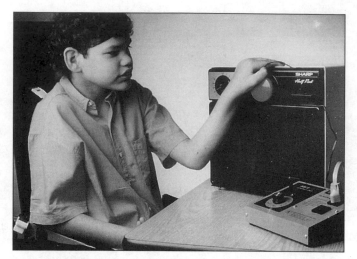

Figure 9-13. This boy controls the microwave oven with a jelly bean switch and adapted timer. (Photo courtesy of AbleNet®, Inc., Minneapolis, MN.)

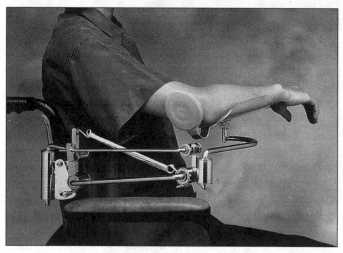

Figure 9-12. The ball-bearing feeder with an elevating arm allows self-feeding and other activities when there is severe loss of upper extremity muscle power. (Photo courtesy of North Coast Medical, Inc., San Jose, CA.)

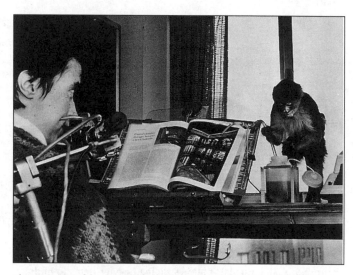

Figure 9-14. This capuchin monkey is setting up the beverage container for his owner. (Photo courtesy of Helping Hands: Simian Aids for the Disabled, Inc.)

Penguin USA. Written for younger readers, focus is on dogs and other pets as helpers as well as therapy.

Degenerative Diseases: Resource Guide. (1991). Bethesda, MD: American Occupational Therapy Association. #4130, $10 AOTA members, $20 non-members. Bibliographies, audiovisuals, resource personnel.

Haldane, S. (1991). *Helping Hands: How Monkeys Assist People Who Are Disabled.* New York: Dutton Children's Books, Penguin. $14.95.

Rehabilitation Engineering Center. *Guide to Controls: Selection, Mounting, Applications.* Palo Alto, CA: Children's Hospital at Stanford. $10. Illustrations and descriptions of the most frequently used commercially available controls.

Amyotrophic Lateral Sclerosis

Hamilton, L. *Why Didn't Somebody Tell Me About These*

Things? Kansas City ALS Patient Services Fund. Ask for loan through local ALS chapter.

Maintaining Mobility and Meals, materials free from the Patient and Community Services Department of the National Office of the Muscular Dystrophy Association.

McGill, F., & Kutscher, L. G. (Ed.). (1980). *Go Not Gently: Letters from a Patient with Amyotrophic Lateral Sclerosis.* Ayer. Out of print, check with library. Letters to a group of friends, dealing with the author's perceptions of her terminal illness.

Also contact the Amyotrophic Lateral Sclerosis Association, which distributes a variety of manuals and a newsletter called *LINK*, listed in *Mealtime Manual*, Chapter 33.

Multiple Sclerosis

Please see Chapter 11.

Muscular Dystrophy

Charash, L., et al. (1991). Muscular dystrophy and other neuromuscular diseases: Psychosocial issues. In *Loss, Grief and Care Series: Vol. 4, Nos. 3 and 4*. New York: Haworth. $34.95.

Schock, N., & Colbert, A. *Ventilators and Muscular Dystrophy*. G.I.N.I., St. Louis, MO., $6. Option of mechanical ventilation for a person with Duchenne muscular dystrophy to improve prognosis for life expectancy. Listed under Post-Polio Syndrome, Appendix C.

Post-Polio

International Polio Network, St. Louis, MO. Publications include *International Polio Directory*. Listing of individuals and organizations. *Polio Network News*, quarterly, $12 consumer, $20 professional. *I.V.U.N. News*, biannual newsletter of International Ventilator Users Network, $8 consumer, $20 professional. *Rehabilitation Gazette*, biannual, $12 consumer, $40 professional. International journal written by people with disabilities. *Handbook on the Late Effects of Poliomyelitis for Physicians and Survivors*, 48-page booklet in dictionary form. $6.75.

Post Polio Syndrome. Post-Polio Awareness and Support Society of British Columbia. San Antonio, TX: Therapy Skill Builders. 29-minute VHS video, $89. Introduces survivors of polio, covers causes, symptoms, and effective management. For caregivers and professionals. **Source:** 522.

Post Polio Video. Sun Coast Media, 29 minutes, $59.95 plus shipping from Accent Special Publications. **Source:** 8. Documents post-polio effects many individuals are now experiencing to help one understand what is happening.

Research and Clinical Aspects of Late Effects of Poliomyelitis, Proceedings of 1986 Warm Springs conference. White Plains, NY: March of Dimes, 10605.

Spinal Cord Injuries

American Occupational Therapy Association. *Practice Guidelines: Spinal Cord*. #1154. Reference tool for managers, third-party payers, and practitioners. Defines evaluation, frequency, duration of treatment, patient care management, and explanation of billing codes. $20 AOTA members, $25 non-members.

Corcoran, P., & Oliare, C. *The Aging Process and People with Spinal Cord Injuries*. Silver Spring, MD: National Spinal Cord Injury Association. $3 members, $5 non-members. Emphasis on preventive measures to avoid and alleviate effects of aging.

Fact Sheets on Spinal Cord Injury. Silver Spring, MD: National Spinal Cord Injury Association. Topics include *What Is Spinal Cord Injury?*; *Spinal Cord Injury Statistical Information*; *What's New in SCI Research?* Free to members, $3 per topic to non-members.

Gadberry, L., & Finke-Fraunheim, T. (1996). *Motivating Life Skill Modules for Individuals With Spinal Cord Injury*. #1164. Bethesda, MD: American Occupational Therapy Association. $35 AOTA members, $47 non-members. Multidisciplinary approach to treating clients with spinal cord injury. Detailed activities include communication, community re-entry, self-care, mobility, and others. Organized for use in group setting in acute care, rehabilitation centers, outpatient, and subacute facilities. Modules contain lesson description, required materials, setup information, skill sheet, and station markers.

Hansen, B. (1993). *Picking Up the Pieces: Healing Ourselves After Personal Loss*. New York: HarperCollins. $14.95. Author who was paralyzed at age 19 offers hope in coping with trauma, rage, denial, and despair to complete the healing process. Available from **source:** 8.

The Homemaker with Weak Upper Extremities. Howard A. Rusk Institute of Rehabilitation Medicine, New York University Medical Center, under a grant from the Campbell Soup Fund. 28 minutes, 16 mm, color/sound. Demonstrates overcoming the loss of function in the upper extremities in meal preparation; kitchen planning for the wheelchair user; selecting equipment for use by quadriplegics. College-age quadriplegic who lives independently prepares two meals and commutes to college. For further information, write Living Media, Inc. **Source:** 332.

How to Live with a Spinal Cord Injury. (1989). Bloomington, IL: Accent. $6.95, plus $2 shipping and handling. Written by a paraplegic, deals with day-to-day activity. **Source:** 8.

Introduction to Spinal Cord Injury. Free from the Paralyzed Veterans of America, Inc.

Laing, I. S. (1995). *A Practical Guide to Health Promotion After Spinal Cord Injury*. Frederick, MD: Aspen. $59. Addresses total health after SCI injury, features patient education hand-outs, illustrations resources on nutritional and sexual health, and stress management.

Maddox, S. (1993). *Spinal Network: The Total Resource for the Wheelchair Community*. Malibu, CA: Miramar. $37.95 plus $5 shipping; #39.95 plus $5 shipping for edition with lay-flat binding. Also available through **source** 8 (add $4 shipping and handling) and **source** 169. Comprehensive *Whole Earth Catalog* for people who use wheelchairs and their families covers many types of neurological diseases although focus is on spinal cord injury. Richly illustrated with resources including news and humor.

Moving Forward: The Guide to Living with Spinal Cord Injury. London, England: Spinal Injuries Association. Equivalent of 25 English pounds plus the amount needed for 4 pounds weight postage. Addresses medical, social, and psychological effects of spinal cord injury, gives practical advice from people with SCI. Step-by-step guide begins right after injury and continues through every stage. Written for clients, family, and caregivers.

NARIC Resource Guide for People with Spinal Cord Injuries and Their Families. (1995, March). Free from the National Association for Rehabilitation Information Center. Periodicals, books, organizations, research centers, funding sources, and database searching. 10 pages.

Phillips, L., (Ed.). (1987). *Spinal Cord Injury: A Guide for Patient and Family*. New York: Lippincott/Raven Press. $18. Primer on spinal cord injuries including physiology, physical implications of injury, resource list, and overview of research.

Rebecca Finds a New Way: How Kids Learn, Play, and Live with Spinal Cord Injuries. (1994). In Touch with Kids Network, Silver Spring, MD: National Spinal Cord Injury Association. $3.50; free to children with SCI.

Spinal Cord Injuries: Resource Guide. Bethesda, MD: American Occupational Therapy Association. #4180, $10 AOTA members, $20 non-members. Bibliographies, audiovisuals, resource personnel.

Spinal Cord Injury Patient Education Resource Manual. (1996). Frederick, MD: Aspen. $169. Annual supplements sent on approval. Medical coverage of body systems, psychosocial management, pain management, independent living strategies, home modification, and assistive technology. Reproducible hand-outs, guidelines, checklists.

Stover, S. L., et al. (1995). *Spinal Cord Injury: Clinical Outcomes from the Model Systems*. Frederick MD: Aspen. $70. Compilation and interpretation of 2 decades of research and data collection on service delivery and outcomes for people with SCI within the Model Spinal Cord Injury Systems Program.

Texas Institute for Rehabilitation and Training publications include *A Monograph: Specialized Occupational Therapy for Persons with High Level Quadriplegia*. (1988). Houston, TX: RRTC in Community Integration with Spinal Cord Injury. $15. Initial treatment at TIRR, functional activities training, community transportation, environmental control prevocational training, resources. *Spinal Cord Injury: A Manual for Healthy Living* (1993). Also available in Spanish. $60. *Compendium for Spinal Cord Injury Educational Resources: Audiovisuals and Unpublished Written Materials* (1994), $50. More than 300 audiovisual resources and 275 unpublished written resources. Send for brochure with additional resources.

Thiers, N. (1994, March). Following patients home. *OT Week*. System for following up patients at home for most effective treatment by the Rehabilitation Institute of Chicago occupational therapists.

Whiteneck, G., et al. (1989). *The Management of High Quadriplegia*. New York: Demos. $74.95. Care of patient with high-level spinal cord injury with complete paralysis below the fourth cervical neurological level. Explores acute care, rehabilitation, discharge planning, and critical lifetime issues. Also available through **source** 169.

Yes, You Can! $9.50 plus $2.50 shipping and handling from the Paralyzed Veterans of America. Available in English and Spanish. Covers daily activities including attendant care and driving.

Please see additional references in Chapter 11 and Chapter 6.

Also see Going Further in Chapter 2 in *Mealtime Manual*.

PERIODICALS

For ordering addresses and rates, see Appendix C in *Mealtime Manual*. For agencies see Appendix C in this guide.

Paraplegia.

Paraplegia News.

Progress in Research. American Paralysis Association. Free. Research on paralysis and spinal cord injury. Address in Appendix C.

Progression. Rehabilitation Institute of Chicago. Newsletter of the RIC Research and Training Center on Prevention and Treatment of Secondary Complications of Spinal Cord Injury. Address in Appendix C.

Rehabilitation: Spinal Cord Injury Update. University of Washington, Rehabilitation Medicine RJ-30, Seattle, WA 98195. Free, 4 issues.

Research Update. Spain Rehabilitation Center, University of Birmingham, RRTC Training Office, Rm. 506, 1717-6th Ave. South, Birmingham, AL 35233-7330.

Spinal Cord Injury Life. Silver Spring, MD: National Spinal Cord Injury Association. News concerning people with SCI, legislation, prevention programs, grants, book reviews, independent living. Free to members, $30 for non-members. Address is in Appendix C.

Spinal Cord Society Newsletter. Focus is on research into a cure for spinal cord injury.

SCI Nursing. American Association of Spinal Cord Injury Nurses, Eastern Paralyzed Veterans Association. Quarterly, $50.

Spinal Network. Miramar. See *Mealtime Manual*.

Topics in Spinal Cord Injury Rehabilitation. Aspen. Multidisciplinary quarterly journal.

10

The Client with Arthritis

Homemaking activities, whether as part of a hospital or a home-based treatment program, must emphasize the following areas:

- Joint protection through selection of correct utensils and handling of activities.
- Proper posture through correct seating, footwear, and ambulation.
- Work simplification and time management to avoid fatigue.
- Proper nutrition.
- Reduction of stress through planning and lifestyle selections. See Chapter 7.

When evaluating a patient with arthritis, all tasks of daily living must be considered. Joint protection techniques are not limited to the hands and hips. Consider the person who spends a good deal of time on the telephone. Grasping the receiver with one shoulder can aggravate arthritis in the neck and shoulder. Not only should the client be sitting with good posture, but the static grip on the phone might be replaced with a speakerphone or headset.

JOINT PROTECTION

Learning correct methods of joint protection is a basic part of the homemaking rehabilitation curriculum when there is rheumatoid arthritis in the hands (Figure 10-1). Educating the patient in joint protection includes demonstrating and reviewing many common tasks, such as closing cabinets and drawers with fingers extended, using a cloth loop to open a refrigerator or heavy doors, pushing up from a chair with the fingers extended, using a sponge rather than a dishcloth, using a dust mitt rather than a cloth—all with the fingers extended. Knives and mixing utensils must be held with the hand completely around the handle, not with the thumb extended. See *Mealtime Manual*, Chapter 2.

Opening containers is one of the most damaging kitchen activities for the person with arthritis in the hands. Most manual can openers place undue stress on the hands and should be replaced with an electric can opener that the patient can operate easily. Test several models to find one with a long, easy-to-operate lever.

A wedge-type jar opener installed at a convenient height eliminates a major source of damaging stress and opens another world of foods (Figure 10-2). **Manufacturer:** 589.

Applying ergonomics to cutting tasks reduces stress on the wrist. The Swedish rehab knife with an angled handle, shown in *Mealtime Manual*, is the second most important tool in the kitchen for saving stress on joints of the hands and wrists (after the jar opener). The angled design transfers stress from the wrist and fingers to the shoulder and reduces the power required to cut up to 80%. Other utensils with large handles may be purchased, or you may add foam cylinders to increase the circumference of the handle and reduce tight finger flexion.

The therapist or home economist must demonstrate new methods of doing tasks to protect joints (Figure 10-3). If a client will not accept a jar opener, then he or she may be taught to open jars with a rubber pad on the bottom and top, turning always toward the thumb or radial side, which means opening it with the right hand and closing it with the left.

Lifting should be done with two hands, adding a second handle to a pan if needed. A pan may be modified for lifting with two hands by adding a plumber's clamp as the second handle. See Chapter 27.

The large, non-stick skillet shown is of medium weight and comes with a solid second handle (Figure 10-4). **Source:** 364.

Recommend that your client purchase milk in half-gallon or smaller cartons (Figure 10-5). Adding a handle provides more secure grip and distributes the weight. **Manufacturers** include 193. Cost is about $2 from housewares stores and mail-order firms. **Sources:** 241, 319, 361, 508, 561B.

Rolling pastry using a French rolling pin, which requires no grasp but is used with the fingers in extension, may even be incorporated as a therapeutic teaching activity for the client with arthritis (Figure 10-6). **Manufacturer:** 20. Pie crust shapers cost about $3 from housewares stores and mail-order firms. **Sources:** 109, 241, 361, 508, 561B.

If stirring or beating with a whisk, moving toward the thumb side reduces the tendency toward ulnar deviation. The therapist can prepare a list of suggestions for the patient to review and follow at home as given in *Mealtime Manual*.

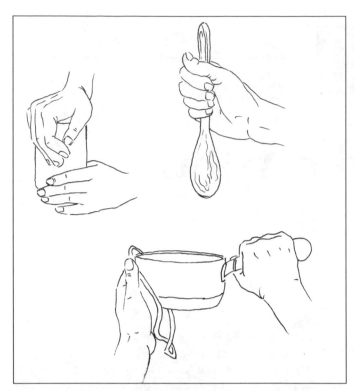

Figure 10-1. Learning correct methods of joint protection is a basic part of the homemaking rehabilitation curriculum when there is rheumatoid arthritis in the hands. (Illustration by G.K.)

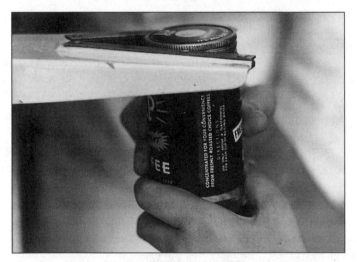

Figure 10-2. A wedge-type jar opener installed at a convenient height eliminates one source of damaging stress. (Jar opener by Zim Manufacturing Company. Photo courtesy of the O.T. Dept., Howard A. Rusk Institute of Rehabilitation Medicine.)

Resting or working orthoses may be indicated to protect or maintain function in the hands of a client with rheumatoid arthritis or osteoarthritis (Figures 10-7A).

Splinting materials that require minimal equipment to use (i.e., hot water, scissors, fasteners) are available from rehabilitation suppliers. **Manufacturers** and distributors include 33, 105, 383, 461, 481, 586. Prefabricated orthoses are also available from reha-

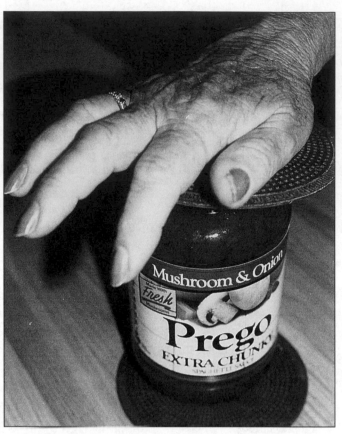

Figure 10-3. The client may be taught to open jars with a rubber pad on the bottom and top, turning always toward the thumb or radial side. (Photo by J.K.)

bilitation firms (Figure 10-7B).

When carpal tunnel syndrome is present, an elastic wrist brace may help relieve pain by stabilizing the wrist and thumb. A variety of braces are available from rehabilitation supply firms. One lightweight, elastic orthosis wraps around the wrist, fastens with Velcro®, and has a strap that partially stabilizes the thumb (Figure 10-8A). Cost is about $8 each. **Sources:** 33, 171.

The elastic Handeze® glove slips over the hand, stabilizing the wrist and hand for light repetitive activity (Figure 10-8B). Cost is about $10 per pair. **Manufacturer:** 520.

PROPER POSTURE

Sitting to work reduces stress on the hips, knees, and feet. If the chair is not properly designed, however, it transfers some of the stress to the back. Raising a chair with a firm cushion or leg extenders lets the person get up without straining. A firm foam cushion also pads a hard chair and reduces pressure on the nerves for the thin patient. A chair with arms divides the effort between the arms and legs when rising or sitting. Adding a lifting cushion reduces stress on the hips and upper extremities.

A lumbar support helps position the back correctly. Office furniture supply companies carry a variety of good postural chairs. See Chapter 14.

requent change of position is important for the person with arthritis. Teach your client to alternate sitting with short periods of

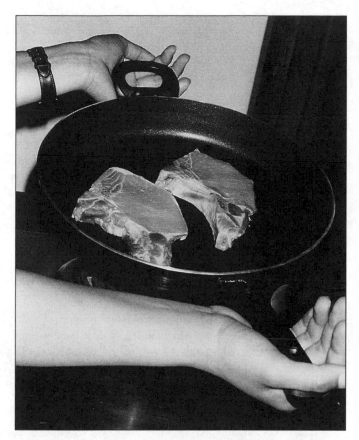

Figure 10-4. This large, non-stick skillet is of medium weight and has a second handle to help distribute weight when lifting. (Wearever® Concentric Air Health Grill. Photo by J.K.)

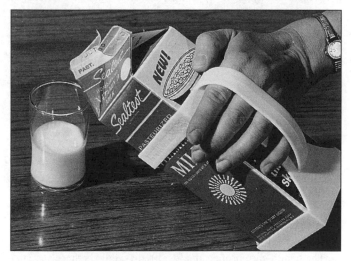

Figure 10-5. Adding a handle provides a more secure grip and distributes the weight. (Photo courtesy of the O.T. Dept., Howard A. Rusk Institute of Rehabilitation Medicine.)

standing and to alternate holding with periods of resting the hands. When setting down a tool, the wrists and fingers should be stretched and relaxed.

Correct shoes translate to better posture. Care of feet with proper fitting shoes for the individual with arthritis allows walking with greater comfort and safety. Foot needs of a patient should

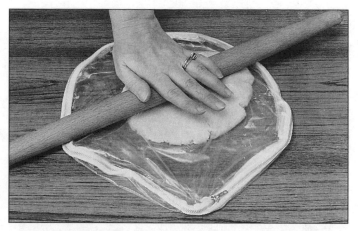

Figure 10-6. Rolling pastry using a French rolling pin, which is used with the fingers in extension, may be incorporated as a therapeutic teaching activity for the client with arthritis. (Photo courtesy of the O.T. Dept., Howard A. Rusk Institute of Rehabilitation Medicine.)

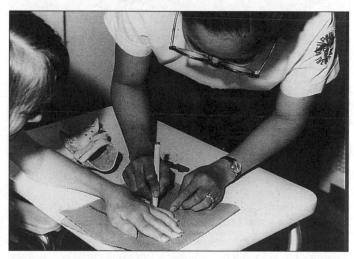

Figure 10-7A. This occupational therapist measures a patient for a resting splint. (Photo courtesy of The Arthritis Foundation, Atlanta, GA.)

be assessed by the physical or occupational therapist in conjunction with ambulation and activities of daily living training. Too often, because of discomfort, the person with arthritis wears non-supportive, loose slippers, which lead to foot deformities as well as accidents. When an occupational or physical therapist is not available, consultation with a physician or podiatrist should be arranged. Some patients require foot orthoses. These may be covered by insurance if prescribed by a podiatrist. New orthotic materials and technology now make fabrication possible and easier by trained occupational and physical therapists. Prefabricated, custom insoles may be quickly adjusted to patients' feet. Contact your local Arthritis Foundation chapter for recommendations. Check information from several companies. **Sources:** 15, 46, 474.

Correct use of an ambulation aid must take into consideration all tasks being done by the patient. If a cane is needed for balance, is it the right height? Does it create pain in the hand, wrist, or arm from pressure on the handle? Does it create problems when carry-

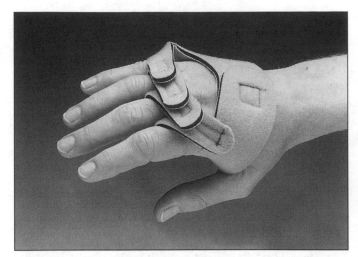

Figure 10-7B. This splint is designed to help prevent ulnar deviation. (Photo courtesy of North Coast Medical, Inc., San Jose, CA.)

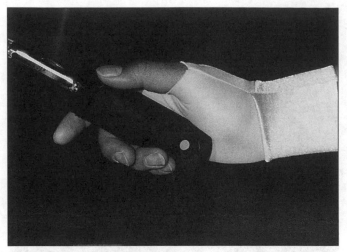

Figure 10-8B. The elastic Handeze® glove is used here with a built-up handle to further reduce stress on the joints. (Gloves by Therapeutic Appliance Group, Woonsocket, RI. Photo by J.K.)

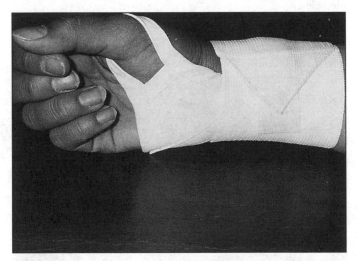

Figure 10-8A. This lightweight, elastic orthosis wraps around the wrist, fastens with Velcro®, and has a strap that partially stabilizes the thumb. (AliMed®, Inc., Dedham, MA. Photo by J.K.)

may need encouragement to do more. A young patient with rheumatoid arthritis, on the other hand, may need assistance in reducing or delegating the number of tasks to be done. See Appendix B for assessment forms and Appendix G for reproducible materials you might share with clients.

There are jobs that a client with moderate to severe rheumatoid or osteoarthritis should consider relegating to someone else. Scrubbing the bathroom, washing windows, cleaning the oven and floors, and outdoor maintenance tasks like shoveling snow and cutting grass are all jobs that might be done by another family member, a hired homemaker, or a chore service. Whether or not finances are a problem, the providing of these services might be an appreciated gift from children or relatives. Willing, inexpensive, hired help is often available through the local senior center and high school employment office. You might also check around the neighborhood or with the housing authority, a church group, or a friend for suggestions of senior citizens or reliable teenagers. See Appendix A.

PROPER NUTRITION

Help with planning a proper diet must take into consideration recommendations from the physician as well as basic good nutritional principles. Extra weight, which adds stress to the lower extremities and increases fatigue, may be addressed through diet. Writing out meal plans is a first step to diet modification. See a sample meal plan form in Appendix G.

The health care professional is often asked, "Is there any special diet that will cure or reduce the effects of my arthritis?" With a disease that has so much pain, this question is natural. The answer is good nutrition to keep the whole system functioning well. Emphasize to your client the need for continued gentle exercise, adequate rest, and outside interests. Encourage the joining of an exercise or support group approved by the local chapter of The Arthritis Foundation or a local hospital for the most up-to-date information on medical advances, as well as a balanced lifestyle. Warn against quacks who thrive on the pain and suffering of those with arthritis.

ing with two hands? A wheeled table, or perhaps a wheeled walker with a basket for carrying items within the home, may be indicated. See Chapter 13. Groceries should be wheeled rather than carried, and loads should be divided into small, manageable weights. See Chapter 26 for suggestions of aids for carrying.

Lifting a walker is stressful on the back, hips, upper extremities, and hands (Figure 10-9). A rolling walker may be indicated for the homemaker who has severe rheumatoid or osteoarthritis. Axillary arm rests reduce pressure on the hands and wrists. **Manufacturers** of rolling walkers include 45, 160, 191, 379, 561. See Chapter 13 and Chapter 30.

WORK SIMPLIFICATION AND TIME MANAGEMENT

Like the individual with low energy, the person with arthritis must determine priorities and eliminate taxing chores. Some older patients, however, are apt to exclude too many jobs and

RESOURCES

Addresses for publishers, periodicals, and organizations are given in Section Four.

PUBLICATIONS

American Occupational Therapy Association. (1996). *Practice Guidelines for Hip Replacement.* Bethesda, MD: Author. $20 AOTA members, $25 non-members. Reference tool for health care facility managers, managed care organizations, third-party payers, OT practitioners. Defines evaluations, frequency, duration of treatment, and gives billing codes explanation.

The Arthritis Foundation publishes a variety of materials for the health care professional working with people with arthritis. Some of these include the *Bulletin on the Rheumatic Diseases*; *A Core Curriculum in Rheumatology* (1989) $10; *Understanding Juvenile Rheumatoid Arthritis* (1987) $50, a manual for health care professionals teaching children with JRA and their families, combines 14 topics with associated teaching plans; plus educational booklets on managing pain, activities, stress, pain, and fatigue. Patient education materials also include a series on various diseases, a health professional sampler, a self-management series, and a series in Spanish. Send for full catalog. Also see Periodicals in *Mealtime Manual* for magazine *Arthritis Today.*

The Association of Rheumatology Health Professionals is an interdisciplinary organization with a national office as well as regional chapters. The group has produced many publications based on patients' needs. The Canadian Arthritis Society also publishes a variety of materials. Write both groups for current publications' catalogs.

Arthritis: Resource Guide. Bethesda, MD: American Occupational Therapy Association. #4050, $10 AOTA members, $20 non-members. Bibliographies, audiovisuals, resource personnel.

Brattstrom, M. (1987). *Joint Protection and Rehabilitation in Chronic Rheumatic Disorders* (2nd ed.). Frederick, MD: Aspen. $43. Assessment techniques and strong emphasis on patient education. Treatment for specific joints, joint protection, technical aids. Illustrated pages for teaching as well as patient instruction sheets.

Chang, R. (Ed.). with Lee, P. (1996). *Rehabilitation of Persons With Rheumatoid Arthritis.* Frederick, MD: Aspen. $66. Team care, exercise for person with rheumatoid arthritis, psychological components, nutrition, adaptive equipment, social supports and community resources, tools for multidisciplinary evaluation and assessment.

Eades, M. D. (Series Editor: McMillan, C. S.). (1992). *If It Runs in Your Family: Arthritis—Reducing Your Risk.* New York: The Philip Lief Group, Bantam Doubleday Dell. $9. Preventive measures, activities to keep fit, importance of good nutrition, resources.

Fernandez-Madrid, F. (1984). *Treating Arthritis: Medicine, Myth, and Magic.* New York: Insight Books, Plenum. $22.95. Types of arthritis, role of nutrition in arthritis, recommendations for patient education.

Joint Preservation Techniques for Patients with Rheumatoid Arthritis. (1992). New York: Demos. $5 single copy, 10 for $30, 50 for $100. Designed for clinic- or hospital-based program. Provides carry-over of prescribed treatment programs including medication, joint preservation techniques, home exercise programs, and use of orthotic devices.

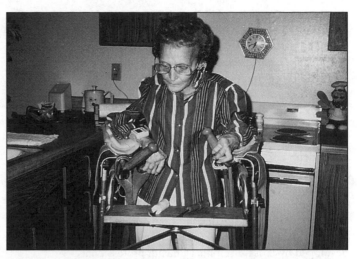

Figure 10-9. Axillary arm rests on this roling walker reduce pressure on the hands and wrists. (Photo courtesy of the O.T. Dept., Rancho Los Amigos Medical Center.)

Liang, M. H., & Logigian, M. K. (1992). *Rehabilitation of Early Rheumatoid Arthritis.* Boston: Little Brown. $32.50. Techniques to maintain and improve function in patients, including accurate assessment of joint impairment, rehabilitation of surgically treated joints, prevention and management of fatigue, psychosocial concerns, patient education.

McIlwain, H. H., et al. (1991). *Winning with Arthritis.* New York: Wiley. $14.95. Comprehensive treatment plan, types of arthritis, controlling stress and back pain.

Melvin, J. (1995). *Osteoarthritis: Caring for Your Hands*, Order No. 1127; and *Rheumatoid Arthritis: Caring for Your Hands*, Order No. 1128. Both from Bethesda, MD: American Occupational Therapy Association. Client education guides describe symptoms and problems, splint-wearing protocols, exercises, joint protection techniques, and activity modifications. $4.50 each AOTA members, $5.50 each non-members.

Melvin, J. L. (1989). *Rheumatic Disease in the Adult and Child: Occupational Therapy and Rehabilitation* (3rd ed.). Philadelphia: F.A. Davis. $49.95. Therapy for joint disease, psychological considerations in patient education and treatment, drug therapy, major rheumatic diseases, arthritis in children and adolescents, evaluation methods including hand pathodynamics, home assessment, activities of daily living, joint protection and energy conservation instruction, orthotic treatment, surgical rehabilitation.

Phillips, R. H. (1991). *Coping with Lupus: A Guide for Living with Lupus for You and Your Family.* New York: Avery. $9.95. Written by a psychologist, focus is on importance of emotions, support groups for family, stress relievers, and a realistic approach to an altered lifestyle.

Phillips, R. H. (1989). *Coping with Osteoarthritis: A Guide for Living with Osteoarthritis for You and Your Family.* New York: Avery. $9.95.

Phillips, R. H. (1988). *Coping with Rheumatoid Arthritis: A Guide for Living with RA for You and Your Family.* New York: Avery. $9.95.

Platt, J. (1991). *Daily Activities After Your Hip Surgery.* Bethesda, MD: American Occupational Therapy Association.

Available in English (#1110) and Spanish (#1110-A). $4 AOTA members, $5.20 non-members. Teaching guide for clients at home after hospitalization; illustrates proper techniques for dressing, bed positioning, bathing, car transfers, and housekeeping.

Platt, J. V., & Begun, R. (1992). *Daily Activities After Your Total Knee Replacement*. Bethesda, MD: American Occupational Therapy Association. $4.50 AOTA members, $5.50 non-members. Describes in detail correct ways for knee patients to sit, lie in bed, climb stairs, bathe, make toilet transfers. Stresses use of assistive equipment. Large type and illustrations.

Primer on Rheumatic Diseases (10th ed.). (1993). Atlanta, GA: Arthritis Foundation/ $25. Concise summary of rheumatic diseases.

Spiera, H., & Oreskes, I. (Eds.). (1991). *Rheumatology for the Health Care Professional*. St. Louis, MO: Warren H. Green. $42.50. Therapeutic approaches to major rheumatic diseases as developed by cross-disciplinary health professionals.

Williams, R. (1995). *Carpal Tunnel Syndrome*. Bethesda, MD: American Occupational Therapy Association. Order No. 1118. $4.50 AOTA members; $5.50 non-members. Demonstrates therapeutic strategies and exercises for managing carpal tunnel syndrome, including office chair exercises, tool selection, and conservative therapeutic management that may be applied to needs of clients with arthritic conditions.

Also see Going Further in *Mealtime Manual*, Chapter 2.

PERIODICALS

Arthritis and Rheumatism. Official Journal of the American Rheumatism Association. Monthly.

Arthritis Care & Research, the Official Journal of the Association of Rheumatology Health Professionals. Quarterly, news of regional chapters, current research, abstracts of literature, and announcements of upcoming regional and annual meetings as well as educational programs.

AUDIOVISUALS

Feeling Good With Arthritis. CD308, $25. Infovision, produced in cooperation with the American College of Rheumatology. 60-minute VHS video discusses how nutrition, exercise, the right medications, and a positive attitude can help clients feel better. Includes light exercises. **Source:** 280.

The Homemaker with Arthritis. Howard A. Rusk Institute of Rehabilitation Medicine, New York University Medical Center. Produced under a grant from the Campbell Soup Fund. 28 minutes, 16 mm, color/sound. Stress-saving techniques and selection of proper equipment in meal preparation and kitchen planning. For further information, write Living Media, Inc. **Source:** 332.

Joint Protection Techniques. 19-minute VHS video. Y13 Productions. Occupational therapist shows client with arthritis in hands how to cope with pain and frustration. Introduces techniques that minimize discomfort, making daily tasks in dressing, cooking, and the bathroom more manageable. Patient is encouraged to develop own solutions to problems as they occur. Shows coping with repetitive motions at home and office, and how simple aids can help. Cost is $99 plus $6 shipping and handling. **Source:** 588.

Knee Replacement Therapy, 17:37 minute VHS video, and *Hip Replacement Therapy*, 21:40 minute VHS video. Both from Y13 Productions. Patient with knee replacement works with physical therapist, starting prior to surgery and immediately after as he is attached to the CPM machine. Depicts normal pain levels, then shifts to helping patient regain balance, ambulatory skills, using a walker and a cane on stairs and level surfaces. Patient with hip replacement works with physical and occupational therapists, from right after surgery to time of hospital discharge. She starts in hospital room with physical therapy evaluation and explanation of precautions, shifts to mobility skills, then to occupational therapy for learning skills to continue at home, with dressing and using bathroom. Cost is $99 each plus $6 shipping and handling. **Source:** 588.

Recovering from Hip Replacement Surgery. A/V Health Services, Inc. 30-minute VHS by Cindy Collett, OTR, focuses on helping patient resume daily and household routines. Cost is $69. **Source:** 65.

11

The Client with Incoordination

Incoordination is a symptom of many diseases, including multiple sclerosis, muscular dystrophy, traumatic brain injury, cerebral palsy, Huntington's disease, and Parkinson's disease. It may also be a factor in weakness and aging. Paralysis agitans, or Parkinson's disease, is a slowly progressive, organic affliction that usually occurs in the fifth or sixth decade of life. It is characterized by a rhythmical tremor of resting muscles and slowness of movement with difficulty maintaining balance in advanced states.

Vestibular disorders are really disturbances in balance; but because they affect coordination and safety, they are included here. Meuniere's disease, for example, is caused by disturbances in the middle ear concerned with equilibrium. Frequent sudden attacks result in loss of consciousness, severe vertigo, nausea, and vomiting. Ataxia, secondary to the vestibular dysfunction, photophobia, and decreased endurance additionally affect the patient.

THE CLIENT WITH MULTIPLE SCLEROSIS

Each individual with multiple sclerosis is different. The combination of symptoms presents a unique patient profile. Fatigue is a characteristic feature of multiple sclerosis. Add to this weakness, incoordination, and visual problems. Weakness or paralysis may be hemiparetic, paraparetic, or quadriparetic. Progression of the disease may be rapid or very slow over a period of years. Remissions occur as well as exacerbations when the client's condition quickly worsens. Sensory symptoms include parathesia, numbness, and objective sensory loss of pain, touch, and temperature. On evaluation, there may be astereognosis of the hand. Bladder dysfunction may be transitory, or severe and permanent.

Incoordination is often present in the upper extremities as an ataxic intention tremor. It may be mild, severe, or vary from day to day. In latter stages of the disease, the tremor may extend to the head. Ataxia and loss of sensation are also present in the lower extremities, so that the client must be able to see her feet in order to ambulate safely. Difficulty in balance is often present.

Visual problems include nystagmus (constant movement of the eyes), diplopia (double vision), or temporary loss of vision.

Often, the patient with multiple sclerosis seems neurotic, but there is a real neuropsychological reaction to multiple sclerosis as well as cognitive losses, which result in emotional disturbances. The individual may be highly euphoric with extreme optimism or deeply depressed. Medication can control reactions but usually has side effects, some of which decrease balance and increase cognitive problems. Teaching relaxation and stress-reduction techniques is often a better way to help the patient cope with fatigue and mood swings.

Homemaking rehabilitation for multiple sclerosis patients requires application of principles in many areas: energy conservation, overcoming incoordination and weakness, protection of hands from heat and cold, visual training for safety, and stress-reduction techniques for fatigue and emotional disturbances. The National Multiple Sclerosis Society distributes materials and has clinics and support groups through local chapters.

TRAINING TECHNIQUES FOR THE HOMEMAKER WITH INCOORDINATION

Your patient may experience ataxia, or tremors, when trying to carry out a task. When moving the extremity during a rest period and without purpose, the tremor may be absent. Frustration only increases the ataxia. Part of homemaking training includes relaxation techniques, such as teaching the patient to let the whole body relax before attempting a motion. Some of the techniques described in Chapter 7 may help. During early training, you might set up non-breakable objects on a counter or tray, then have the patient practice lifting and stacking them while concentrating on relaxing. Teach the patient to change position frequently to avoid stiffness in the upper and lower extremities.

Side effects of medication to reduce incoordination or tremors affect performance in the kitchen and other tasks of daily living. These include, but are not limited to, confusion, dizziness, blurring of vision, and increased difficulty with balance.

Encourage the patient to sit to work. This helps reduce prob-

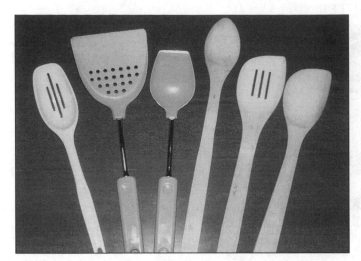

Figure 11-1. Plastic, nylon, Teflon-coated, and wooden utensils help protect finish and reduce scratching of pans. (Photo by J.K.)

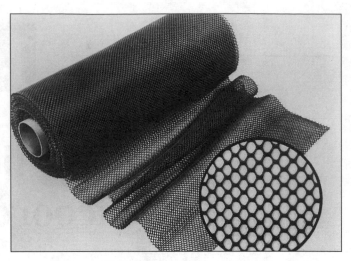

Figure 11-2. Non-slip materials may be purchased in rolls, then cut to size. (Neotex® Protective Mesh Matting photo courtesy of Research Products Corp., Madison, WI.)

lems of impaired balance, slow movement, and poor hand coordination. A swivel chair, without casters, may be placed next to the work area. The patient can then sit safely and swing into position. Postural changes (transferring from sitting to standing and bending) should be made slowly to maintain balance, and in the case of Meuniere's disease to minimize the labyrinthine effect.

UTENSILS AND KITCHEN TASKS

Some patients who have incoordination but no weakness, such as those with cerebral palsy, find it easier to work with heavier utensils. These must be non-breakable. Commercial strength pots like those manufactured by Caphalon are a good choice. See *Mealtime Manual*, Chapter 1.

Plastic, nylon, Teflon-coated, and wooden utensils help protect finish and reduce scratching of pans (Figure 11-1). Make sure that the attachments to the handles are strong enough to take strong pressure. Check handle construction.

Stabilizing objects with a friction material allows concentration on the task and reduces spills (Figure 11-2). Non-slip materials, such as Neotex® Protective Mesh Matting, Dycem®, Medigrip®, Posey Grip™, or Grip Liner™, may be purchased in rolls, then cut to size. **Manufacturer** of Dycem®: 178; of Medi Grip®: 554; of Neotex®: 442; of Posey Grip™, 413; of Grip Liner™: 452. Contact your local durable medical equipment supplier. See Chapter 8. Coating handles and bases with Plasti-Dip also reduces slipping. See Chapter 9.

Some aids used for the person with the use of one hand can help the individual with incoordination. Many of these devices keep the other hand out of the way when cutting or help with holding when mixing. Recommend non-breakable dishes like Corelle by Corning or Melamine. Use a cutting board with sides to prevent food from scattering. See Chapter 8.

Products produced for commercial use more readily sustain the tough treatment sometimes given to utensils by people with incoordination (Figure 11-3). The cup shown has a wide, curved handle that stabilizes the thumb for easier grasping. **Source:** 453.

An oral medicine holder may be used as an adapted measuring spoon for liquids like vanilla or vinegar. Squeezing then releasing the bulb on the holder brings liquid to desired level. Re-squeezing it over the bowl or other container releases the ingredient. It may be necessary to change some ingredients to small containers that have wider openings. See the oral syringe in Chapter 2 .

Scissors mounted on a block allow the person with severe incoordination or use of one hand to open packages with greater safety and ease than using a knife. If grasp is weak, loop-handled, spring-opening scissors may be attached to the block. **Manufacturer:** 191. **Sources:** 1, 14, 33, 279, 343, 383. See *Mealtime Manual*, Chapter 27. The block may be placed on non-skid material. If cutting paper or fabric, the block may be left free to slide across the counter.

Organize kitchen storage so that one item can be picked up at a time and other things will not be knocked down while reaching. Add narrow, tiered shelves as well as pull-out shelves. Removing cupboard doors eliminates excess motions. Keep utensils, dishes, and food grouped near the place they will be used to reduce walking and carrying. A lazy susan maximizes space. See *Mealtime Manual*, Chapter 14.

Correct lighting is important to permit safe handling of tasks. For the patient with multiple sclerosis and visual involvement, lighting must maximize residual sight and not increase visual problems. For the Meuniere's client, lighting should be kept low but adequate.

Turning around quickly may upset balance, so teach your client to move slowly and to use a wheeled cart to transport items. Gather all items before sitting to work. Avoid bending if this upsets balance; instead, use a long handled dustpan and brush and a reacher.

SELECTING APPLIANCES

An electric stove is safer than a gas stove for a person with incoordination. Even better when there is marked loss of control in upper extremity function is a microwave oven. It should be used with plastic or non-breakable containers. See *Mealtime Manual*, Chapter 20 under microwave ovens and accessories, and Chapter

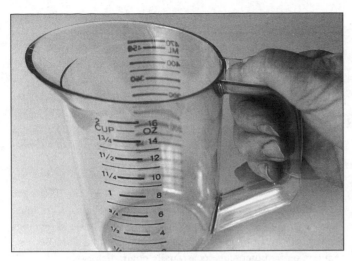

Figure 11-3. This cup has a wide curved handle that stabilizes the thumb for easier grasping. (Measuring cup from Rubbermaid® Commercial Products, Inc., Winchester, VA. Photo by J.K.)

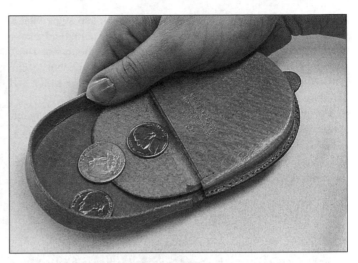

Figure 11-4. The coins are held within the rim of this horseshoe purse for easier selection. (Photo courtesy of the OT Department, Howard A. Rusk Institute of Rehabilitation Medicine.)

28 in this guide. The patient must be instructed to request help when the microwave's glass tray needs to be removed for cleaning. To reduce both spilling and the need for cleaning up, demonstrate how to partially fill containers and then cover them, as well as how to judge cooking times so foods do not overflow.

Retrieving foods from a side-by-side refrigerator freezer is easier than a top and bottom unit. If the laundry appliances are on another floor, the family may want to consider installing a compact unit on the main floor. See Chapter 25.

When using portable appliances, select solidly constructed items. A can opener that remains on the counter, rather than a handheld one, is safer. It may be pushed against the back of the counter or placed on non-skid material to stabilize it. A standard countertop model mixer is more reliable than a portable mixer. An instant hot water heater, like the Hot Shot® (see Chapter 20 in *Mealtime Manual*) eliminates carrying hot water to and from the stove.

Special switches permit the person with severe incoordination to operate appliances and share in the experience of food preparation. Adapted switches are available from several companies. **Sources:** 4, 294, 418, 506, 516, 532. See Resources for publications on using technology and switches for those with severe disabilities. Uses of switches are shown in Chapter 2, Chapter 9, and Chapter 27.

The client who has Parkinson's disease may find voice volume markedly decreased. This increasingly leads to social isolation, even from the family, and limits the ability to communicate in an emergency. Speech therapy can help improve both articulation and amplification. In some cases, a voice amplifier for talking in-person and on the telephone is needed. One answer is a small microphone worn on the lapel or front of a shirt with the amplifier on the table or in a pocket. **Sources** include 337, 430.

A purse with sides helps keep money from spilling when one is shopping (Figure 11-4). The purse can be attached to a cord that slips in the pocket so that it is easier to retrieve. Cost is about $6 from variety stores and mail-order firms. **Sources:** 361, 495, 508, 561B.

EATING AIDS

Problems in self-feeding caused by incoordination include loss of control, not only of the extremities and body but of the mouth and throat. If not addressed, difficulty in swallowing and chewing may lead to malnutrition. Because some drugs designed to decrease incoordination tend to dry the mouth, a solution of salt or sodium bicarbonate may be recommended. Commercial mouthwashes containing alcohol are contraindicated because they exacerbate the problem of dryness. Some individuals with Parkinson's may be on special low-protein diets, and consultation with a dietician will assist both the patient and family to plan nutritionally balanced meals.

Explain to the family as well as the patient that whether at home or away, dining should be a relaxing activity; the person handles it better when adequate time is allowed. If chewing and swallowing are affected, recommend six small meals a day with the same amount of food as three meals. See Chapter 4.

At the table, the client may find that using a swivel spoon, a plate with a rim or plate guard, or built-up handles on utensils makes a meal more relaxing. See Chapter 22 *Mealtime Manual* and Chapter 4 in this guide. A plate with a warming section will keep food heated when eating is very slow. A mug with a large handle or a straw may be used for drinking. One-way straws help the person who has difficulty swallowing or maintaining a sucking pattern. When eating out, the client should take along adapted eating utensils, then order items that are easy to handle or ask to have them cut in the kitchen.

Reduction of stress is important for all patients, but when there is incoordination it becomes a factor that physically affects performance. Incorporating relaxation techniques into homemaking tasks and using energy-conservation methods reduces anxiety and increases the functional level. This is especially important for the person with vestibular disorders. Relaxation techniques that consist of tensing and releasing all body muscles plus a 20-break daily for pure relaxation or meditation should be built into the daily schedule.

The person with vestibular or balance disorders may also have some dietary concerns, including decreased salt and sugar intake. Other dietary factors include distributing food and fluid intake evenly throughout the day, drinking adequate amounts of fluid, avoiding caffeine-containing substances, limiting alcohol to one glass of wine or beer a day, avoiding foods containing MSG, and avoiding aspirin-containing medications and cigarettes.

For other ideas on training and equipment, contact the organization involved with your client's disability (cerebral palsy, muscular dystrophy, head injury, vestibular disorders, brain tumor, Parkinson's) for information, materials, support groups, and possible funding. See Appendix C.

RESOURCES

Addresses for publishers, periodicals, and organizations are given in Section Four. Also see *Mealtime Manual*, Chapter 1.

PUBLICATIONS

Levin, J. & Scherfenberg, L. (1987). *Selection and Use of Simple Technology in Home, School, Work, and Community Settings*. Minneapolis: AbleNet®, Inc. **Source:** 4.

Cerebral Palsy

Dolan, M. (1994, winter). Aging with cerebral palsy. *Accent on Living*, pp. 54-56.

Sinkiewicz-Mercer, R., & Kaplan, S. (1989) *I Raise My Eyes to Say Yes*. Boston: Houghton Mifflin. $17.95. Woman with quadriplegic cerebral palsy describes life in an institution and entry into community living at age 28.

Schleichkorn, J. (1983). *Coping with Cerebral Palsy*. Austin, TX: Pro-Ed. $28. Aids parent-therapist relationship by answering questions not usually discussed in a therapy session. **Source:** 423.

Multiple Sclerosis

Bhasin, C. (1995, August). Understanding MS. *Team Rehab*. Guidelines for ordering a wheelchair for a client with MS.

Buxbaum, R., & Frankel, D. *Maximizing Your Health*. Massachusetts Chapter of the Multiple Sclerosis Society. $6.25 from the National Multiple Sclerosis Society, New York. Program of graded exercise, meditation, and stress management (by Joan Borysenko and Herbert Benson) for a person with multiple sclerosis.

Carroll, D., & Dorman, J. (1993). *Living Well with Multiple Sclerosis: A Guide for Patient, Caregiver and Family*. New York: HarperCollins. $12.

Jensen, K., et al., (Eds.). (1988). *Mental Disorders and Cognitive Deficits in Multiple Sclerosis*. New York: Demos. Focuses on impairment of intellectual function and other mental disorders with multiple sclerosis; gives a prophylactic approach to management.

Kalb, R., & Scheinberg, L. (1992). *Multiple Sclerosis and the Family*. New York: Demos. $21.95. How MS impacts the family; resources to help effectively manage lives in the presence of multiple sclerosis.

The National Multiple Sclerosis Society provides a variety of information on exercise programs, and family relationships when there is MS and when there is loss of vision. Free publications include: Sarnoff, J., with Dosich, D. (1993). *Food for Thought: MS and Nutrition*; Frankel, D. (1993). *Living with MS*; Sanford, M.E.,

& Petagan, J. H. (1994). *Multiple Sclerosis and Your Emotions*; Minden, S., & Frandel, D. (1995). *Plaintalk: A Booklet About MS for Families*; Giesser, B. (1991). *Positive Nutrition*; Bain, L, & Shapiro, R. T. (1994). *The Rehabilitation Outlook*; La Rocca, N. G., with King, M. (1995). *Solving Cognitive Problems*;Jaffee, C. et al. (1992). *Someone You Know Has Multiple Sclerosis: A Book for Families*. Illustrated for reading to children; Holland, N. (1995). *Taking Care: A Guide for Well Partners*; Rogers, S. (1995). *Things I Wish Someone Had Told Me: Practical Thoughts for People Newly Diagnosed with Multiple Sclerosis*.

Rosner, L., & Ross, S. (1992). *Multiple Sclerosis: New Hope and Practical Advice for People with MS and Their Families*. New York: Prentice Hall, Random House. $11. Book makes complex material accessible to lay people, including emotions and relationships, needs to be read with other literature in the field because chapters on treatment are occasionally contradictory.

Shapiro, R. T. (1991). *Neurorehabilitation: Volume 4—Multiple Sclerosis: A Rehabilitation Approach to Management*. New York: Demos. $21.95. Neurology of MS, physical and occupational therapy, speech, and swallowing disorders. Available also from **source** 8.

Parkinson's Disease

American Parkinson Disease Association, Inc. Free pamphlets and booklets on starting a Parkinson's disease support group, nutrition, coping: Johnson, M. *Let's Communicate: A Speech and Swallowing Program for Persons with Parkinson's Disease* (includes eating safely and dietary recommendations); *Young Parkinson's Handbook* (nominal fee), hospitalization, living will, and durable power of attorney for health care. Quarterly newspaper.

Parkinson's Disease. (1993). *Harvard Health Letter*,16-page booklet, $6.50 from Dept. PD, Box 380, Boston, MA 02117.

The National Parkinson's Disease Foundation. Quarterly. Publications on handling daily activities, suggestions for eating, research, social involvement, caregiving, book reviews. See list in *Mealtime Manual*, Chapter 1, Going Further. Additional publications include *Fighting Back Against Parkinson's: One Woman's Winning Battle* (1995); Dorros, S., & Dorros, D. (1995). *Patient Perspectives on Parkinson's: A Series of Essays*.

Parkinson's Disease Update. Newsletter with coverage of medical, social, and psychological aspects. See Periodicals.

Pierce, J. R. (1990). *A Patient's Perspective: Living with Parkinson's Disease*. New York: Demos. $12.95. Symptom descriptions, psychological mechanisms for overcoming depression, handling daily living activities, importance of exercise, medication and side effects, locating support groups.

Robinson, M. B., with the Occupational Therapy Department, Burke Rehabilitation Center, White Plains, NY. (1989). *Equipment and Suggestions to Help the Patient with Parkinson's Disease in the Activities of Daily Living*. New York: American Parkinson Disease Association. Free. Ideas for increasing function and independence throughout the house. List of American Parkinson Disease Association Information and Referral Centers.

Vestibular Disorders

Greuel, H. *Sudden Deafness, Vertigo and Tinnitus*. Available through Vestibular Disorders Group. Working with the patient who has vestibular disorders, including relaxation exercises, changes in lifestyle, biofeedback methods, and relaxation techniques.

On the Level: Quarterly Newsletter of the Vestibular Disorders Association. $15 includes annual membership.

AUDIOVISUALS

Growing Up Capable. (1992). 9-minute VHS video, with 7-page viewer guide. Minneapolis: AbleNet. $38. Designed for families, teachers, and therapists. Focuses on children gaining increased independence through use of specially designed and affordable switches, control units, and mounting systems for toys, games, appliances, computers, and communication systems. **Source:** 4.

The Homemaker with Incoordination: Handicapped Homemaker Series. Howard A. Rusk Institute of Rehabilitation Medicine, New York University Medical Center, under a grant from the Campbell Soup Fund. Demonstrates equipment used in meal preparation by a homemaker with cerebral palsy. Sequences include planning a dinner party, shopping, and kitchen tasks, such as cutting and chopping foods, handling containers and appliances, cooking and clean-up, setting the table, and serving. Careful selection and safe use of equipment is emphasized. For further information, write Living Media, Inc. **Source:** 332.

VO—Staying Even. Dramatization of most major problems faced by people with vestibular disorders including coping strategies, family and community support. *V-C Can What I Eat Affect the Way I Feel?*; *V-D How Can Physical Activity Help?* with Judi Grucella, physical therapist. Each videotape costs $8 for a one-week period from the time it is received. To rent these or for a full list, contact the Vestibular Disorders Association.

12

The Client Who Has an Amputation

The need for retraining in kitchen and other household activities differs whether working with individuals with an upper or lower extremity amputation. The person with an upper extremity (UE) amputation must learn to use the prosthetic arm to perform tasks requiring dexterity and coordination as well as to carry and lift objects. The person with a lower extremity (LE) amputation requires strengthening of ambulation skills as well as balance to stand and perform activities.

In one area, however, both UE and LE amputees have the same need—that is to work through their own self-concepts, to become comfortable with and accepting of their artificial limbs.

The role of the health care professional differs depending on the point that the client has reached in rehabilitation. Early treatment involves dressing and hardening of the stump, including desensitizing massage. Physical and occupational therapists work with the patient to increase range of motion, strength, and endurance before the limb is fitted. Even in home care programs, the patient may not yet have a final prosthesis and may be learning to do things with one hand, with a wheelchair, or on crutches. All amputees need to learn and follow hygiene as outlined in *Principles for all Amputees*. See reproducible page in Appendix G.

UPPER EXTREMITY AMPUTEE

Depression affects the client's ability to adjust to a prosthesis, especially when the cosmetic appearance of an arm and hand does not match one's self-image. The patient should be involved in the selection of all terminal devices. While hooks are the most versatile terminal devices, the body-powered prosthetic hand, complete with rings and watch, is sometimes preferred, especially by women. Helping a patient adjust to using both types is part of training in homemaking as in other areas.

If the patient goes through a rehabilitation program, he or she learns to handle controls of the prosthetic arm through shoulder movement at that time. Opening and closing the terminal device is usually the first operation taught. The therapist then moves up the limb, teaching the remainder of the controls. There are

patients, especially those with long, below-elbow amputations, who learn to function basically one-handed and prefer a passive glove without the added straps and controls.

Practical matters include the most efficient ways to hold objects or secure utensils while working. The sound arm or hand becomes the dominant extremity; the artificial limb is used as an assist. Teaching how to protect the terminal device from hot water, burns, and stains is another concern. Practice in cutting, opening containers, hand mixing, and carrying various sized objects should all be part of upper extremity training. Techniques for working with one hand may be adapted to the needs of the person with an upper extremity amputation.

See *Mealtime Manual*, Chapter 1, and in this guide, Chapter 8 .

Development in prosthetics continues. An electrically operated, robotic terminal device allows for specific hand movements. It is mainly used in industrial settings for manipulating tools and looks like the less expensive devices.

The myoelectric arm, which picks up electrodes through nerve impulses implanted in muscle sites, eliminates around-the-body strapping.

The Utah artificial arm is lightweight and free from cables (Figure 12-1A,B). Developed originally at the University of Utah, the modular artificial arm and hand system for above-elbow amputees permits sensitive control of both the elbow and the hand using only two muscles. Electrodes are placed on the skin where they sense the electrical activity of the muscle. Some retraining of the patient's muscles is needed to develop strength and control. The myoelectric hand control may be interchanged with a body-powered terminal device. For further information, contact **source** 369.

The Steeper powered gripper is an electric terminal device with wide-opening, rubber-lined jaws to handle large items, like cups and jars, and the hard tips that are preferred to pick up small items (Figure 12-2). The gripper is smooth on the outside so that it can be easily pushed into a pocket to remove keys or a wallet, something difficult to do with the rubber glove on a powered hand. A right-angle step on the palmar side lets one push on a lever, box, or object with a right-angle edge. **Source:** 318.

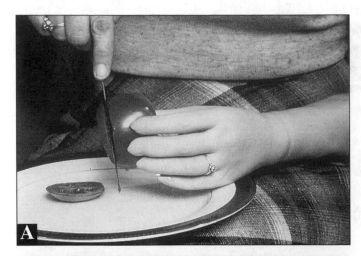

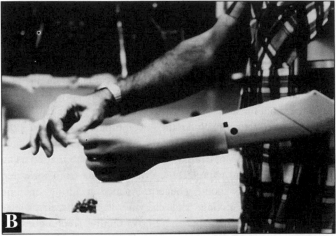

Figure 12-1A,B. The Utah artificial arm is lightweight and free from cables. (Photos courtesy of Motion Control, Inc., Salt Lake City, UT.)

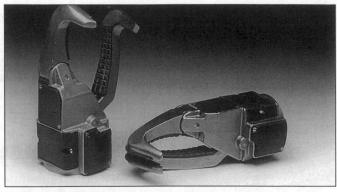

Figure 12-2. This Liberty Technology unit weighs only ¾ pound, so is light enough to allow myoelectric control for an amputee using a conventional elbow, yet provides up to 13 pounds of grip. (Photo courtesy of Liberty Technology, Hopkinton, MA.)

LOWER EXTREMITY AMPUTEE

Selection of a prosthesis must take into account the lifestyle of the client. A sedentary person requires a different type of prosthesis than one who hikes and jogs. Therapists who do not treat amputees on a frequent basis may be surprised at advances in prosthetics. Weight-activated knee systems require shifting weight when sitting down. New ankle prostheses, such as the Tru-Foot from College Park Industries, Inc., incorporate up to seven actions that mimic motion of the anatomical foot. **Source:** 127.

Basic ambulation skills for the lower extremity amputee are usually taught in physical therapy. Learning to look where the foot is being placed avoids many falls. This may seem simplistic, but not looking is the major cause of falls. Mastering standing and walking activities in the home may be done with the help of an occupational therapist. Learning to bend and reach items stored in the kitchen, handling a broom, dustpan, or vacuum cleaner, scrubbing the floor, carrying items, lifting laundry or groceries, and driving are all skills that the patient may have to acquire. To prevent overuse of the uninvolved leg, a therapist must monitor the patient to make sure that the patient puts equal pressure on the prosthetic and non-prosthetic leg.

The use of a cane or crutch during inclement weather or when balance feels uncertain, as when in a crowd of people, may be recommended. Family members and friends should be taught to respect the need for the individual to maintain standing balance and not make sudden moves that will upset him or her. An amputee may find the best way to counteract this is to grab on to a stable object.

Finding a relaxed way to sit reduces pressure on the stump. A high stool may be more comfortable than a lower chair. Using a wheeled table is safer than carrying a load in one's arms when balance is not steady.

The McBuddy allows a lower extremity amputee to work with good stability when not wearing a prosthesis (Figure 12-3A,B). The adjustable height support works for above- or below-knee amputations, is suitcase portable, may be used at the kitchen or bathroom sink, even with an easy chair, or in the car. For further information, contact **source** 349.

Finding a suitable car for driving with a lower extremity prosthesis may take some testing and adaptation. The foot-well design is often too cramped. See Chapter 30 for resources, such as General Motors, Ford, Chrysler Corporation, and the *AAA Disabled Driver's Mobility Guide*.

Occasionally, a lower extremity amputee will not be fitted with a prosthesis. This is usually due to poor circulation, as in diabetes. Ensuring the best sitting posture and distribution of pressure is still paramount to minimize the chances of further skin breakdown. Special cushions may be indicated. See Chapter 16.

If ordering a wheelchair for a lower extremity amputee, the axle must be moved back about 1½ inches to counterbalance the weight shift caused by loss of a lower extremity. Conversion kits are available from wheelchair supply firms. An extended Swingaway Stump Support for a lower extremity is available from **source:** 222B.

RESOURCES

Addresses for publications, periodicals, and organizations are given in Section Four.

PUBLICATIONS

The American Amputee Foundation, Inc., (AAF) a non-profit organization, assists in meeting the information and referral needs

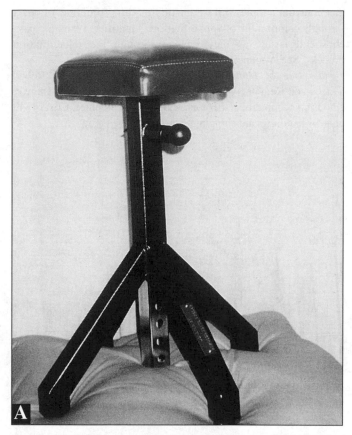
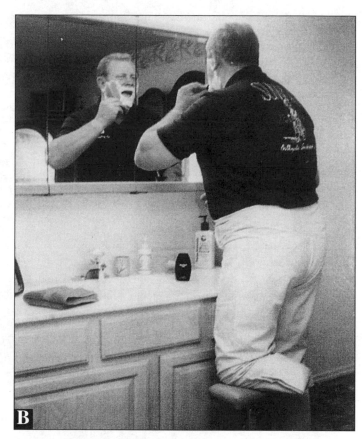

Figure 12-3A,B. The McBuddy allows a lower extremity amputee to work with good stability when not wearing a prosthesis. (Photos courtesy of McBuddy, Whitehall, MT.)

of amputees. Their *National Resource Directory* has listings of organizations for amputees as well as other disabilities, publications, sources of advanced prostheses, and a wealth of information for any health care professional or person with a disability, $25. The AAF also distributes amputee-related publications, such as *Crutches on the Go*, $3; *Hygienic Problems of the Amputee*, $2; *Handbook for Lower Extremity Amputees*, $7.50; *Observations on Phantom Limb Phenomena*, $2.50; add 10% for postage. Send for full list, which includes videos, see below.

The American Orthotic and Prosthetic Association has two free brochures. *Orthoses and Prostheses and the Older Adult: Staying on the Move* offers answers on prosthetic care, maintaining independence, physical activity, and paying for treatment. *Orthoses and Prostheses for Children: Growing Up Independent* gives advice on building a positive self-image and obtaining a properly fitting device. Send a self-addressed, stamped envelope for a copy of each.

Amputee Coalition of America. Organization for amputees. Publishes magazine *In Motion*.

Karacoloff, K., Hammersley, C., & Schneider, F. (1992). *Lower Extremity Amputation: A Guide to Functional Outcomes in Physical Therapy* (2nd ed.). Frederick, MD: Rehabilitation Institute of Chicago Publication Series, Aspen. $65.

Mooney, R. J. (1995). *The Handbook for New Upper Extremity Amputees, Their Families, and Friends*. Lomita, CA: Mutual Aid Amputee Foundation.

Orthotics/Prosthetics: Resource Guide. Bethesda, MD: American Occupational Therapy Association. #4290, $10 AOTA

members, $20 non-members. Bibliographies, audiovisuals, resource personnel.

Sabolich, J. (Ed.). *You're Not Alone: The Personal Stories of Forty Amputees*. NovaCare Sabolich Prosthetic and Research Center. **Source:** 386.

Wilson, A. B., Jr. (1989). *Limb Prosthetics* (6th ed.). New York: Demos. $19.95. Surgical approaches to amputation, devices currently available, special considerations in care of elderly amputees and of children, care of prostheses, functional capacities of amputees. Available from **source** 8.

Winchell, E. *Coping with Limb Loss*. New York: Avery. $14.95.

PERIODICALS

Please see Going Further, *Mealtime Manual*, Chapter 3.

In Motion. Mutual Aid Amputee Foundation. Designed for the consumer with an amputation and professionals.

Orthotic and Prosthetic (O & P) Business News. Semi-monthly publication focuses on new products, services, events, and tech tips of practical applications.

AUDIOVISUALS

Amputee Therapy. Y13 Productions. 26.57-minute VHS video. Follows patient from hospital room after surgery to gym with mobility issues, stump wrapping, and prosthesis fitting. Former patient and a physical therapist talk with patient. Demonstrates effective ways to employ crutches and canes in daily activities.

Cost is $99 plus $6 shipping and handling. **Source:** 588.

Life without a Limb. 50 minute VHS video for amputees and their families, support groups, and health care professionals. $34.95 plus 10% for postage, from the American Amputee Foundation, Inc.

The Process of Psychological Adaptation to Limb Loss. 1982. 28-minute VHS, $50. Available from RRTC in Community Integration for Individuals with Spinal Cord Injury. Concerns that confront people with traumatic limb loss from time of onset through completion of rehabilitation. Identifies 10 major psychosocial issues as they change through the rehabilitation process. See Appendix C.

The Use of Upper Extremity Prostheses. Dynamic Rehab Videos and Rentals. 49-minute VHS video, 1988, by Art Heinze, who is an occupational therapist and bilateral amputee. Cost is $49 plus $4 handling and shipping. **Source:** 179.

The Client Who Requires an Ambulation Aid

A patient who is having difficulty walking must be fully evaluated by a therapist. This assessment will determine if there is a need for ambulation training, changes in gait patterns, or the addition of ambulation aids. Falls are one of the most devastating accidents that affect the older individual's life. See Chapter 1 and Chapter 24.

Fitting of an ambulation aid and training are major concerns of the professional health care worker. A client must be able to ambulate safely within the home or extended care facility. If this is not possible, an aid or use of a wheelchair is mandated.

Standard aids for ambulation including canes, crutches, and walkers are discussed in *Mealtime Manual*, Chapter 4. If, however, there is marked involvement of the upper extremities that limits range of motion or reduces strength, adaptation of the ambulation aid or an alternate method may be necessary. Pressure on the brachial plexus will cause nerve damage if the patient cannot keep weight off the axillary rests of crutches. A switch to Lofstrand or forearm crutches may be indicated. When the wrists and hands are affected by arthritis, built-up and specially molded handgrips for canes or crutches distribute pressure on the hands more evenly and reduce pain.

CANES

The Fenix walking stick has a molded handgrip that supports the whole palm, distributing weight and increasing comfort (Figure 13-1A,B). It is particularly suitable for the patient with arthritis who may complain of pain in the thumb, wrist, elbow, and shoulder when using a regular cane. The handle angles to suit the degree of mobility in the patient's shoulder, elbow, and wrist. Designed by Sweden's Ergonomic Design Group. **Manufacturer/ Source:** 191.

A large orthopedic handle on a quad cane will allow the hand to grip in a more natural manner. It adjusts for left- or right-handed use. A positive spring-lock button adjusts height in one-inch increments. Cost is about $25 and up. **Manufacturers** include 191, 294B, 336, 454. **Sources** include

11, 14, 198, 205, 343, 383, 420, 461. A quad cane with a forearm crutch is available from **source** 461.

The Momentum Supercane™ has a built-in lower handgrip that assists the individual in standing up from a bed or chair, and it has a centered line of force for optimal stability and balance (Figure 13-2). The unique geometric shape flexes when it hits the ground, reducing shock to the wrist and shoulder. High-density foam handgrips are ergonomically contoured to provide added gripping comfort. Cane adjusts and comes in standard to tall sizes at a cost of about $45 each. **Sources:** 21, 98, 383. Note: cane is not recommended for people with Parkinson's disease or a tendency to lose balance when leaning forward. User must have good trunk balance and be assessed for safety and usefulness of this cane under supervision of therapist.

Forearm supports for canes, Lofstrand, and axillary crutches are available from hospital suppliers (Figure 13-3). **Manufacturers** include 454, 499. **Sources:** 33, 161, 461. Cost is about $75 a pair for axillary crutches, $112 and up for armrest crutches, and $120 for a quad cane/forearm crutch. Padded cuffs for Lofstrands are also available from 161.

Soft covers for crutch handgrips attach with Velcro® and provide more comfort when hands are affected by arthritis or weakness. Cost is about $16 per set. **Sources:** 161, 461.

WALKERS

A walker provides a portable base of support for the patient with poor balance and/or weak lower extremities to ambulate more safely. The patient using a walker, however, should be carefully evaluated for specific needs. Weight, width, handle height, and pressure on hands all affect performance and safety. The button or mechanism for folding a walker when going to and from appointments may be difficult for a client with weak hands or arthritis to manage.

Walker designs range from rigid to folding models, nonwheeled to two-, three-, or four-wheeled designs and allow customizing of unit to a client. Often, the weight of a walker becomes a major factor with constant lifting. Wheeled walkers

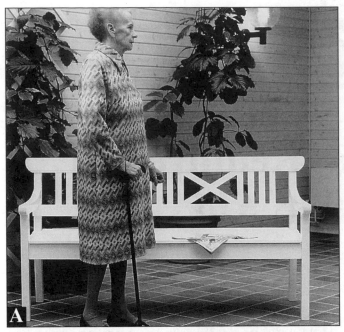

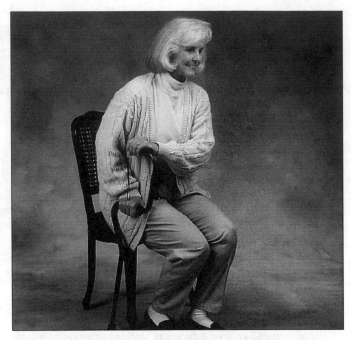

Figure 13-2. The Momentum Supercane™ has a built-in lower handgrip that assists the individual in standing up from a bed or chair. (Photo courtesy of North Coast Medical, Inc., San Jose, CA.)

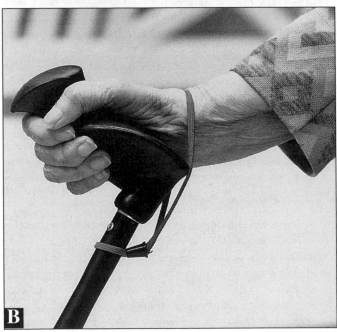

Figure 13-1A,B. The Fenix walking stick has a molded handgrip that supports the whole palm, distributing weight and increasing comfort. (Photos courtesy of Etac USA, Inc., Waukesha, WI.)

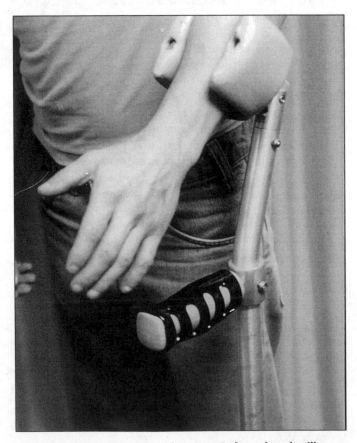

Figure 13-3. Forearm supports for canes, Lofstrand, and axillary crutches are available from hospital suppliers. (Photo courtesy of Danmar Products, Inc., Ann Arbor, MI.)

eliminate hoisting for each step. A forgetful or unstable patient, however, is not a safe candidate for a wheeled unit. A person with Parkinson's disease, for example, often cannot control forward motion. A fold-down seat provides a resting place when the patient tires. Before using, an evaluation is necessary to determine safety of this accessory with the individual patient.

The arms of the chair or the edge of the bed, not the walker, should be used for support when sitting down or rising. A higher seat, about 20 inches, is easier to get out of, and arms are recommended. Do not use a walker on more than two steps, and even this will require training.

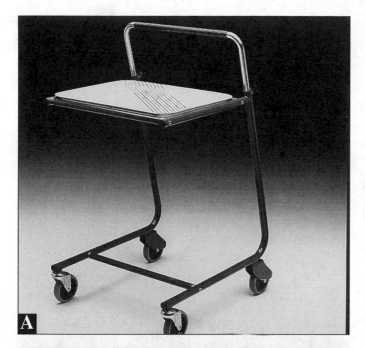

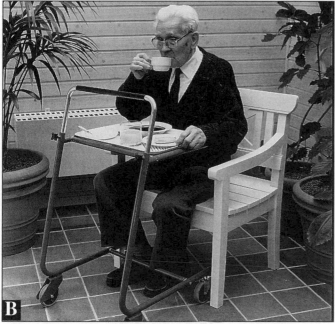

Figure 13-4A,B. This walking table may be used as an ambulation aid, tea trolley, or bed table. (Photos courtesy of Etac USA, Inc., Waukesha, WI.)

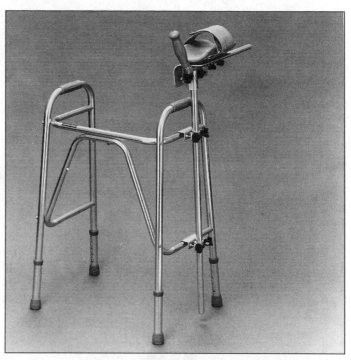

Figure 13-5. A forearm support on a walker allows a person with marked loss of function or severe arthritis in one arm to ambulate by holding the built-up hand grasp. (Photo courtesy of AliMed®, Inc., Dedham, MA.)

When prescribing walkers or ambulation aids, new and adapted products allow greater mobility and independence for a wider range of clients. A walking table may be used as an ambulation aid, tea trolley, or bed table (Figure 13-4A,B). Balanced for safety and stability, the "Walking Matilda" provides support for a newly ambulating patient and assists when rising from a seated position. The total width of 20.8 inches allows passage through almost any doorway. For further information, contact **manufacturer/source** 191.

A forearm support on a walker allows a person with marked loss of function or severe arthritis in one arm to ambulate by hold-ing the built-up hand grasp (Figure 13-5). If there is marked spasticity in the arm or poor trunk balance, it is not suitable. Walkers may also be adapted with two forearm rests. In such cases, a clip rather than Velcro® is recommended for easy release. **Manufacturers** include 454, 499. **Sources:** 33, 336.

Large-diameter, cushion-tired wheels on the Nova Rollator permit outdoor as well as indoor use (Figure 13-6A,B). A unique braking system increases security and confidence. Handles adjust for both width and height. The seat is a standard feature. Accessories include a shopping basket and transparent tray. It weighs about 16 pounds and folds for travel. For further information, contact **manufacturer/source** 191.

The Avant Rollator is completely adjustable to suit a patient's dimensions (Figure 13-7A,B). A main adjustment matches it to the patient's height and sets the height of the seat. The unique strap brakes take very little power to apply, either for slowing or for parking. When seated, the curved handle supports the user's sides and back. The seat, with its hand cut-out, flips up easily when not in use so one can "step in" to the walker. This allows closer approach to kitchen counters and grocery shelves. Wheels and tires are molded together for tough outdoor use. A basket and crutch or cane holder are optional accessories. For further information, contact **manufacturer/source** 191.

The Wenzelite™ walker may allow the client with severe lower extremity involvement to walk limited distances with adequate support (Figure 13-8). Walker may be pulled up under a bed or chair for better mechanical advantage when rising or sitting down. Optional forearm supports adjust forward and backward; a ratchet lever then locks the forearm support into

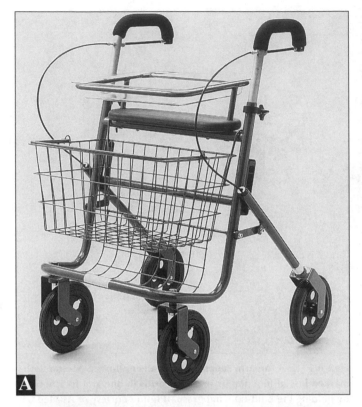

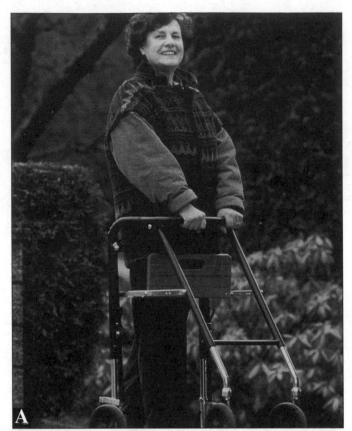

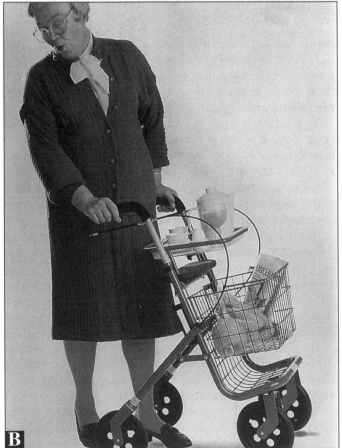

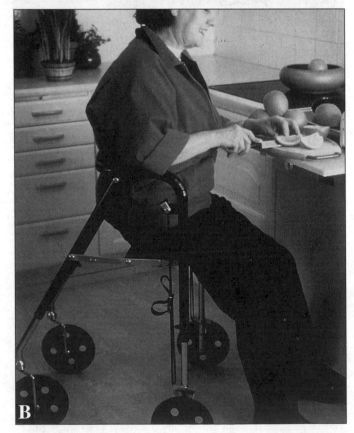

Figure 13-6A,B. Large-diameter, cushion-tired wheels on the Nova Rollator permit outdoor as well as indoor use. (Photos courtesy of Etac USA, Inc., Waukesha, WI.)

Figure 13-7A,B. The Avant Rollator is completely adjustable to suit a patient's dimensions. (Photos courtesy of Etac USA, Inc., Waukesha, WI.)

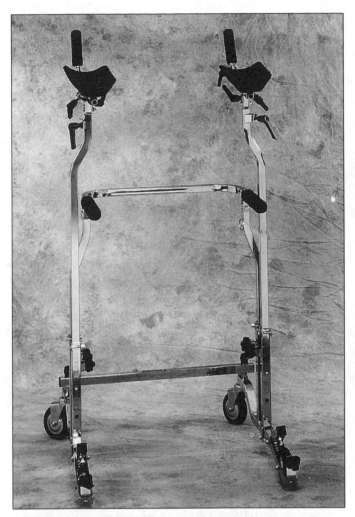

Figure 13-8. The Wenzelite™ walker may allow the client with severe lower extremity involvement to walk limited distances with adequate support. Walker may be pulled up under a bed or chair for better mechanical advantage when rising or sitting down. Optional forearm supports, as shown here, adjust forward and backward. (Photo courtesy of Wenzelite Medical Supply Co., Brooklyn, NY.)

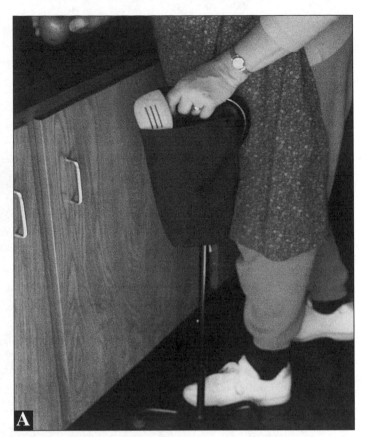

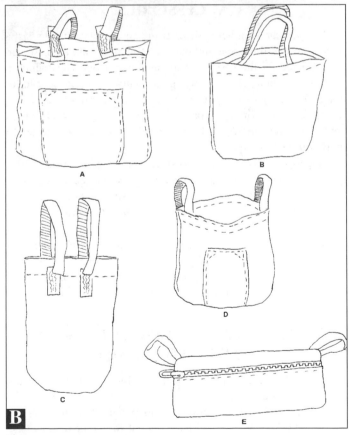

Figure 13-9A,B. Canvas bags come in various styles for use with a walker, quad cane, crutches, wheelchair side pocket, or back handles of a wheelchair. (Bags by the Bag Lady, West Stockbridge, MA. Photo by J.K. Illustration by G.K.)

the desired configuration. An optional transverse handle bar allows use with one hand. Other accessories include an IV holder, an oxygen tank holder, a basket, and a self-storing retractable seat. The unit moves as the patient pushes it, but placing full weight on the unit stops forward movement. This may render the design a safer alternative to a regular walker for a client with overflow motion, such as patients with cerebral palsy and Parkinson's disease or marked weakness such as with amyotrophic lateral sclerosis. A Dial-A-Brake adjustment knob provides resistance on one or both rear wheels to help control speed or an asymmetrical gait pattern. Height of handrails on adult model adjusts from 40 to 47 inches. The folding walker shown is approved by Medicare in cases where a patient is unable to use a regular pick-up walker due to obesity, neurological disorders, or restricted use of one hand, Code E0147. For Medicaid reimbursement, use Code E1399, sent with medical justifications for prior approval. The Wenzelite pediatric models include

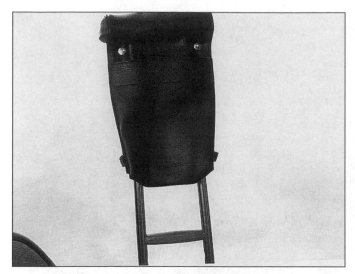

Figure 13-10. A bag may be fitted on an axillary crutch for carrying light items. (Photo courtesy of AliMed®, Inc., Dedham, MA.)

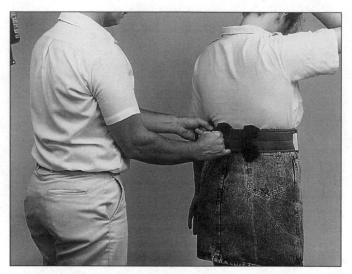

Figure 13-11. For the health care professional working with a patient using an ambulation aid, a walking belt with handholds increases safety, especially during the initial learning period. (Photo courtesy of Sammons/Preston, Inc., ©1992 Bissell Healthcare Company.)

a standard anterior walker and a posterior model that allows the child to stand more upright and does not interfere with stride. **Manufacturer:** 569.

Other rolling walker **manufacturers** include 45, 336, 379, 395, 445, 454, 499, 561. Please see Chapter 30.

ACCESSORIES

Aids for carrying items while using an ambulation aid assist a patient around the home and outside. The client should, however, be evaluated for the best unit and cautioned about overloading it. Canvas bags in a variety of styles are lightweight and flexible for items like eyeglasses, purses, tissues, and cordless phones. A wheeled cart is more appropriate for moving large items like food containers and pans. See Chapter 26 in this guide and Chapter 16 in *Mealtime Manual*.

Canvas bags come in various styles for use with a walker, $11; quad cane, $6; crutches, $6; wheelchair side pocket, $11; or back handles of a wheelchair for patients who use chairs to ambulate or want to carry more items, $11 (Figure 13-9A,B). **Manufacturers:** 19, 29, 70, 126.

A bag may be fitted on an axillary crutch for carrying light items (Figure 13-10). The person using crutches to ambulate should, however, balance any but a very light load by dividing the weight between two bags. **Source:** 33.

WALKING WITH A CLIENT USING AN AMBULATION AID

For the health care professional working with a patient using an ambulation aid, a walking belt with handholds increases safety, especially during the initial learning period (Figure 13-11). Aides and others working with the patient should be taught to use the walking belt. **Sources** for walking belts include 1, 383, 461.

Use your legs and bend your hips when helping a patient rise. Do not use your back! Walk close to the patient on his or her

involved side, because that is the side toward which the patient usually falls.

Walk behind the patient going upstairs, in front of him or her going down, and caution him or her to go slowly, checking balance on each step.

PRINCIPLES FOR AMBULATION

Teaching the rules of ambulation to your client will increase safety. They are listed in Appendix G and may be photocopied.

STANDING WITH WEAK LOWER EXTREMITIES

A patient with moderate weakness in the lower extremities may find it comfortable to stand and work in the kitchen part of the time if provided with a sling hooked to the counter (Figure 13-12). The support braces his or her back; a pillow may be added for additional comfort at the front. The pillow is attached to the cabinet with adhesive-backed Velcro® or Poly-Lock®, so it may be removed when not in use. Walking aids are stored within reach. In providing this aid, attention must be given to storage of most needed utensils and foods to avoid walking back and forth. A cart may be used to gather needed items ahead of time.

RESOURCES

Addresses for publishers, periodicals, and organizations are given in Section Four.

PUBLICATIONS

Goodman, W. (1989). *Mobility Training for People with Disabilities: Children and Adults with Physical, Mental, Visual and Hearing Impairments Can Learn to Travel.* Springfield, IL: Charles C. Thomas. $32.75.

Product Report: Walkers, D14390, 1992. Free from AARP Fulfillment, EE0220. Describes and compares in detail various types of walkers plus accessories.

Also see the *Home Rehabilitation Guide* by Paul A. Roggow, Debra K. Berg, and Michael D. Lewis, listed in Appendix F. Information on crutch walking, proper use of canes, and walker ambulation.

AUDIOVISUALS

How to Be Almost Happy on Crutches. Introduced by Hereward S. Cattell. 21-minute VHS. $30. How to adjust crutches, walk, get in and out of chairs and bed, handle stairs, carry, use elevators and escalators, simplify kitchen and bathroom chores. **Source:** 1.

Independence Skills (For Seniors). Y13 Productions. 9-minute VHS video. Physical therapist teaches a senior citizen correct way to use ambulation aids, including fitting and using a walker on level surfaces, car transfer with a walker, using a cane on level surfaces and stairs. $99 plus $6 shipping and handling. **Source:** 588.

Using a Cane, Crutch or Walker. Y13 Productions. VHS video. Instructs patient, aides, and family members about correct use of ambulation aids. Demonstrates non-weight-bearing and partial weight-bearing; shows how to adjust aid to correct height. $99 plus $5 handling. **Source:** 588.

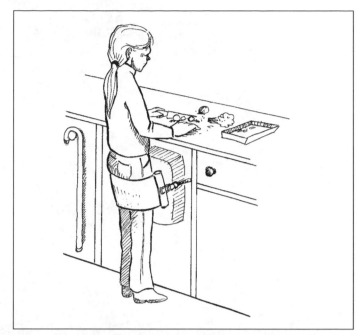

Figure 13-12. A patient with moderate weakness in the lower extremities may find it comfortable to stand and work in the kitchen part of the time if provided with a sling. Walking aids are stored within reach. (Illustration by G.K.)

14

The Client with Back Pain or Chronic Pain

Pain accompanies many disabilities. Thirteen percent of all Americans have their lives disrupted by constant pain. This distress reduces motivation to do for oneself. The patient's goals and your treatment plans in homemaking, ambulation, or any other activity is affected by your client's tolerance for, or control of, pain.

Nutrition may be disrupted because the individual does not feel like eating, considers it too tiring (painful) to fix food, or finds food unappetizing because of the side effects of medication. Using quick, easy-to-fix recipes and preparing foods ahead for "bad days" may be incorporated into a treatment program. Excess weight increases back pain and may have to be approached through individualized meal planning training.

Medication may be used to reduce pain but is not a final answer. Side effects create their own problems, such as reduced cognition, decreased balance or dizziness, increased or decreased appetite, depression, and lack of safety awareness. Check a drug reference book to ascertain what side effects may be experienced. See Appendix F. These effects must be addressed when training the patient in meal preparation as in other tasks.

Courses, audiovisuals, and books can help teach your client how to prevent back pain by using correct posture and body mechanics. Emphasizing the importance of daily exercises to strengthen the back and ensuring that the patient fits these into his or her everyday schedule is part of home management.

Several organizations offer materials to aid in the treatment of patients with chronic pain. The American Chronic Pain Association has support groups throughout the country and distributes a workbook for people not near a chapter. Their relaxation tapes provide a way to begin self-control of pain. They should be used under the guidance of a health care professional. See Resources.

The National Chronic Pain Outreach Association, Inc., is a non-profit organization established to help people regain control of their lives. It operates an information clearinghouse for health care providers as well as pain sufferers. Their educational publications and cassette tapes cover a wide range of pain management topics. *Lifeline*, their quarterly newsletter, focuses on coping tech-

niques, developments in pain management, book reviews, and personal profiles. They also offer seminars or lectures and help form local chronic pain support groups.

The most common ailment today is headaches. More than 45 million Americans seek the help of a physician to stop severe headaches. Add to this 16 to 18 million more who have migraine headaches. If a patient's head pain interferes with completing daily activities, a visit with the physician is indicated. The National Headache Foundation distributes materials for training by health care professionals and by oneself.

Headaches are caused by many factors: poor nutrition, bad sleeping posture or habits, incorrect breathing patterns, medication side effects, high blood pressure, allergy, or tension. Once the reason is known, it may be alleviated by incorporating relaxation, proper breathing, and posture training as well as good nutrition into the homemaking program. A patient who is sensitive to tyramine may find that avoiding foods containing this substance alleviates the headaches. See Resources for a tyramine-free cookbook.

Types of pain vary, but teaching your patient certain principles will help reduce almost any pain during meal preparation tasks:

- Conserve energy whenever possible. Sit to work in a proper chair.
- Re-do storage to avoid bending, twisting, and lifting as much as possible.
- Choose the best time of the day to do chores that require effort. This may be following a relaxation tape session or during a specific period after medication.
- Draw up a meal plan for the week that includes foods prepared ahead of time and enough flexibility that menus may be switched around.

SAVING THE BACK

Exercises prescribed by the physician or physical or occupational therapist are an essential part of any client's daily back program. When making out a daily schedule, exercises should be written in at a time selected by the patient. Relaxation techniques

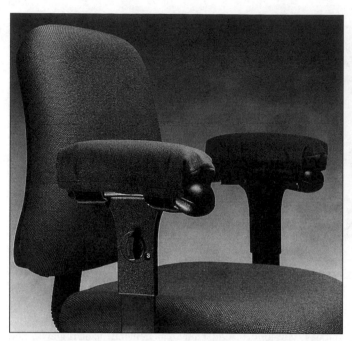

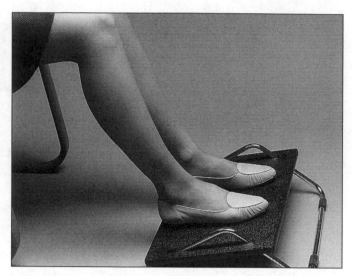

Figure 14-2. An angled footstool helps reduce pressure on the back when sitting for long periods of time. (Photo of WorkMod footstool courtesy of North Coast Medical, Inc., San Jose, CA.)

Figure 14-1. This office chair has a curved back and higher arm rests to allow the upper extremities to relax while working. (Work Mod Chair photo courtesy of North Coast Medical, Inc., San Jose, CA.)

are also a part of a back program. Using methods in Chapter 7 will relieve stress and help your patient cope with back and chronic pain. If a back brace has been recommended by the patient's physician, assess how it is helping the patient and whether he or she wears it regularly. If he or she does not, find out why. Modifications may be required.

Teaching body mechanics is a crucial part of the health care professional's job with the homemaker who has back pain. Just as for the worker in industrial rehabilitation, the homemaker must apply principles of body mechanics. A reproducible page of "Be Good to Your Back—Using Principles of Body Mechanics" is given in Appendix G.

Teaching your client how to stand, move, sit, lift, and carry will take into consideration the whole body, emotional status, and daily physical requirements. Evaluation will also consider clothing and footwear that may interfere with correct body mechanics.

The chair in which your client sits to work should meet the size and contour of his or her body, allowing the torso to rest on the proper muscles. Proper fit means the chair will adapt to the user's movement and maintain the S-curve, which is necessary to support the lumbar vertebrae and relieve pressure on the disks. Seat depth should be long enough to support the thighs, but not so long that it impedes circulation in the lower legs. Chair arms reduce stress on the back when rising or sitting down. The feet should be flat on the ground or supported by a footstool. A cushion, if used, should be firm but not hard. Soft cushions allow the body to sink and put pressure on the hip joints. If reaching forward creates tension or pain, a tilt function in the chair may be considered.

If more back support is needed, lumbar back supports are available from durable medical equipment dealers. **Manufacturers** include 69, 293, 388, 542. A contoured seat insert or cushion may

be indicated to provide additional ischial, sacral, and hip support as well as coccyx relief. **Manufacturers** include 186, 293, 388, 448, 541, 542. Cost is about $50 and up. For additional information on back and seat supports, please see Chapter 10 and Chapter 16.

Ergonomically designed office chairs for sitting at a table and draftsmen's stools for sitting at a standard height counter come with or without arms, height adjustment, and tilt tension and may be used in the kitchen. Prices range from about $60 and up from local stores or by mail. **Sources:** 211, 219, 225, 258.

An office chair that has a curved back and higher arm rests allows the upper extremities to relax while working (Figure 14-1).

When sitting on a stool or chair where the feet do not reach the ground, a footstool should always be used (Figure 14-2). An angled footstool helps reduce pressure on the back when sitting for long periods of time. Hips are flexed to relax tired back muscles. Stools are available from office supply and self-help firms. **Manufacturers** include 69. **Sources** include 383.

Teaching tips to help reduce stress on the back include the suggestion that when standing the client keep one foot on a low stool while preparing meals or doing other tasks. This reduces both the curve in and strain on the back.

A posture support belt may be recommended for use when doing any lifting or bending, such as when cleaning and doing laundry. The belt provides lower back and abdominal support, spreading the base of support over a larger area of the lower back, limits pelvic flexion, and creates awareness of proper body mechanics. **Sources:** 1, 21, 161. Cost is about $40 and up.

Your client should be taught to wheel rather than carry items, using carts and dollies. For the ambulatory patient, an upright vacuum is better for the back than a canister cleaner. When lifting is necessary, the load should always be within the client's pain limitations and done using correct body mechanics. When going to work or grocery shopping, check the type of bag your client uses. If the weight is carried forward or is too heavy, modifications may have to be made. A special back-saver bag shifts the load to lessen stress and pressure on the back, shoulders, and neck. Cost is about $20 and up from mail-order firms. **Sources:** 69, 171, 382. An alternate answer is a small backpack.

RESOURCES

Addresses for publishers, periodicals, and organizations are given in Section Four.

PUBLICATIONS

ACPA Member Workbook and Relaxation Tapes. Rocklin, CA: American Chronic Pain Association. Workbook for people without a chapter of ACPA nearby. Explains what chronic pain does and how one can regain control. Member Manual is $20 for members, $35 for health professionals. Tape #1 (Pain Relief and Breath Relaxation) and Tape #2 (Autogenic Relaxation and General Relaxation) are $10 each for members, $20 for health professionals.

American Occupational Therapy Association. (1996). *Practice Guidelines: Back*. Bethesda, MD: Author. $20 AOTA members, $25 non-member. Reference tool for health care facility managers, managed care organizations, third-party payers, OT practitioners. Defines evaluations, frequency, duration of treatment, billing codes explanation.

Back Owner's Manual: A Guide to Care of the Low Back. (1991). San Bruno, CA: Krames. Illustrated, shows evolution and causes of back pain, physician's role, body mechanics, and exercise program. Hand-out to patient with therapist's supervision. **Source:** 308.

Body Mechanics Resource Library. Gays Mills, WI: Country Technology. $79.95. 114 reproducible cards relate to patient's real-life activities, including housework, child care, and gardening. Kit includes principles of posture, positioning, movement, lifting, and two activity and pain checklists to assess activity level, define treatment plans, monitor and document progress. **Source:** 148.

Cailliet, R. (1988). *Low Back Pain Syndrome, Pain Series* (4th ed.). Philadelphia: F.A. Davis. $18.95. Functional anatomy, posture, diagnosis, therapeutic approach, prevention of recurrence, disk disease, and chronic pain.

Caudill, M. A. (1995). *Managing Pain Before It Manages You*. New York: Guilford. $18.95. Body-mind connections, relaxation and exercise techniques, coping and communication skills, setting goals, effects of nutrition and medication, ergonomics.

Diamond, S., et al. (1990). *Headache and Diet: Tyramine-Free Recipes*. Madison, CT: International Universities Press. $24.95. Mechanisms of a headache, types and treatments, diet-precipitated headaches and their causes. Outlines clinic's tyramine-restricted diet and menu, gives tyramine-free recipes. **Source:** 284.

Duckros, P. N., et al. (1995). *Taking Control of Your Headaches: How to Get the Treatment You Need*. New York: Guilford. $14.95. Team of headache experts gives step-by-step treatment program that takes into account all factors that can affect headaches. Allows clients to collaborate in their own treatment, reduce medication, and find the best professional care.

Hanson, R. W., & Gerber, K. E. (1992). *Coping with Chronic Pain: A Guide to Patient Self-Management*. New York: Guilford. $30. Differentiates between biomedical and biopsychological treatment approaches to pain, the client taking primary responsibility for change in the latter. Techniques include cognitive distraction, imagery, relaxation techniques, and biofeedback for use in inpatient and outpatient settings.

The Headache Handbook and *How to Talk to Your Doctor About Headaches*. Chicago: National Headache Foundation. Send $.55 postage on a self-addressed envelope.

McCormack, G. L. (1993). *Pain Management: Mindbody Techniques for Treating Chronic Pain Syndromes*. San Antonio, TX: Therapy Skill Builders. $60. Author feels that traditional pain management creates patient dependency. Stresses that chronic pain treatment must be holistic and multidisciplinary, directed at the whole person. It should allow the patient to develop self-empowerment techniques to take control of both his or her life and pain.

McIlwain, H. H., et al. (1994). *Winning with Chronic Pain: A Complete Program for Health and Well-Being*. Amherst, NY: Prometheus. $12.95. Signs of chronic pain, control and prevention techniques, specific exercises.

Mandell, P., et al. (1989). *Low Back Pain: A Historical and Contemporary Overview of the Occupational, Medical and Psychological Issues of Chronic Back Pain*. Thorofare, NJ: SLACK Inc. $40.

Melnik, M. S. (1994). *Understanding Your Back Injury*, #1117. Bethesda, MD: American Occupational Therapy Association. $4.50 members, $5.50 non-members plus handling. Consumer guide to use as workbook for monitoring progress; illustrates correct body mechanics in kitchen, bathroom, driving, sitting, lifting, and carrying. Space for therapist to add specific comments pertaining to individual's needs.

Pain Management Patient Education Manual. Frederick, MD: Aspen Reference Group, Aspen. $159. Ready-to-use patient teaching materials in large print: instructions, procedures, exercises, guidelines, charts, diagrams, and other tools. Also covers pain assessment, reimbursement, and communication tips. Annual supplements sent on approval for review.

Pain Management: Resource Guide. (1991). Bethesda, MD: American Occupational Therapy Association. #4140, $10 AOTA members, $20 non-members. Bibliographies, audiovisuals, resource personnel.

Saxon, S. V. (1991). *Pain Management Techniques for Older Adults*. Springfield, IL: Charles C. Thomas. $24.95.

Self Care for Your Back. Chicago: Patient Education, Encyclopedia Britannica Education Corp. Program includes two videocassettes (¾-inch U-Matic, ½-inch Beta, or ½-inch VHS), *Patient Take-home Booklet* and detailed *Instructor's Guide*. $450. Sent on approval for 15 days. **Source:** 188B.

Skevington, S. M. (1996). *Psychology of Pain*. New York: Wiley. Author presents pain in a social context, the biological mechanisms of pain, measurement of painful sensations, memories and images of pain, the consultation process, and coping mechanisms.

Stacy, C. B., et al. (1992). *Living with Persistent Pain*. Yonkers, NY: Consumers Reports® Books. $18.95. Disorders that cause pain, treatment options from surgery and physical therapy to psychological help and pain-clinic approach. Places to contact for assistance and additional information.

Tepperman, P. S., & Roberts, F. (1993). *Sit Up and Take Care of Your Back*. Toronto: ObusForme® Ltd. Booklet from inventor of ObusForme® back support and a physiatrist illustrate back protection techniques. Available in combined English/French edition. **Source:** 388.

Traines, M. A. (1995). *Occupational Therapy in the Relief of Foot Pain*, #1126. Bethesda, MD: American Occupational Therapy Association. $4.50 members, $5.50 non-members plus handling. Consumer guide shows how occupational therapists evaluate and treat foot pain, provides definitions and illustrations of common problems. Simple modifications that can help correct problems and may eliminate more expensive treatments. Teaches client how to adjust activity/work; gives techniques for properly fitting shoes and modifying footwear.

You and Your Back. (1977). South Deerfield, MA: Channing L. Bete. $1.25 per copy. Illustrated booklet discusses common problems, gives basic exercises, suggestions to avoid chronic strain and how to lift, and tips for working. **Source:** 114.

AUDIOVISUALS

Back Pain (Lower Back) at Time of Diagnosis™ . (1996). New York: Time Life Medical, Patient Education Media, Inc. Video program and work booklet. $25. 30-minute color VHS. Available from Info Vision. **Source:** 280.

Body Mechanics—Lower Back Care. 14-minute VHS video from Y13 Productions. Patient, physical and occupational therapists progress through bending, lifting, standing, and using simple aids on extended driving. Begins with refresher course on posture. $99 plus $6 handling and shipping charge. **Source:** 588.

For additional resources and examples of back supports and aids, see *Mealtime Manual*, Chapter 5.

CHAPTER

15

The Client with Loss of Sensation

Safety precautions are paramount when your client has loss of sensation, as in multiple sclerosis, diabetes, peripheral neuropathies, or spinal cord injury. The following items should be checked:

- Pipes under sink are insulated to protect legs from burns. Faucet handles do not heat up. If they do, an insulated cover for the pipes and a new faucet unit or turning handle is necessary.
- Handling of hot pans must be completely safe. If weakness is present with loss of sensation, teach the individual how to slide, rather than lift, pots. The range top should have an adjoining surface to which a pan may be slid. Insulated mats eliminate lifting. **Sources:** 306, 453.
- Potholders should always be used. Make sure they are heavy enough to completely protect the hands from the heat. Slip-on mitts are usually best and may also be used when handling frozen or very cold items.
- Pan handles and utensils used to mix at the stove must be of stay-cool materials or your patient reliable enough to always use mitts.
- A lapboard used with a wheelchair should have a raised edge to prevent spilling on lap.
- Hot pans or casseroles should be transported on a cart rather than carried if there is any weakness in the arms
- When holding or carrying a pan or utensil, your client must always watch movements. If not watching, grip may be released.
- When washing dishes, the client should learn to gauge water temperature. If the heat bothers hands, insulated latex gloves or delegation of the task to a dishwasher and other members of the family may be recommended. Textured palms on the gloves increase safety when holding dishes. See Chapter 17 in *Mealtime Manual*. Anti-scald devices for installation on sink and other faucets in the home are available through plumbing suppliers. When the unit recognizes a scalding temperature, the water flow is reduced to a trickle. Units like the pushbutton UltraFlo, see *Mealtime Manual*, preset water temperature.

Flameguard™ mitts are made of 100% cotton fabric treated to resist and retard fire, and they are water repellent (Figure 15-1). The wide mitt with extra-thick cotton padding protects hands from heat up to 400°F. Mitts come in 10.5-, 13-, 15-, 17-, and 24-inch lengths. They are available from restaurant suppliers and gourmet kitchen firms. A baker's pad with a wrist strap and steam barrier for use when poor coordination or weakness makes using a mitt difficult, a terry sleeve to protect the forearm, Teflon™ or silicone handle covers for metal cookware, and insulated rubber gloves are available from the same company. **Manufacturer:** 403B. Cost is about $11 to $16 for set of two mitts, depending on length, and about $6 for a set of handle covers. **Source:** 306.

The Hot Hand is a silicone, rubber-molded hand protector (Figure 15-2A,B). It was originally designed for safely gripping hot beakers, flasks, and bottles in a laboratory. The rubber-studded gripping surface holds a pan handle firmly, minimizing the chance of slipping when sliding to and from a stove. A person with loss of sensation may also use the Hot Hand to protect skin from contact with frozen or cold surfaces. Two end pockets fit fingers and thumbs of any size. **Sources:** 343, 347. Cost is about $11 per pair from laboratory, hospital, and self-help supply firms.

Cool Handles™ are rubber, heat-resistant covers (up to 500°F) that slip over the handles of pans (Figure 15-3). Dishwasher safe, they come in three sizes to fit most one- to 10-quart pots and pans. **Manufacturer:** 451B. Cost is about $3.50 to $5.50 each from housewares stores. **Source:** 347.

If a client is forgetful, you might consider Hot Pot Decals. Applied to any surface, these heat-sensitive decals change to expose the word "hot" when they reach 135°F. The warning vanishes when the item cools. A sheet of four stickers is $2 with a self-addressed, stamped envelope sent to the Burn Prevention Group. **Source:** 103.

When removing toast or hot biscuits and bagels from a toaster, wooden toast tongs should be used to prevent burning hands on either the toaster or the food. Cost is about $2 and up from variety stores and mail-order firms. **Manufacturers** include 20.

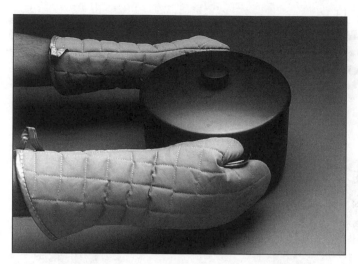

Figure 15-1. Flameguard™ mitts are treated to resist and retard fire, and are water repellent. (Photo courtesy of Parvin Manufacturing Co., Los Angeles, CA.)

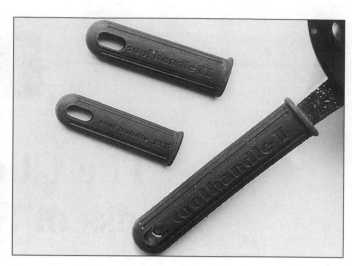

Figure 15-3. Cool Handles™ are rubber, heat-resistant covers (up to 500°F) that slip over the handles of pans. (Cool Handles™ by Rowoco®, Woodbridge, IL. Photo by J.K.)

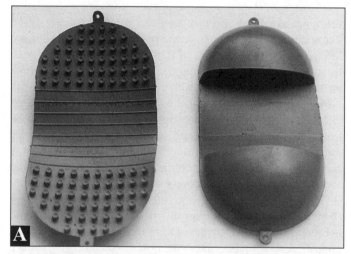

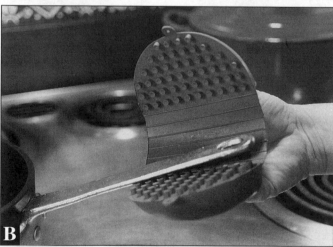

Figure 15-2A,B. The Hot Hand is a silicone, rubber-molded hand protector. (Hot Hand from Maddak, Inc., Pequannock, NJ. Photos by J.K.)

CHAPTER 16

The Client Who Uses a Wheelchair

Basic use of a wheelchair is taught to a patient while in the hospital or rehabilitation center. The chair should be prescribed with correct measurements, seating modifications, and accessories. It must then be checked carefully with the patient upon delivery that it meets all needs, including proper posture and mechanics. Before discharge, the individual should usually be able to handle the chair, including propelling and safely transferring to and from it.

This is the ideal. More often, a patient returns home with a poorly fitting chair or has not learned how to propel and transfer safely. Even remembering to lock the brakes is often ignored. It is even possible that difficulty in doing tasks related to home management stems from improper seating. If the chair is not satisfactory, the first step is to contact the hospital. Determine if the chair is rented or purchased and complain loudly. Request that the durable medical equipment (DME) representative meet with you and assess the chair. Deficiencies can be remedied with determination and are often funded by insurance or Medicare.

In some cases, the client who has not been hospitalized requires immediate use of a chair so he or she receives a temporary chair from a DME firm, loan closet, or other source. Then, it is your responsibility to refer the patient to a professional who is trained to evaluate wheelchair needs, usually an occupational or physical therapist. If this is not possible, the best answer is to work with the DME representative. Deficiencies in wheelchair prescription and fit can be remedied with the changes often funded by insurance or Medicare. Resources on wheelchair assessment are given at the end of this chapter.

Evaluation and prescription of a wheelchair must include several components:

- What type of seating system offers the best postural support for the patient? This takes into account weakness, deformities, and uncontrolled motions, such as athetosis of patients with cerebral palsy. Movement patterns of the upper extremities and trunk must be considered.
- What type of mobility base allows the patient to optimally function within his or her environment? Space requirements

and activities to be performed, as well as physical abilities of the client, must be assessed.

Proper seating in a wheelchair is important for several reasons: It maximizes trunk stability, prevents deformities and skin breakdown, allows efficient use of the arms, helps normalize tone in the body, facilitates normal movement patterns, and provides maximal comfort.

Proper seating position in a wheelchair normally is head over pelvis; lumbar section of back in slight extension; hips and knees both at a 90° angle; and feet in a neutral position, usually at 90° to the ankles (Figure 16-1). This position may be changed for several reasons, including hip flexion contractures, trunk instability that requires the person to sit with a slight posterior lean, and the need of positioning to reduce athetoid or other motions.

Wheelchairs have become more user friendly and adaptable. The standard, heavy regular or desk arm chair that may or may not fold for transport has largely been replaced with chairs that change with the consumer's needs.

The Invacare Ride-Lite wheelchair has removable desk arms, adjustable swingaway foot rests with calf supports, and a padded back and seat cushion (Figure 16-2). **Source:** 285.

The Swede Elite wheelchair of durable titanium weighs only 21 pounds (Figure 16-3). The upholstery conforms to the user's needs with a backrest that adjusts in contour as well as angle. Rear wheels may be set in 11 different positions for perfect balance; alternate wheel sizes are available for rear wheels and casters. **Source:** 191.

Manufacturers of wheelchairs include the following (addresses are given in Appendix E:

- Damaco Freedom on Wheels (158)—manual and powered.
- Etac USA, Inc. (191)—manual and powered.
- Everest & Jennings Inc. (192)—manual and powered.
- Freedom Designs, Inc. (214)—manual.
- Gendron, Inc. (220)—manual.
- Invacare Corp.® (285)—manual and powered.
- Iron Horse Productions, Inc. (287)—manual.
- Kendall-Futuro® @ Co. (303)—manual.

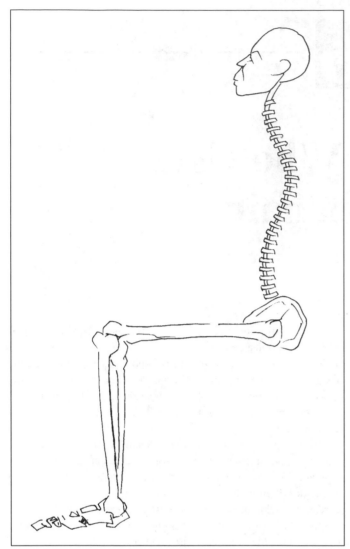

Figure 16-1. The proper seating position in a wheelchair is exhibited here. (Illustration by G.K.)

- Kushall of America (311)—manua.l
- La Bac (313)—manual and powered, with high backrests.
- Lumex® Inc. (336)—manual.
- Motion Designs, Inc. (370)—manual.
- Motovator (371)—manual.
- Permobil (408)—manual and powered.
- Production Research Corp. (425)—manual and powered.
- Redman, Inc. (436)—manua.
- Sunrise Medical (499)—Guardian and Quickee manual and powered, reclining power chair.
- Theradyne (517)—manual and powered.
- 21st Century Scientific, Inc. (54)—powered, including powered glider-type chair.
- Wheelchairs of Kansas, Inc. (570)—extra large chairs, manual and powered.

Assessing a client for a wheelchair requires careful measuring and testing. A client assessment form designed for use with modular type seat and back cushions is given in Appendix G. (Used with permission of Jay® Medical Ltd.) **Source:** 293.

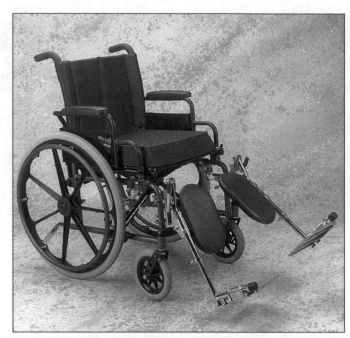

Figure 16-2. This Invacare Ride-Lite wheelchair has removable desk arms, adjustable swingaway foot rests with calf supports, and a padded back and seat cushion. (Photo courtesy of Invacare Corp., Elyria, OH.)

Correct positioning in the wheelchair begins with stabilization of the pelvis; then stabilization of the upper torso and shoulders. Third are the lower extremities and, finally, the head.

The diagnosis of each patient must be taken into account. With the spinal cord injured individual, for example, the paralyzed trunk tends to collapse under gravity, and there is a lack of sensation. Quadriplegics have limited movement of the upper extremities and may not be able to do push-ups or shift position in their chairs. Supports may be added to accommodate problems such as poor trunk balance, kyphosis, or hip flexion contractures.

The wheelchair seat should normally be solid. A soft-sling seat increases kyphosis and posterior pelvic tilt. This may lead to back pain, spinal deformities, and tissue trauma over extended periods of time. Solid seats or solid seat inserts are available from most distributors. Some come with drop hooks so that the seat may be lowered or adjustable brackets to allow tilting of the seat to attain the correct angle of hip flexion. If your client is sitting for long periods of time for homemaking or other activities, the seat needs a layer of foam or gel cushioning to avoid skin breakdown.

The Isch-Dish™ takes pressure off the ischials and tailbone by suspending them over an open contoured pocket (Figure 16-4). Body weight is distributed along the broader, more pressure-tolerant areas of the femurs. The open pocket of the wheelchair cushion ventilates away heat and perspiration to reduce skin breakdown and promote healing. The contoured pocket centers the pelvis and limits pelvic rotation, which discourages slouching. Construction includes high-impact plastic base, anti-slip mat, machine washable Cordura cover, and a variety of pocket sizes to fit individual users. A Dura-film covered foam core is available for incontinence protection. Weight is about two pounds; the Isch-Dish Thin for those who are at low risk of pressure sores or want a cushion for a hemi-

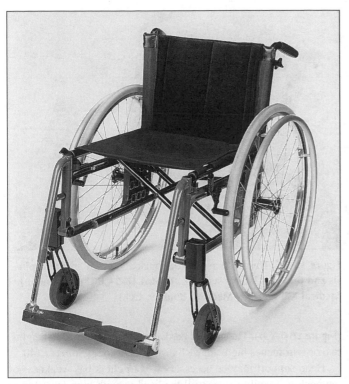

Figure 16-3. This Swede Elite wheelchair is made of durable titanium. (Photo courtesy of Etac USA, Inc., Waukesha, WI.)

chair or office or car seat is even lighter. Cost is about $165 and up depending on model. Call for name of DME dealer nearest you. **Manufacturer:** 186.

Therapists now specialize in the practice of therapeutic seating and positioning. If you have a complex problem and want to find a seating specialist in your area, contact RESNA. Address is in Appendix C.

A wheelchair back may be straight or contoured. Contoured inserts provide additional lateral support to the torso as well as comfort. Lateral trunk supports give stability when balance is poor, improve circulatory and respiratory function, and may be indicated for patients with spinal cord injuries, amyotrophic lateral sclerosis, advanced Parkinson's disease, or geriatric problems. A small, rolled towel or lumbar pad helps achieve proper alignment of the spine. It also helps the patient retract the shoulders and reduces head drop.

Solid seats and backs do not allow the posterior shifting required by a spinal cord injured patient for adequate stability and function. A contoured seat with a posterior tilt-in space gives the correct postural alignment. Patients with cerebral palsy, muscular dystrophy, and other neuromuscular diseases also function better with customized seating, sometimes with tilt and recline options. Maximal proximal support is essential for the individual with a weak, hypotonic trunk.

A variety of cushions and backrests are available in modular design for custom seating. A simulated seat may be designed, allowing the patient to interact with it before finalizing design. This gives an opportunity to modify the seating for best posture and movement patterns. Companies providing adaptive seating systems include Freedom Designs, Inc. (214), Jay® Medical Ltd.

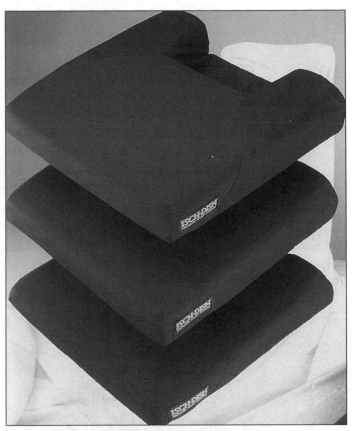

Figure 16-4. The Isch-Dish™ takes pressure off the ischials and tailbone by suspending them over an open contoured pocket. (Photo courtesy of Embracing Concepts, Inc., Rochester, NY.)

(293), Pin Dot Products (410), Signature 2000™ (475), and Varilite by Cascade Designs, Inc. (110).

A modular seat and back allow individualized positioning of the patient in a wheelchair (Figure 16-5A,B,C). The therapist is able to determine exact needs before ordering. The diagram shown of the modular seat shows separate forms that may be combined to create a customized modular seat. The custom modular back allows for severe kyphosis and provides lateral support. **Source:** 293.

Wheelchair cushions designed to provide pressure management, postural stability, and comfort also are **manufactured** by Action Products (17), Flofit (207), Iskra Med (288), Roho®, Crown Therapeutics, Inc. (448), Special Health Systems (487), Spenco Medical Corp. (489), SupraCor (502), and Ulti-Mate® (541). Wheelchair seating systems and cushions are normally covered by Medicare and insurance.

Full arms on wheelchairs provide support for the person with poor trunk balance and assist with transfers. If trunk balance is not a problem, desk arms are preferred, because they allow closer approach to lowered work surfaces. Make sure that patient's shoulders are not hunched, which is a sign of too-high wheelchair arms. Adjustable-height arms allow better positioning.

When an individual has poor lateral or trunk balance in the chair, additional support may be required. Having to rest one's arms on the arm rests reduces function and efficiency. Lateral supports leave the upper extremities free to perform tasks. **Sources** include 24, 25, 125, 214, 292, 395.

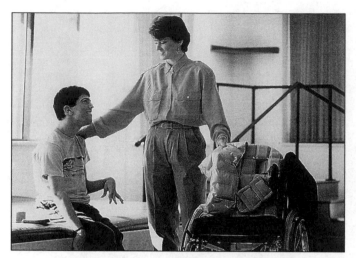

Figure 16-5A. A modular seat and back allow individualized positioning of the patient in a wheelchair.

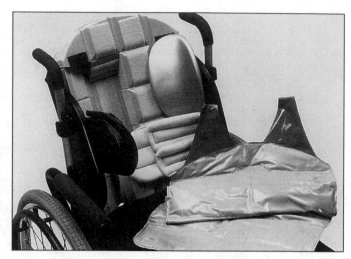

Figure 16-5C. This custom modular back allows for severe kyphosis and provides lateral support. (Photos 16-5A,B,C courtesy of J Medical Kid Kan, Jay Medical, Boulder, CO.)

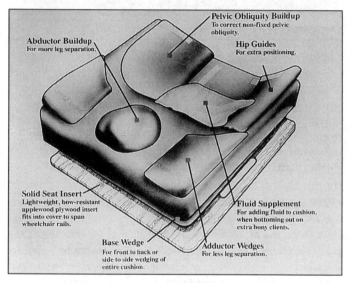

Figure 16-5B. This diagram of the modular seat shows separate forms that may be combined to create a customized modular seat.

A lateral support swings out of the way while transferring, then pivots back and locks into position to provide trunk support (Figure 16-6).

A pelvic stabilizer may be indicated for the patient with increased lower extremity tone and poor trunk balance. Hip or thigh inserts attached to the arm rests or seat of the wheelchair give lateral support. Abductors help position thighs. **Sources: 14, 25, 125, 205, 413.**

Leg rests come in a variety of styles, with or without padded calf supports, heel loops or straps, and adjustable foot rests. Leg rests should always be swingaway and removable. The patient who tends to have edema or swelling in the lower extremities may require elevating leg rests to be used when sitting for long periods of time.

Heel loops position paralyzed feet on foot rests and protect them from slipping off and being injured.

Extruded plastic heel loops are soft enough to crush down under pressure but "spring back" and do not lose form like nylon webbing

(Figure 16-7A,B). They do not harden in cold weather. Two heights, two or four inches high, are each eight inches long. **Source: 140.**

Head support may be necessary if your client has weakness of the neck or inability to control the head as with high level spinal cord injuries, spina bifida, muscular dystrophy, cerebral palsy, advanced Parkinson's disease, and amyotrophic lateral sclerosis. Head supports are **manufactured** by 24, 25, 125, 161, 214, 574. A padded collar head support is worn with a transparent chest support to help maintain good posture in the wheelchair (Figure 16-8).

The supportive positioning device has been designed for use with wheelchairs, geriatric chairs, and recliners (Figure 16-9). It slips over the backrest on chairs with 16- to 20-inch wide seats to provide lateral trunk support and reduce fatigue and restraints. Of fire retardant expanded vinyl with foam filled side bolsters, cost is about $130 and reimbursable under Medicare. **Source: 50.**

A lapboard is an essential accessory for functional use of a wheelchair in the kitchen and around the home. A variety of commercial styles are available through durable medical equipment firms. Some of these fasten with Velcro®; others have attachments that do not extend very far and do not support the outer edge of board very well. Attachments on any lapboard must be assessed for safety before being used as a carrying aid in the kitchen. The weight of a heavy pan on the outer edge of an improperly secured board can cause the board to slant downward. The client must also be able to remove and put on the lapboard independently. Exceptions might be the person with limitations in range of motion or marked weakness in the upper extremities, or the client with dementia to whom the board serves as a functional control.

When there is loss of sensation in the lower extremities, being able to see the position of one's legs is important (Figure 16-10). An acrylic lapboard allows a clear view and lets the wheelchair user more carefully propel himself or herself without hitting his or her feet. The high rim keeps items from rolling off, and in the kitchen helps prevent spills. **Sources: 14, 21, 25, 140, 198, 214, 383, 434, 461, 483.**

A lowered lapboard conserves energy when working. A plan for constructing one that may be adapted to fit upholstered full or

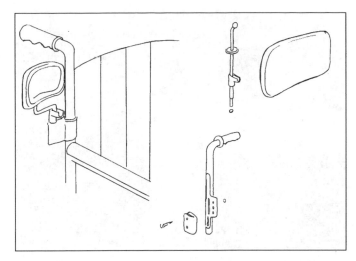

Figure 16-6. This lateral support swings out of the way while transferring, then pivots back and locks into position to provide trunk support. (Illustration by G.K.)

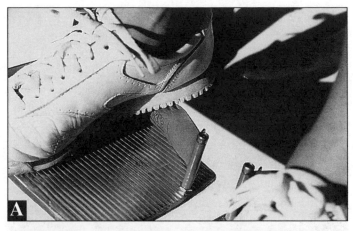

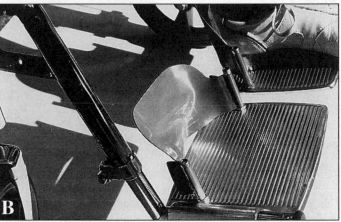

Figure 16-7A,B. These extruded plastic heel loops are soft enough to crush down under pressure but "spring back" and do not lose form like nylon webbing. (Photos courtesy of Consumer Care Products, Inc., Sheboygan, WI.)

desk arms is given in Appendix G. (Designed at the Howard A. Rusk Institute of Rehabilitation Medicine.) It is not appropriate for tubular arms.

Bracket sets for fabricating lapboards to meet your clients' needs are available through **sources** 25, 140, 518.

The Cam-Lever lock tray mounting hardware system is a lightweight method of securing a tray to the arms of a wheelchair or other mobility aid (Figure 16-11). The eight sub-components fit on all trays with 5/16-inch slot-outs or may be used with a universal mounting pad for custom-made trays lacking slot-cuts. **Source:** 140.

Wheelchair gloves or cuffs of leather and mesh with Neoprene palmar pads and Velcro® closures help protect the palms from burns and blisters when the person using the wheelchair is propelling extended distances or outdoors with the chair. A variety of gloves, including leather or mesh and leather, with Neoprene pads and Velcro® closures are available from self-help and rehabilitation supply firms. **Manufacturers** include 244, 489. Cost is about $12 per pair and up. **Sources:** 1, 11, 343, 383, 461, 489.

Quad cuffs by Harness Designs, Inc., are made for extended wheelchair propulsion (Figure 16-12). They have a fingerless, thumb-loop design that is easy to put on and take off. The double-stitched, rubber push surface provides good friction. Although designed for heavy use, these gloves might be helpful for the person who finds wheeling a chair hard on sensitive palms. **Source:** 244.

If your client lives in a residence where doors are narrow or very tight for passing through in a wheelchair, a narrowing device may be installed on some wheelchairs that have permanent arms. **Source:** 220.

POWERED CHAIRS

The individual with severe loss of upper extremity strength, arthritis, or a chronically low energy level may wish to consider a powered chair. This commitment to an expensive vehicle requires careful evaluation of total design, including the fitting factors dis-

cussed earlier plus consideration of different types of controls. Powered chairs are sometimes funded by agencies and insurance companies, especially if the patient is going to school, is employed, or is a full-time homemaker raising a family. Modifications in the home and in transporting the client must be evaluated. Because powered chairs are heavy, the client may need ramps or a lift to enter and leave a residence or other building. Transporting the person in a powered chair is easier with van transport or wheelchair accessible buses. See Chapter 30.

An alternative to a powered wheelchair is a "portable" power unit that attaches to the chair. If only required for longer distances, it may be removed to allow the patient to increase manual power within the home, thus maintaining or even increasing strength in the upper extremities. On some units, a patient with weak upper extremities will need assistance to lift off the batteries and rear unit because of weight and the fact that the unit is attached to the back of the wheelchair, or he or she must propel the manual chair with the power unit still attached. See *Mealtime Manual*, Chapter 7.

The Roll-Aid does not need to be lifted on and off a wheelchair and adapts to fit most standard collapsible wheelchairs (Figure 16-13A,B). The person rolls over the unit until the attachment system locks onto the chair, then it is ready to drive away under power. To return to manual control, a release cord is pulled, and the individ-

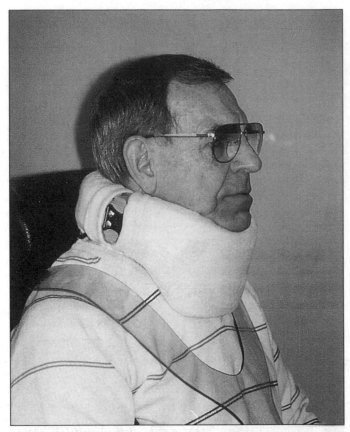

Figure 16-8. This padded collar head support is worn with a transparent chest support to help maintain good posture in the wheelchair. (Photo courtesy of Danmar Products, Inc., Ann Arbor, MI.)

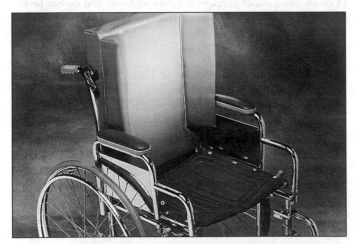

Figure 16-9. This supportive positioning device is designed for use with wheelchairs, geriatric chairs, and recliners. (Photo courtesy of Anna-Dote™, Inc., West Middlesex, PA.)

ual rolls away from the unit. If purchasing a new wheelchair, a straight bar frame is recommended because it affords increased ground clearance with the Roll-Aid attached. The unit folds to fit in most car trunks. The heaviest section weighs 35 pounds. Cost is about $2000 and up. **Source:** 493.

Two other **manufacturers** of units that convert a manual to a powered chair are Damaco (158), shown in *Mealtime Manual,*

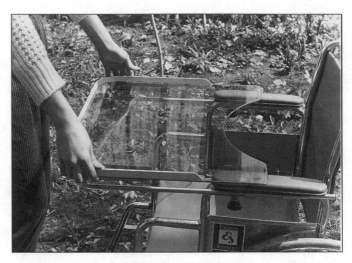

Figure 16-10. An acrylic lapboard allows a clear view and lets the wheelchair user more carefully propel himself or herself without hitting his or her feet. (Photo courtesy of Consumer Care Products, Inc., Sheboygan, WI.)

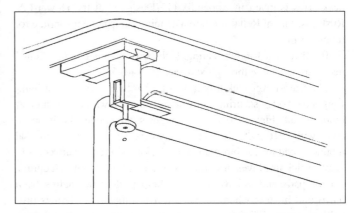

Figure 16-11. The Cam-Lever lock tray mounting hardware system is a lightweight method of securing a tray to the arms of a wheelchair or other mobility aid. (Cam-Lever Lock Tray Mounting Hardware from Consumer Care Products, Inc., Sheboygan, WI. Illustration by G.K.)

Chapter 7, and Gendron (220), which makes Solo II, a power unit that can replace the large rear wheels of most manual wheelchairs.

One of the most common problems that arises with a powered wheelchair or scooter is difficulty in maintaining battery charges. The best answer when problems arise is to call a DME representative, unless you or a member of the patient's family have technical knowledge. A reference listed at the end of this chapter gives basic background on understanding and using wheelchair batteries.

ELECTRIC SCOOTERS

If endurance, trunk balance, and upper extremity strength and control are adequate, an electric scooter may be a lighter weight, less expensive, powered alternative. Selecting to use a scooter, however, requires careful evaluation to determine the appropriateness for the specific client. If trunk balance is poor and endurance limited, the scooter will require a customized seat with solid arms to ensure safety. If hand function and upper extremity range of motion are limited, a joystick control may be indicated. If cognition or vision is poor, then "license" to drive a scooter may be limited. If lower extremities are weak, transfer training to and from the scooter will be necessary. With all these caveats, scooters are popular solutions that increase independence and social interaction. Optional features include seating that swivels and locks, power seat lift options, baskets, and joystick alternates.

Articles evaluating scooters appear frequently in magazines like *New Mobility, Team Rehab,* and *Accent on Living*. Evaluation must take into consideration the factors for wheelchairs discussed earlier as well as the size of the base of the scooter in relation to floor space and layout of the client's residence. Some scooters require more turning space than a narrow hall may allow. Scooters are Medicare-approved durable medical equipment for which clients can apply for reimbursement with the Medicare Certificate of Medical Necessity. See sample in Appendix G. Form must be completed by a specialist in neurology, orthopedics, rheumatology, or physical medicine.

Clients may be able to use a compact electric scooter in their homes (Figure 16-14). The swivel seat allows the patient to turn toward the counter and dishwasher, or swivel to play the piano when kitchen cleanup is done. Removable accessory baskets carry groceries, laundry, and other items. **Source:** 47.

The design of most scooter seats may not be safe for the person with poor trunk balance and increasing spasticity, as with multiple sclerosis. More manufacturers of scooters have recognized this need, especially for people with multiple sclerosis and muscular dystrophy, so they are including customized seating possibilities.

Manufacturers of electric scooters include the following:
- Amigo Mobility International (47)—Adapt-a-Seat frame permits building of customized seat with a variety of cushions.
- Bruno Independent Living Aids (100)—customized seating available.
- Electric Mobility (183)—adjustable adaptive seating frame available.
- Optiway Technology, Inc. (392)—unit with multiple seat adjustments, i.e., adjustable seat height, seat depth, back angle, and back height.
- Ortho-Kinetics, Inc. (394).
- Pride Health Care, Inc. (420).

When selecting a table for wheelchair or scooter accessibility, the legs or supports must allow the foot rests and chair to roll under (Figure 16-15). Wheelchair arms vary slightly in height but are usually about 29½ to 30 inches. **Manufacturers** of tables to meet wheelchair specifications include 294B, 484.

Accessible, ergonomically designed work stations for art or computer work may be adapted for wheelchair kitchen use. Height is adjustable, foot space is open for the chair, and extra storage units may be added where needed. The cost of a table with an oak plastic laminated top and adjustable height from 23¾ to 34¾ inches is about $490 and up, depending on size and features. Check with local office supply stores, and make sure that surfaces are heat-, water-, and stain-proof. See Chapter 25.

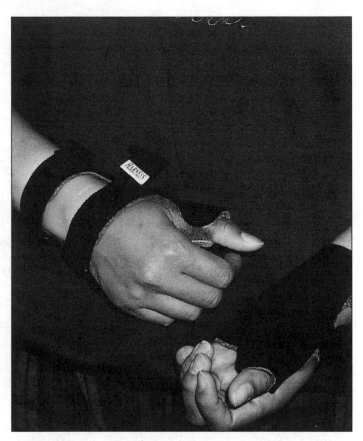

Figure 16-12. These Quad cuffs are made for extended wheelchair propulsion. (Gloves by Harness Design, Inc., Champaign, IL. Photo by J.K.)

STANDING AIDS

More frequently, clients who use wheelchairs are asking about units that will allow them to stand in the kitchen or elsewhere to work, to improve circulation and muscle tone, or to increase social interaction (Figure 16-16A,B,C,D). Wheelchair standing units, such as the Levo from Kushall, 311; the Stand-Aid, 493; and the Moto-Stand (28) allow this. Once standing, the user can move from place to place in the kitchen, home, school, workplace, or elsewhere. When standing, the client can reach cabinets and items for which the home might otherwise have to be modified. With the Moto-Stand there is a "lean down" feature that allows the person to lower to the floor, pick up items, or even pat the dog. Physical benefits include improved circulation, reduction of pressure ulcers, muscular spasms, contractures, osteoporosis, as well as bladder and intestinal therapy. The standing unit also reduces stress on caregivers who find it difficult to lift a client as heavy or heavier than themselves. Most units allow the user to stand and be supported by back panel and sling if needed, with a single switch. Units are adjustable for the client's height.

Standing equipment must be evaluated carefully with both the client's physician and physical and/or occupational therapist in terms of the client's muscle power, overall physical condition, and ability to use upper extremities as efficiently while standing as when supported in a wheelchair. Most systems fold to fit in an automobile trunk. Insurance companies will cover standing

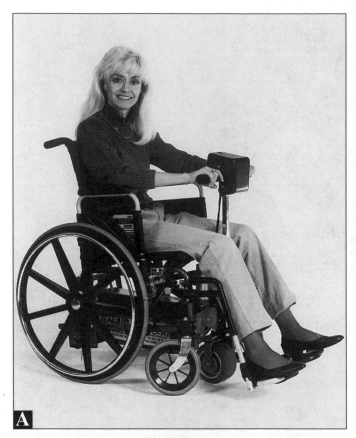

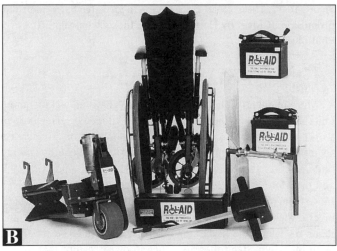

Figure 16-13A,B. The Roll-Aid does not need to be lifted on and off a wheelchair and adapts to fit most standard collapsible wheelchairs. The unit folds to fit in most car trunks. (Photos courtesy of Stand Aid of Iowa, Inc., Sheldon, IA.)

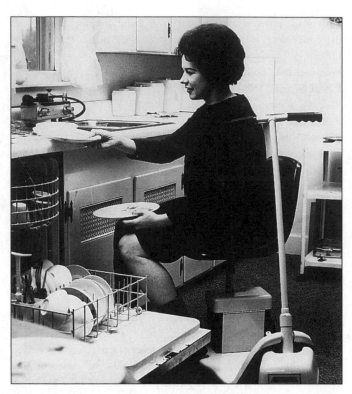

Figure 16-14. This woman uses a compact electric scooter within her home. (Photo courtesy of Amigo® Mobility International, Inc., Bridgeport, MI.)

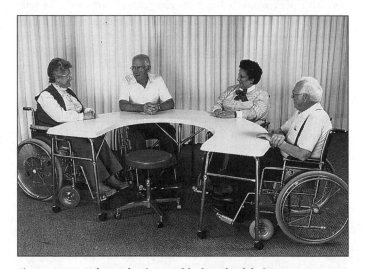

Figure 16-15. When selecting a table for wheelchair or scooter accessibility, the legs or supports must allow the foot rests and chair to roll under. (Photo of AdjusTables™ courtesy of Space Tables, Inc., Minneapolis, MN.)

systems only if considered a medical necessity and will consider the preventive maintenance of good circulation and skin condition versus the costs of hospitalization when there is skin breakdown. Cost for manual units is about $4600 and up, plus accessories or modifications; for electric $7000 and up. For further information, write sources given above. A free video showing a motorized standing unit in use is available from 493. Also see Chapter 2.

RESOURCES

Addresses for publishers, periodicals, and organizations are given in Section Four.

PUBLICATIONS

Bergen, A. F., et al. (1992). *Positioning for Function: Wheelchairs and Other Assistive Technologies: Strategies for*

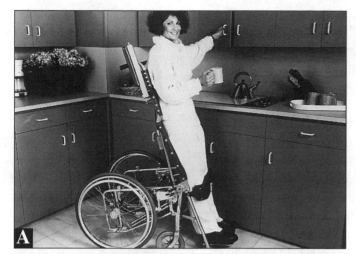

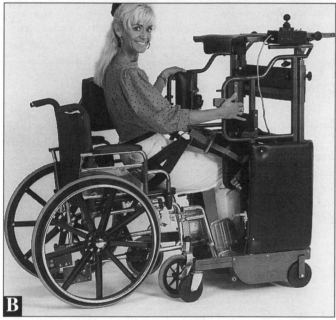

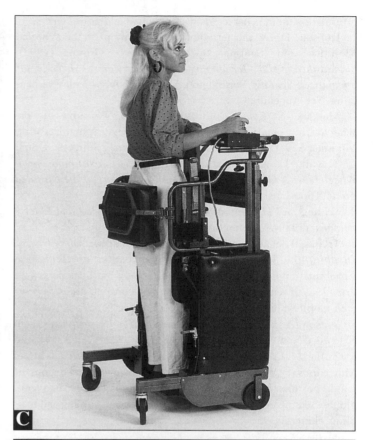

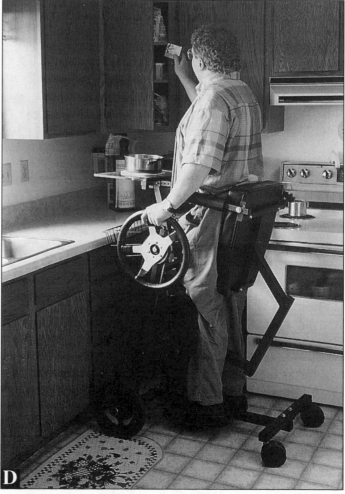

Figure 16-16A,B,C,D. Clients who use wheelchairs are frequently asking about units that will allow them to stand in the kitchen or elsewhere to work, to improve circulation and muscle tone, or to increase social interaction. Wheelchair standing units, such as (A) the Levo from Kuschall, 311; (B,C) the Stand Aid, 493; and (D) the Moto-Stand (28) allow this. (Figure 16-16A courtesy of Kuschall USA, Camarillo, CA.; Figure 16-16B,C courtesy of Stand Aid of Iowa, Inc., Sheldon, IA.; Figure 16-16D: Moto-Stand from The Advanced Technology Corp., Kansas City, MO.; photo courtesy of AliMed®, Inc., Dedham, MA.)

Assessment and Intervention. White Plains, NY: Valhalla Rehabilitation Pub., Ltd. $49.95 plus $3.50 handling. Seating, wheeled mobility, switches, augmentative communication devices, construction plans, and case studies.

Cheever, R., & Garee, B. (Eds.). (1987). *Wheelchair Batteries.* Bloomington, IL: Accent. $3.50. Selecting, using, and recharging batteries. **Source:** 8.

A Guide to Wheelchair Selection: How to Use the ANSURES-NA Wheelchair Standards to Buy a Wheelchair. Washington, DC: Paralyzed Veterans of America. $9.50. 53-page guide provides information on the characteristics of manual and power chairs.

Hobson, D., & the terminology task group of the Wheeled Mobility and Seating Special Interest Group. (1992). *Standardization of Terminology and Descriptive Methods for Specialized Seating.* Washington, DC: RESNA. $12 plus $2 handling. See Appendix C.

Maddox, S. *Spinal Network: the Total Resource for the Wheelchair Community* (2nd ed.). Malibu, CA: Spinal Network, Miramar. $29.95 wire-bound, $27.95 paperback. **Sources:** 8, 363.

Mayall, J., & Desharnais, G. (1995). *Positioning in a Wheelchair: A Guide for Professional Caregivers of the Disabled Adult.* Thorofare, NJ: SLACK Inc. $25.

Seating and Mobility Needs of Severely Disabled and Elderly Persons. (1989). Washington, DC: RESNA. $5.

Trefler, E., et al. *Seating and Mobility for Persons with Physical Disabilities.* San Antonio, TX: University of Tennessee Rehabilitation Engineering Program, Therapy Skill Builders. $39. Principles of seating for clients of all ages, concentrations on powered mobility, diagnosis-specific information.

Wilson, A. B., Jr. (1992). *Wheelchairs: A Prescription Guide* (2nd ed.). New York: Demos. $19.95.

Zollars, J.A. *Special Seating: An Illustrated Guide.* Minneapolis: Otto Bock. More than 300 original illustrations of sitting postures, assessment procedures, simulation teaching techniques, seating component options. $64 plus $7 shipping and handling. **Source:** 395.

PERIODICALS

New Mobility. Address under Periodicals in *Mealtime Manual.*

Pin Dot News. Free subscription from Pin Dot Products offers in-depth information on seating problems. The company also offers seating seminars. **Source:** 410.

Spinal Network Extra. Quarterly magazine for the wheelchair community. Address under Periodicals in *Mealtime Manual.*

Team Rehab. Detailed articles on wheelchair seating and adaptations. Free to professionals.

AUDIOVISUALS

Advanced Wheelchair Skills. 10-minute video from Y13 Productions. Correct techniques for getting off the ground, car transfers, negotiating curbs. $99 plus $6 handling fee. **Source:** 588.

Trefler, E. *Decision-Making Therapeutic Guidelines for Seating and Positioning* and *Matching Client Needs with Specialized Seating Options*; Norgaard, M. *Matching Client Needs with Powered Mobility*; and Silverman, M. *Eclectic Approach to Seating.* Cost is $25 per tape, or set of four for $90 from Pin Dot Products. **Source:** 410.

Your Guide to Buckles and Belts. Styles of belts for wheelchairs, how to select, mounting methods, innovations. Also includes gait belts. $39.95 from Thompson Video Productions. **Source:** 525.

CONTINUING EDUCATION

Courses on wheelchair fitting for health care professionals and medical equipment dealers are given by several manufacturers. Etac USA, Inc. (191) offers two types of courses: a one-day course for therapists and a three-day wheelchair fitting certification course for dealers and therapists. Jay Medical Ltd. (293) offers a wheelchair fitting course. Pin Dot Products (410) has a three-day course on providing wheelchair seating for the physically challenged. For further information, contact the companies directly.

The Client Who Has Chronic Obstructive Pulmonary Disease

Chronic obstructive pulmonary disease (COPD) is characterized by pulmonary insufficiency due to a limited airflow. Two main diseases are pulmonary emphysema and chronic bronchitis. Cystic fibrosis is a third respiratory disease, affecting the life activities and expectancy of its victims, who are often children. Others include bronchiectasis and interstitial lung disease. There are well over 15 million Americans who suffer from asthma but can learn to live safely with proper treatment and management. Additional millions suffer from allergic rhinitis, which may be continual or seasonal, and may be dangerous when combined with chronic lung diseases.

Treatment of a client with lung disease should be multidisciplinary with the dual goals to improve life and to reduce periods of inactivity or hospitalization by:

- Decreasing respiratory symptoms and complications.
- Encouraging self-management and control of the condition.
- Increasing physical stamina and performance through graded exercise done on a regular basis.
- Improving emotional well-being and reducing stress.
- Maintaining optimal levels of health through good nutrition, a healthy environment, and exercise.

COPD is a progressive illness. The patient fatigues quickly with physical exertion. This increases to the point where simple tasks of daily living may have to be adjusted to the minimal level of activity. The client may be on intermittent or continual oxygen, and even with this have periods of exacerbation requiring hospitalization. Chapter 8 in *Mealtime Manual* details suggestions that may be incorporated into a COPD client's treatment program.

Conserving energy is paramount when working with the COPD client. The principles for working with a low-energy patient apply here. See Chapter 19. Setting priorities for basic tasks is necessary, including eating, personal hygiene, and self-grooming.

Shortness of breath and fatigue may interfere with the patient's ability to eat a balanced diet. The amounts and type, as well as the timing, of meals must be planned into a schedule acceptable to the individuals. A dietician associated with a pulmonary rehabilitation program can provide counseling on nutrition and practical suggestions for shopping and methods of preparing food and eating. Diet plans with several small meals a day, nutritional supplements, or enriched foods may be developed when fatigue, shortness of breath, or poor appetite interfere with good nutrition.

Heat in a room, weather temperature, air pressure, and personal stress all contribute to increased difficulty in breathing. Relaxation techniques as described in Chapter 7 are a good way to start a session. Therapy and nursing sessions should be coordinated. The COPD patient should receive postural drainage and other treatments as well as help with daily dressing and bathing well enough in advance of a home management or therapy session to be rested.

A patient with COPD may also have asthma or allergies that contribute to respiratory distress on a periodic or continual basis. When making a home assessment, the therapist notes general cleanliness as well as air quality. Patients should be cautioned to keep windows closed so pollen does not enter the house during periods when the pollen count is high and, when possible and needed, to use air conditioning, which filters incoming air. Air-filtration systems to reduce pollen and dust in the air may be especially helpful for people with asthma and allergic rhinitis. Discuss units with a local durable medical equipment supplier or contact the American Lung Association or the Asthma and Allergy Foundation of America. **Manufacturers** of air-filtration systems include 381. Low-pile carpets and vacuum cleaners that have maximal sealing, suction, and high-efficiency particulate air (HEPA) filtration are recommended. **Manufacturers** of vacuums with these features include 359, 393. Individuals who have asthma and allergic rhinitis may be able to do housecleaning with more ease if they wear a particle mask, which is available from hardware stores and some pharmacies. The patient with moderate to severe respiratory distress should not remain in a room while it is being cleaned.

When home maintenance or modifications are planned, the client will often require an alternate living situation while activities like carpentry or painting are occurring. The client who is using continual oxygen must not cook with a gas stove because of the danger of combustion. Studies of women with allergies using gas stoves, moreover, have found an increase in wheezing and breathing problems. The suspected culprit is nitrogen dioxide, a pollutant emitted by gas burners. In the research, men did not have this link but still must switch to electric cooking and avoid barbecue grills if using oxygen.

For all cooking, the kitchen area should be well-ventilated, with additional fans added if needed. The client should be taught to rest and sit in a cooler part of the kitchen while food is simmering, rather than hovering over a burner. When warm and non-humid weather allows, kitchen windows may be kept open. A microwave oven and training in its use provide an excellent alternative to cooking with heat. The microwave oven may be placed in a position that eliminates bending. It also allows the use of lightweight dishes and reduces energy expenditure in cleaning up.

When traveling by automobile, special situations may affect the client with COPD or asthma. The individual and the family must be aware of the increased difficulty in breathing when there is inadequate ventilation in the car or when the car becomes overheated while sitting, as when someone leaves the client in a parked car and goes on an errand that takes longer than expected. Again, during high pollen count periods, air should be allowed to filter into the car through the ventilating or air conditioning system. They also should be aware of the possible danger of an airbag, which can stifle breathing when suddenly inflated in case of an accident. A small, portable, battery-powered fan may be carried for times when still, humid air increases breathing difficulty. See fan in *Mealtime Manual*, Chapter 8.

The therapist working with clients with COPD should consult with the respiratory therapist when questions arise about equipment and patient needs. Lighter weight oxygen units, valves that conserve oxygen so smaller tanks can be used for a longer period of time, and portable oxygen concentrators for travel may offer increased possibilities and freedom to your patients.

An oximeter will allow monitoring of the oxygen level in the blood of a patient with COPD on a periodic basis. It is recommended that an oximeter not be left with the patient. As levels fluctuate markedly, an individual who has his own oximeter, rather than being reassured, tends to check more and more frequently and as a result becomes increasingly stressed. One manufacturer of respiratory care equipment is LifeCare, **source** 322.

RESOURCES

Addresses for publishers, periodicals, and organizations are given in Section Four.

PUBLICATIONS

American Academy of Allergy Asthma and Immunology. Publications include *Making the Most of Your Next Doctor Visit*, which assists patients in tracking medications, symptoms, and situations that trigger attacks, includes chart to record episodes over a 4-week period.

American Allergy Association.

The American Lung Association distributes a well-illustrated, free booklet, *Help Yourself to Better Breathing*, for handing out to patients, as well as other pamphlets on COPD.

Asthma and Allergy Foundation of America.

Astry, D. (Director). (1996). *The Health House Workbook*. Minneapolis: American Lung Association, Minneapolis Affiliate. Homeowner's manual/journal when planning a house or remodeling project with a healthier indoor environment. Design considerations, air pollution primer, mechanical systems, filtration, heating systems, maintenance tips, handling of cleaning and waste.

Bach, J. R. (1996). *Pulmonary Rehabilitation: The Obstructive and Paralytic Conditions*. Philadelphia: Hanley & Belfus. $69.95. Details rehabilitation for patients with COPD and for paralytic syndromes.

Davis, M., et al. (1995). *The Relaxation and Stress Reduction Workbook* (4th ed.). Oakland, CA: New Harbinger. Section on breathing for health and relaxation that may be adapted to client's treatment program.

Haas, F., & Sheila S. (1990). *The Chronic Bronchitis and Emphysema Handbook*. New York: Wiley. $14.95. Helps patient to understand disease and lead a full, more productive life. Explains COPD and the respiratory system, treatment and therapy, gives techniques for life, work, and travel, and further resources from support groups and books to institutions specializing in lung disease treatment.

Hannaway, P. J. (1994). *The Asthma Self-Help Book* (2nd rev. ed.). Salem, MA: Lighthouse Press. $13.95 plus $2 handling. Technical aspects, management between the family, the environment, and physician.

Lankow, E. (1917, republished). *How to Breathe Right*. Pomeroy, WA: Health Research. Series of breathing exericese.

Morris, K., & Hodgkin, J. E. (1996). *Pulmonary Rehabilitation Program Administration and Patient Education Manual*. Frederick, MD: Aspen. $129. Total approach including administration forms, lesson plans, and reproducible patient education materials.

National Heart, Lung, and Blood Institute. Government sponsor of research in respiratory diseases.

National Jewish Center for Immunology and Respiratory Diseases. Publications for people with COPD. Request brochure.

Prevention Magazine Editors. (1983). *The Allergy Self-Help Book*. Emmaus, PA: Rodale. $21.95.

Shayevitz, M. B., & Burton R. (1985). *Living Well with Emphysema and Bronchitis: A Handbook for Everyone with COPD*. New York: Bantam Doubleday Dell. $15.95.

Simpson, C. (1995). *Coping with Asthma*. New York: Rosen. $15.95. Teenagers learn that with proper treatment asthma is completely manageable.

Weiss, J. H. (1994). *Breathe Easy! Young People's Guide to Asthma*. New York: Magination Press, Brunner/Mazel. $10.

PERIODICALS

American Journal of Respiratory and Critical Care Medicine. American Lung Association.

American Review of Respiratory Diseases. American Thoracic Society.

Batting the Breeze. Seminole, FL: Emphysema Anonymous, Inc.

Second Wind. Torrance, CA: Little Company of Mary Hospital.

New Directions. National Jewish Center for Immunology and Respiratory Medicine.

The Pulmonary Paper. For health care professionals.

The Client with Complete or Partial Loss of Vision

Aids and techniques to help the client with loss of vision are discussed in *Mealtime Manual*, Chapter 9.

When working with the patient with loss of vision, the greatest tool for the health care professional is awareness of the services available for those with loss of or low vision. More than 500 agencies for the blind are located in major U.S. cities. The first place to check is your State Society for the Blind. It may have trained staff who will come to the home and do an evaluation and training program with your patient.

Training for working with people who are blind or have severe loss of vision is part of many health care professionals' programs (Figure 18-1). It is an inservice seminar you might develop for the staff at your agency or institution as a future service to patients.

The American Foundation for the Blind distributes publications for the blind. The Lighthouse Inc. distributes aids and publications; its catalog on equipment is a valuable resource. **Source:** 326. The National Federation of the Blind, which is listed in Appendix C, also has a catalog listing a variety of homemaking and other aids. The Talking Book program from the Library of Congress includes taped cookbooks as well as books on self-care and how to manage without sight.

More than 11 million people in the United States do not see well enough to function normally without the use of low-vision aids. They are not blind, but require assistance and comprise the second largest group of people with disabilities in our country. The National Association for the Visually Handicapped deals with the partially sighted, providing education, equipment, and visual aids information. It distributes large-print and recorded books, organizes self-help and support groups, and has a lending library.

Other groups that provide services and distribute materials to people with loss of vision include the following. Addresses are given in Appendix C, in Section II unless otherwise noted.
- American Academy of Ophthalmology.
- American Brotherhood for the Blind.
- American Council of the Blind, Inc.
- American Diabetes Association.

- American Ophthalmological Society.
- American Optometric Association.
- American Printing House for the Blind.
- Association for Macular Diseases, Inc.
- Association for Radio Reading Services.
- Better Vision Institute.
- Blind Rehabilitation Programs of the Veterans Administration.
- Blinded Veterans Association.
- Bureau for Blind and Visually Handicapped, Rehabilitation Services Administration, Department of Education.
- Gladys E. Loeb Foundation.
- The Lighthouse National Center for Vision and Aging.
- Lions Club International.
- National Association for Visually Handicapped.
- National Braille Association, Inc.
- National Diabetes Information Clearinghouse.
- National Eye Care Project.
- National Eye Institute—Scientific Reporting Section.
- National Federation of the Blind.
- National Library Services for the Blind and Physically Handicapped. Section 1.
- National Society to Prevent Blindness.
- Research to Prevent Blindness, Inc.

These are only a sample of agencies and organizations serving individuals with visual loss. Check references in your library for other local services, such as sight-saver bills from the utility company or extra large checks from the bank.

KITCHEN ORGANIZATION AND PLANNING

An organized kitchen promotes safety and efficiency while working. Once the floor plan is set up and learned by the patient, furniture or other things should not be moved around without the client's knowledge and agreement. Principles include the following:

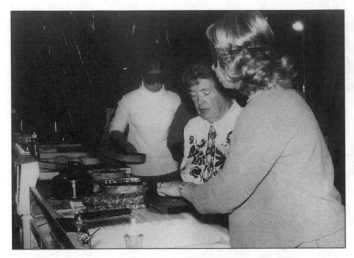

Figure 18-1. Training for working with people who are blind or have severe loss of vision is part of many health care professionals' programs. (Photo courtesy of ACTION®, Washington, DC.)

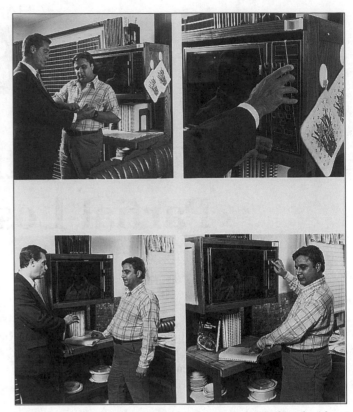

Figure 18-3. The Braille overlay for the controls combined with a Braille cookbook make this man an independent "novice" chef. (Photo courtesy of Whirlpool® Corp., Benton Harbor, MI.)

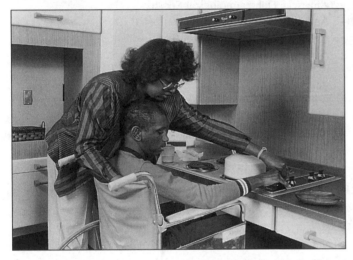

Figure 18-2. The personal management instructor at this facility for the multi-handicapped blind teaches use of an electric cooktop. (Photo, the Conklin Center, Madison, FL., courtesy of Whirlpool® Corp., Benton Harbor, MI.)

- Eliminate all protuberances that could be bumped into, tripped on, or knocked over. This includes cupboard doors, knick-knacks on shelves, and small scatter rugs.
- If there is a tendency to splash water on the floor while at the sink, a flat-edged rubber floor mat prevents skidding.
- Set up a specific cooking area where the homemaker is in close physical contact with basic utensils and foods.
- Plan a specific place for each tool, eliminating those not used, and reinforce to the family as well as the patient the importance of returning them to the right place.
- Use drawer dividers as points of reference when looking for a tool.
- Check knife storage, and add a coil- or slot-type safety holder if needed.
- In cupboards, add dividers so one pot or pan at a time may be

retrieved. For foodstuffs, use tiered or helper shelves so foods do not have to be stacked.
- Use pull-out shelves to bring items within reach.
- If cupboard doors could cause an accident, encourage patient to remove them and if desired replace with cloth or bamboo curtains.
- Adapt stove controls, if necessary, with tactile markers to locate temperature settings. Electric stoves are preferred to gas; microwaves are safest.
- If matches must be used, teach the patient to use long matches and/or to light them before turning on the gas, then to douse them in water. Emphasize and re-emphasize the need to wear short or tight sleeves, to keep arms away from flame, and to never reach over a pan that is cooking.

Setting temperature controls is an essential task for independent meal preparation (Figure 18-2). Teaching setting as though the knob were a clock, and adding tactile marks to the stove and dial simplifies the operation for people with loss of vision.

A Braille overlay for microwave oven controls combined with a Braille cookbook can make a blind patient an independent "novice" chef (Figure 18-3).

A guard ring for electric range tops keeps pots in place and prevents accidents (Figure 18-4). It is good for people with loss of vision, incoordination, or use of one hand. Three spring tabs fit over the edge of the present ring. **Sources:** Gladys E. Loeb Foundation, 347.

Large, bold numbers on contemporary kitchen equipment aid the person with limited vision (Figure 18-5). Bright colors are eas-

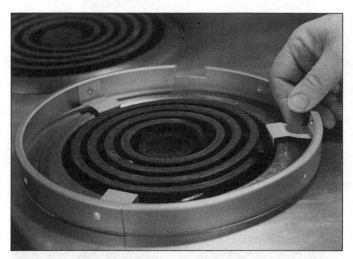

Figure 18-4. This guard ring for electric range tops keeps pots in place and prevents accidents. (Guard ring from the Gladys E. Loeb Foundation, Inc., Silver Spring, MD. Photo by J.K.)

ier to locate in a kitchen cabinet.

A no-spill chopping board folds in the middle to form a channel (Figure 18-6). This lets the person with loss of vision or limited use of hands guide the food into a dish or pan. Of lightweight polyethylene, it is dishwasher safe and folds to 5 inches by 15 inches for storage. **Distributor:** 290. **Source:** 361. Cost is about $7.

The tines on a meat holder provide a guide for slicing meat when vision is poor or when there is incoordination (Figure 18-7). The fingers are kept out of the way. Cost is about $13. **Sources** include 326, 334, 347, and the National Federation of the Blind.

A pan with a locking lid allows the person with loss of vision or with the use of one hand to drain foods while keeping hands away from the hot water (Figure 18-8). Pans with locking lids are not available in regular stores but from firms that specialize in self-help equipment for those with limited vision. **Sources** include 326, 334, 347, and the National Federation of the Blind.

Additional kitchen aids for individuals with loss of vision, which are available through firms listed above, include liquid level indicators, adjustable slicing knives, an auto fork that when squeezed pushes the food off the tines, pie cutter guide, as well as graduated measuring cups and spoons, egg rings, egg separator, rice cooker, sewing aids, and more.

Raised, lined paper makes it possible for a person with limited or no vision to make notes for others to assist in shopping and other activities.

Equipment designed to speed kitchen tasks for people with normal sight may be adopted for use with vision loss (Figure 18-9). An egg slicer quickly cuts mushrooms. A hamburger press with sides that define the size or a pasta measurer with holes to determine the amount of dry pasta per serving are two other examples. **Manufacturer** of latter items: 180.

Gourmet cooking firms often sell devices that help any pastry maker roll out an even thickness of dough (Figure 18-10). Rubber rolling pin rings slip over the ends of the rolling pin and keep the thickness even across the dough. A set of three pairs in

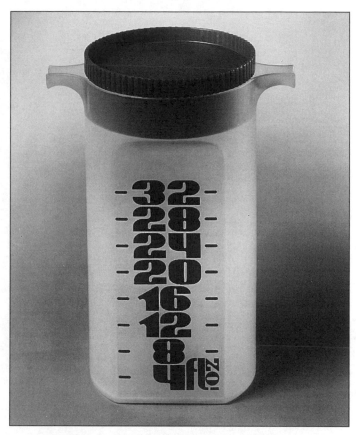

Figure 18-5. Large, bold numbers on contemporary kitchen equipment. (Photo courtesy of Copco.)

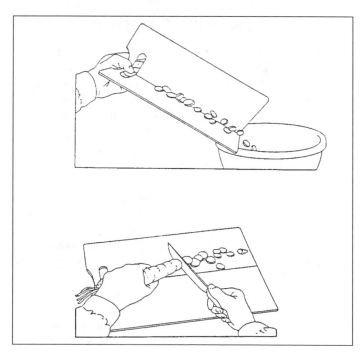

Figure 18-6. This no-spill chopping board folds in the middle to form a channel. (Photo courtesy of J.H. Smith Co., Inc., Greenfield, MA.)

$1/4$-, $3/16$-, and $1/8$-inch thickness costs about $6. **Sources:** 334, 361.

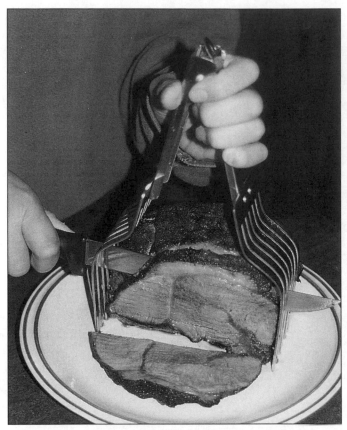

Figure 18-7. The tines on this meat holder provide a guide for slicing meat. (Photo by J.K.)

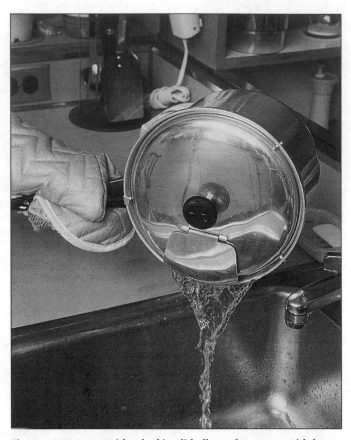

Figure 18-8. A pan with a locking lid allows the person with loss of vision or with use of one hand to drain foods while keeping hands away from the hot water. (Photo courtesy of the O.T. Dept., Howard A. Rusk Institute of Rehabilitation Medicine.)

IDENTIFYING FOODS

Fresh foods are easy to identify by touch and smell. For packaged items, weight, sound, and smell become the clues. Shake before you bake! Practice identifying, shaking, and listening to foods. Rice has a different sound and box shape than pasta. Corn oil sounds different than vinegar when shaken. Syrup has a distinctively shaped bottle and smell. Spices and herbs have unique aromas. Braille labels and tape codes help identify some foods, although older individuals who lose their sight often find it hard to learn Braille or tape codes. Small, plastic forms of food also help identify items as does writing with glue or raised printing. Location and having help putting items away are other solutions. If the patient has partial vision, a wide-tipped marking pen may be used to code the foods, such as a "T" for tomato soup, "BB" for baked beans. Most elderly patients have a limited amount of food supplies, so organization is easier than for a large family.

Ways of marking cans and food containers include large, raised letters, Braille tapes, and magnetized symbols or shapes of the food (Figure 18-11). Elastic bands attached to shapes allow use with cans or boxes. Plastic forms may be used from children's toy food sets.

TECHNIQUES

- Begin training with one-dish, familiar meals.
- Let the patient cook something he or she knows by heart.
- Tactile discrimination should be part of training, such as making apple pie, a fruit cup, or preparing vegetables.
- Making cookies increases ability to measure, divide into portions, and develop mental visualization when placing dough on pan.
- No idea should be beyond the reach of the cook, and family members or guests can help with last-minute details. In fact, making traditional dishes lets the family learn how independent a person can be without sight. (A therapist worked with an 83-year-old woman who baked apple pies as part of home care therapy. She also made cookies for her grandchildren and cheesecake for the holidays. It was in the kitchen where she really felt free.)

Some companies that distribute aids specifically for people with loss of vision include the following: Bausch & Lomb (78)—magnifiers and readers; Edmund Scientific Company (181)—magnifiers, microscopes, telescopes; Eschenbach Optik of America (190)—magnifiers, with and without illumination; Independent Living Aids, Inc. (279)—full range of self-care, homemaking, and communication aids; Lighthouse Enterprises (326)—full range of self-care, homemaking, and communication aids, large-print and braille publications; LS&S Group (334)—full range of self-care, homemaking, and vocational aids; Maxi-Aids (347)—self-care, homemaking, vocational aids; Science Products (466)—self-care, homemaking, vocational aids; Telesensory (513)—wide range of communication aids; and Whirlpool Corporation (571)—Braille, large-type, and audio instructions and cookbooks.

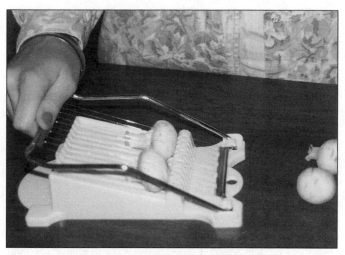

Figure 18-9. Equipment designed to speed kitchen tasks for people with normal sight may be adopted for use with vision loss. (Photo by J.K.)

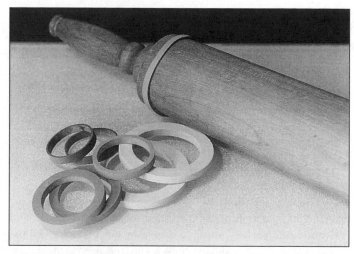

Figure 18-10. These rubber rolling pin rings slip over the ends of the rolling pin and keep the thickness even across the dough. (Photo by J.K.)

GUIDE DOGS

The person with loss of vision who has an interest in and affinity for animals and wants to be more independent might consider a guide dog. The dog helps in getting around and serves as security within the home. The dog is trained to notice danger, such as fire, and alert the owner. The cost of training a dog is often covered by donations. A number of schools train dogs and individuals. Among these are Guide Dogs for the Blind, Guide Dog Foundation, Guiding Eyes for the Blind, International Guiding Eyes, Leader Dogs for the Blind, and Pilot Dogs. Addresses are in Appendix C. You can also contact your State Society for the Blind for the best local referral.

RESOURCES

Addresses for publishers, periodicals, and organizations are given in Section Four. Note: all books from the American Foundation for the Blind are ordered through American Book Service, **source:** 39.

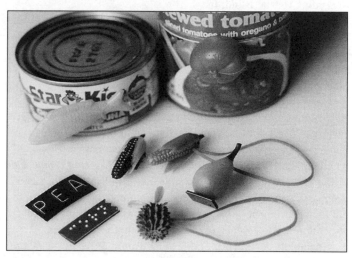

Figure 18-11. Ways of marking cans and food containers include large, raised letters, braille tapes, and magnetized symbols or shapes of the food. (Idea from the Gladys E. Loeb Foundation, Silver Spring, MD. Photo by J.K.)

PUBLICATIONS

The American Foundation for the Blind distributes a catalog of publications including training manuals, a listing of services for the blind and people with low vision, some of which are given below. Send or call for the current edition of the Publications Catalog.

The American Association of Retired Persons provides materials for more than two million visually impaired Americans. These include audiotapes of their most requested consumer publications and *Modern Maturity* through Talking Book libraries. More than two dozen titles of their consumer publications are arranged in the following series: Medical Care, Housing and Living Arrangements, Financial Matters, Health and Nutrition, and Long Term Care. AARP also works with the Association of Radio Reading Services (ARRS), producing programs on living independently. See Resources in Chapter 1 Aging and Vision.

AFB Directory of Services for Blind and Visually Impaired Persons in the United States (24th ed.). New York: American Foundation for the Blind. ISBN 0-89128-242-4, $75, plus shipping and handling. Available in print or on cassette—15/16 ips. Almost 3000 local, state, regional, and national services with program name, address, telephone number, contact person, and service descriptions.

Bailey, I., & Hall, A. (1990). *Visual Impairment: An Overview*. New York: American Foundation for the Blind. ISBN 0-89128-174-6. Common forms of vision loss and their impact on the individual. Photographs simulate how people with various types of loss of vision see. Describes adaptive techniques, devices, resources, and services for professionals, people with vision loss, and their families.

Belivieau, M., & Smith, A. J. (Eds.). (1980). *The Interdisciplinary Approach to Low Vision Rehabilitation*. New York: American Foundation for the Blind. Order Code: 389.005, $47 from the National Clearing House for Rehabilitation

Materials. Addresses primary concerns in low-vision service delivery including pathology of the eye, training considerations for the client, and psychosocial aspects of low vision.

Cockerman, P. W. (1987). *Low Vision Questions and Answers: Definitions, Devices, Services* (rev. ed.). New York: American Foundation for the Blind. ISBN 0-S9128-196-7, 25 copies, $35 plus shipping and handling. Request single copy from local agencies.

Curtis, P. (1982). *Greff: The Story of a Guide Dog.* New York: Lodestar Books, Penguin. $9.95. Early life and rigorous training of a dog who becomes a guide to a young individual.

Dickman, I. R. (1983). *Making Life More Livable.* New York: American Foundation for the Blind. ISBN 0-9128-115-0. $16.95 plus shipping and handling from American Book Service or **source** 190. Large-print. Simple adaptations for the home and environment of visually impaired adults and older people. 54 illustrations examine the home, room by room, raising common questions: How can I tell what a can contains? How can I dial the phone? How can I use my workshop? Can I continue to sew? Simple to ingenious ideas. Also available on cassette from Recording for the Blind, Inc.

The Eyes Have It. Washington, DC: American Association of Retired Persons, Health Advocacy Services Program Department. Free. Excellent patient education publication. Explains how the eye works, describes four major types of vision loss that affect older people, gives tips on care of eyes, sources for help.

Family Guide to Vision Care. American Optometric Association. Free with self-addressed, stamped, business-sized envelope. Care of eyes from developmental through working and mature years. Symptoms of problems with recommendations.

Greenblatt, S. L. (Ed.). (1991). *Meeting the Needs of People with Vision Loss.* Lexington, MA: Resources for Rehabilitation. $24.95. Emphasizes interdisciplinary communication and cooperation leading to improvement of service delivery. Covers older adults, diabetics, children, adolescents, psychosocial issues. Case studies.

Greenblatt, S. L., (Ed.). (1989). *Providing Services for People with Vision Loss: A Multidisciplinary Perspective.* Lexington, MA: Resources for Rehabilitation. $19.95. How various professionals can work together to provide coordinated care for people with vision loss. Also available on cassette.

Griffin-Shirley, N., & Groff, G. (1993). *Prescriptions for Independence: Working with Older People Who Are Visually Impaired.* New York: American Foundation for the Blind. ISBN 0-89128-244-0, $24.95 plus shipping and handling. Hands-on book of practical suggestions for preparing meals, handling money, etc. Establishes framework for looking at daily problems, increasing options for independence. Includes directions for making simple aids; resources for information, and products.

Handbook for Senior Citizens: Rights, Resources and Responsibilities. Baltimore: American Brotherhood for the Blind. $7. Practical experience and advice for older people who lose their vision. Appendices give references for obtaining local services.

Hearing Impaired/Visually Impaired: Resource Guide. (1991). Bethesda, MD: American Occupational Therapy Association. #4100, $10 AOTA members, $20 non-members. Bibliographies, audiovisuals, resource personnel.

Huebner, K. M., & Swallow, R. M. (Eds.). (1987). *How to Thrive, Not Just Survive: A Guide to Developing Independent*

Life Skills for Blind and Visually Impaired Children and Youths. New York: American Foundation for the Blind. $9.95.

Jose, R. T. (Ed.). (1983). *Understanding Low Vision.* Houston, TX: Lighthouse of Houston and University of Houston. $49. Framework for understanding impact of low vision on functioning, learning, and psychosocial status.

Living with Low Vision: A Resource Guide for People with Sight Loss (4th ed.). (1996). Lexington, MA: Resources for Rehabilitation. $43.95. Large-print directory of services, products, and publications to allow clients to keep reading, working, and enjoying life. Chapters for children and elders, self-help groups, laws affecting people with sight loss.

Mendelsohn, S. (1989). *Financing Adaptive Technology: A Guide to Sources and Strategies for Blind and Visually Impaired Users.* New York: Demos. $24.95. Public and private sources of equipment for handicapped individuals. Ways to gain access and develop needed funding.

Orr, A. L. (1992). *Vision and Aging: Crossroads for Service Delivery.* New York: American Foundation for the Blind. ISBN 0-89128-216-5, $39.95 plus shipping and handling. Overview of service delivery systems in the aging and blindness fields; policy and service questions that will demand national attention. Fifteen chapters by experts cover physiological, psychological, social aspects of aging and visual impairment, low vision, rehabilitation, orientation and mobility services, long-term and community-based care, gives resources.

Rehabilitation Resources Manual: VISION (4th ed.). (1993). Lexington, MA: Resources for Rehabilitation. $39.95. Desk reference for providers, librarians, and others to make effective referrals. Case vignettes.

Ringgold, N. P. (1991). *Out of the Corner of My Eye: Living with Vision Loss in Later Life.* New York: American Foundation for the Blind. ISBN 0-89128-193-2 (large-print); ISBN 0-89128-211-4 (cassette—1 7/8 ips), $19.95 each. Order from American Book Service. Personal account of vision loss and adjustment, including initial reaction, accommodations in order to continue indoor and outdoor activities and to regain dignity and independence. Extensive resource section.

Smith, E. (1982). *A Guide Dog Goes to School.* New York: William Morrow.

Whirlpool® Corp. began offering Braille, large-type, and audio-cassette formats to visually impaired customers using their appliances several years ago. They now also produce laundry, dryer, and range cooking guides and microwave cookbooks for general sale. Materials available include the following:

Whirlpool Micro Menus Cookbook. Tested with 600-700 watt microwave ovens, contains basic microwave cooking directions, tips, and more than 220 recipes, $20 (6 volumes) in Braille, $15 (1 volume) large-type, $30 audio cassette (8 cassettes in album holder).

The Whirlpool Microwave Cooking Guide. For use with 400-500 watt microwave ovens, outlines basic microwave techniques, and includes simple-to-prepare recipes. $5 for Braille or large-type editions.

The Cooking Guide. Generic information about cooking with electric ranges—choosing correct pans, diagnosing common baking problems, roasting, broiling, saving energy. $4 in Braille or large type.

Also available are a *Laundry Guide*, $3 in Braille or large type and a *Dryer Guide*, $2 for Braille or large type.

To receive an order form and price list, write Whirlpool® Corp., Appliance Information Service. **Source:** 571.

Willoughby, D., & Duffy, S. (1989). *Handbook for Itinerant and Resource Teachers of Blind and Visually Handicapped Students*. Baltimore: National Federation of the Blind. $20. Coping with all types of travel, teaching Braille, understanding medical assessments.

Younger, V., & Sardegna, J. (1992). *One Way or Another: A Guide to Independence for the Visually Impaired and Their Families*. San Jose, CA: Sardegna Productions. Psychological adjustment, family dynamics, acquiring ADL skills, technology and adaptive aids, in-home orientation, and mobility training. Check your local library.

For additional references, see Chapter 1 and Chapter 6.

PERIODICALS

AFB News. New York: American Foundation for the Blind. National newsletter, 5 issues per year.

Long Cane News. New York: American Foundation for the Blind. Biannual newsletter for orientation and mobility specialists.

Update, a quarterly newspaper free from the National Vision Research Institute. Reports on latest breakthroughs in vision research, eye health, and safety.

AUDIOVISUALS

Aging and Vision: Declarations of Independence. American Foundation for the Blind, order through American Book Center. ISBN 0-89128-220-3/VHS format, $39.95; ISBN 0-89128-276-9/PAL format, $49.95 plus handling costs. An 18-minute, color, personal look at five older people who have coped successfully with visual impairment and live active lives. Inspirational and practical.

Blindness: A Family Matter. American Foundation for the Blind, order through the American Book Center. ISBN 0-S9128-229-X/VHS format, $19.95; ISBN 0-S9128-271-S/PAL, $29.95 plus shipping and handling. Effects of an individual's loss of vision on a family and how family members can play a positive role in the rehabilitation process. Interviews with three families and with newly blinded adults in a rehabilitation program.

The Seven-Minute Lesson. American Foundation for the Blind. Order through the American Book Service. ISBN 0-S9128-229-7/VHS format, $19.95; ISBN 0-S9128-4/PAL format, $19.95 plus shipping and handling. Seven-minute introduction to the basic techniques used when acting as a sighted guide for a blind or visually impaired person. **Source:** 39.

Out of the Shadows. 16-mm sound film on guide dogs and their training. Free loan from Guide Dog Foundation.

The Eyes Have It. Washington, DC: American Association of Retired Persons. Video or color slides with audiocassette. Free loan includes poster and 50 copies of brochure *The Eyes Have It*. Request 90 days in advance from AARP Scheduling Office. Discusses four major causes of low vision in older people: glaucoma, macular degeneration, diabetic retinopathy, and cataracts.

CHAPTER 19

The Client with Lowered Energy Levels

Low energy is a symptom of many diseases and has varied causes. It may result from weakness or advanced age and can affect the duration of time that a patient can perform a task. It may be emotional, disturbing the ability to organize or even begin activities. It may be physical as with heart disease, rheumatoid arthritis, post-polio syndrome, or chronic obstructive pulmonary disease. As in chronic fatigue and immune dysfunction syndrome, Lyme disease, AIDS, HIV infection, and multiple sclerosis, it may be both physical and emotional. Chronic Fatigue Syndrome (CFS) is now believed to affect some 400,000 people in the United States, according to the CFIDS Association of America. It is at least 20 times as prevalent as the Center for Disease Control originally estimated.

The major symptoms of CFS include exhaustion, lightheadedness, and depression. If a patient has exhaustion accompanied by low fever, sore throat, memory lapses, achiness, headache, and sleep disturbances, a referral to the physician must be made and followed up. These additional symptoms may be due to an immune system problem brought on by a viral infection.

Stress itself also reduces energy. The suggestions given in Chapter 7 may help your patient increase energy and vitality.

Adding to the problem of fatigue is the frequent refusal of family members, friends, and co-workers to accept that there is such a thing as low energy or chronic fatigue. It is important for the patient as well as the whole family to acknowledge this. Mom or Dad can still be a super parent without wielding a vacuum, handling a community job, or baking everything from scratch. In fact, conserving energy to follow family or personal interests and spend quality time is an important aspect that must be emphasized. Rules to Conserve Energy, in Appendix G, may be given to a patient to review with the family and post in a prominent place.

With only so much fuel for handling tasks, the individual must determine how to get the best mileage. The health care professional works closely with a client to develop a workable agenda, showing how to use energy-saving principles and equipment, and scheduling a rest period between activities.

If a client is having difficulty sleeping at night, this decreases energy during the day. Providing guidelines to help one sleep is a first step. If books are not available through your local library, the American Sleep Disorders Association, Association of Professional Sleep Societies, and the National Sleep Foundation will provide helpful material. Suggestions include using the bed only for sleep, trying relaxation techniques such as a warm bath or meditation before bed, and imagining a calming scene that lulls one to sleep. Sleeping medications are not recommended, because they throw the body's clock off, increase lethargy during the day, and may increase emotional problems. Ascertaining if there is a reason for sleeplessness, such as stress or anxiety, may require counseling by a social worker or other health care professional.

Setting priorities is a first step to efficient use of available energy. Writing down the schedule for a day, then for a week provides a baseline. This may take several sessions before becoming finalized. Our client may be a true homemaker, one whose time is hers, or his, to divide and use within the context of the home and needs of the family. More difficult to schedule when there is low energy or chronic fatigue is the woman, or man, who must handle a home and family as well as an outside job. For this person, scheduling and limiting becomes doubly complex. Then add the financial needs and the constraints this puts on choices for better health.

For either group, however, the next step in setting priorities is to break the lists of activities down into categories: "Must do, Ought to do, Would like to do, Will delegate, and Eliminate." The last category may raise the question of force of habit; that is questioning why a job is necessary. For the person with outside employment, cuts in tasks around the home may be easier to make than those required at work. Weekends and any holiday time must then be carefully delineated in order to allow a recuperation of the body and spirit. A reproducible form for beginning the phase of breaking into categories is in Appendix G.

Delegating jobs is the second step and is often hard for a client to do. The person feels it may appear as though he or she

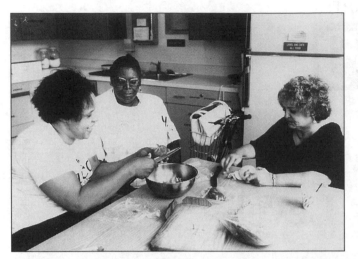

Figure 19-1. Working in a group setting lets clients exchange ideas and reinforces teaching. (Photo courtesy of the O.T. Dept., Rehabilitation Institute of Chicago.)

is giving up. At this point, the family must be brought into the planning process. Young children can help put things away, their own as well as others. In other cultures, they cultivate food and tend animals; here they can learn to set and clear the table, fold and put away laundry, empty wastebaskets, scrub the tub, and cook under supervision. Teenagers can cooperate by taking on more responsible jobs, many of which will stand them in good stead as young adults. For utmost cooperation, everyone should be in on the planning from the beginning. Ordering a job to be done raises hackles; sharing in the decision making strengthens the family. Each person must understand how fulfilling a designated role helps everyone benefit.

When there is no family to help with jobs, outside help may be necessary. Finances often dictate the type of help that can be afforded. In many cases, volunteer programs provide chore service, shopping, or child care services. See Appendix A.

Some jobs cannot be eliminated or delegated. Breaking tasks into manageable steps is the third phase of teaching. Are there certain times of the day that are best, least tiring, or stressful? By testing varied schedules over a period of time, the patient can demonstrate to himself or herself and the therapist that certain jobs are accomplished more easily at selected times of the day, that cleaning one room a day, or doing one load of laundry rather than four in one day, lets one win the race—just like the tortoise.

It is important for the client to realize that some days may require that chores be put on hold, without feeling guilty or stressed. Certain diseases, like arthritis, CFS, and multiple sclerosis, have their ups and downs. The person with chronic obstructive pulmonary disease reacts to hot weather, humidity, and air pollution, so he or she must learn to relegate tasks to clear, cooler days.

Large energy challenges like major shopping and spring cleaning have to be cut down to size and often delegated. These jobs require more reaching, bending, and pushing than most normal daily tasks. They stress joints, muscles, and endurance. If a job cannot be relegated to someone else, the client should work with others on big jobs for two or three days instead of one. Outside

help, such as a chore service or volunteer group to assist, may be the best solution.

Planning an efficient work area is the fourth step. Having a place to sit and rest between phases of the job, keeping the equipment nearby, and using ergonomics, or proper posture and body mechanics, reduces fatigue. Changing position frequently while working reduces fatigue on one set of muscles. Using body mechanics when lifting and rolling instead of carrying conserves energy.

Working in a group setting lets clients exchange ideas and reinforces teaching (Figure 19-1). A low work surface provides a comfortable food preparation area.

If the patient's kitchen is large enough in which to sit down and eat, perhaps trips to and from the dining room can be eliminated. A wheeled cart or a pass-through to the dining room also cuts back on walking and carrying. When remodeling, moving the laundry near the bedroom area may cut out lugging. All individual steps have to be considered and reconsidered. Changing habits is not easy, especially when any sense of guilt or frustration is involved. Small changes conserve energy. If the current set of dishes is too heavy, a lightweight set reduces energy expenditure. A long-handled dustpan and brush curtails bending. An electric scooter extends range. Vertical filing reduces lifting. See Chapter 14, *Mealtime Manual*, and Chapter 25 in this guide.

A low work area with a pull-out board saves lifting for a client (Figure 19-2). He or she can roll the wheelchair under the board to slide items in and out of the microwave oven. Choosing recipes carefully cuts preparation time. Frequently used items can be stored on an accessible lazy susan, or other countertop storage unit.

The fifth step is to find shortcuts. Each little achievement conserves energy, whether preparing meals, cleaning the house, shopping, caring for children, or finding a way to reduce or pare a nonessential at home or on the job. Many books by Heloise, Better Homes and Gardens® and Reader's Digest®, plus family service magazines, give ways to do things faster and easier. These range from faster grooming and easier dressing, to quick cooking and streamlined house cleaning. See Resources at the end of this chapter. With so many women working outside their homes today, articles are widely available in family service magazines on finding extra precious minutes and maximizing one's potential.

County extension agents and home economists are trained to teach work simplification. They have publications that can be shared with or used as training manuals for a client.

Exercise is important even for the person with lowered energy levels and should be incorporated into daily activities. If the possibility exists for sharing exercise time in a community group, this gives the client a chance for expanding horizons, sharing thoughts, and reducing depression. It also will often result in a decrease in fatigue, both physically and mentally, and improve the quality of sleep at night.

Ideas for easing meal preparation include cooking once for two meals, combining convenience foods with fresh foods, utilizing the microwave oven for faster cooking, preparing meals early in the day while feeling energetic, and providing back-up meals for days when energy is low.

When there is weakness in the lower extremities or severe fatigue, use of a powered scooter may be considered. The amount

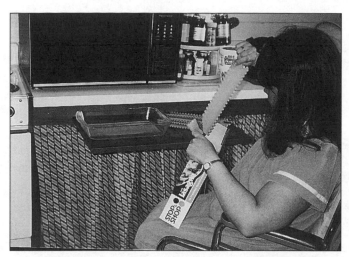

Figure 19-2. This client rolls her wheelchair under the board to slide items in and out of the microwave oven. (Ballard Green, Ridgefield, CT. Photo by J.K.)

it is used should be determined with the doctor or therapist. There must be a balance between maintaining muscle power in the lower extremities and conserving strength for specific tasks. Walking through grocery stores and department stores may be overtaxing. All scooters are battery powered; the main difference is in design of the seats and controls. A scooter may be covered by insurance if prescribed by the physician.

Using a scooter to conserve energy allows more quality time with the family (Figure 19-3). **Source:** 183. See other scooter units in Chapter 25 and Chapter 30.

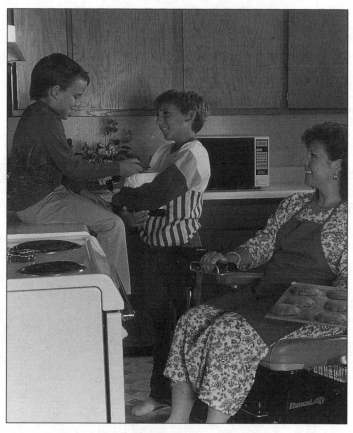

Figure 19-3. This unit, the Rascal, comes with a swivel seat, which is adjustable in height if needed, and has a solid non-tipping base. (Photo courtesy of Electric Mobility, Sewell, NJ.)

RESOURCES

Addresses for publishers, periodicals, and organizations are given in Section Four.

PUBLICATIONS

American Sleep Disorders Association. Free pamphlets include *Insomnia: The Inability to Fall Asleep or Stay Asleep*, (1994, revised); *Restless Legs Syndrome & Periodic Limb Movement Disorder* (1994); *Sleep Hygiene: Behaviors That Help Promote Sound Sleep*. Listed in Section VI.

Bell, D. S., & Donev, Stef. (1996). *Curing Fatigue: a Step-by-Step Plan to Uncover and Eliminate the Causes of Chronic Fatigue*. New York: PutnamBerkley. $6.99.

Bell, D. (1993). *The Doctor's Guide to Chronic Fatigue Syndrome: Understanding and Living with CIFDS*. Reading, MA: Addison-Wesley. $21.

Bell, D. (1991). *The Disease of a Thousand Names: CFIDS*. Lyndonville, NY: Pollard. Emphasis on symptomatology, epidemiology, cause and treatment.

Berne, K. H. (1995). *Running on Empty: Chronic Immune Dysfunction Syndrome* (2nd ed.). Alameda, CA: Hunter House. $15.95.

Better Homes & Gardens® Household Hints and Tips. Des Moines, IA: Meredith. $19.95

Christy, D., & Sarafconn, C. (1990). *Pacing Yourself: Steps to Save Energy*. Bloomington, IL: Accent. $10.95. Co-authors, an occupational therapist, and a client with sickle cell thalassemia give tips from self-care and morning organization to meal planning and preparation, child care, laundry, home planning, travel, physical relations, and psychological issues. **Source:** 8.

The Chronic Fatigue and Immune Dysfunction Syndrome (CFIDS) Association offers information packets and a CFIDS chronicle. Section II.

Conant, S. (1990). *Living with Chronic Fatigue*. Dallas, TX: Taylor. Addresses coping issues. **Source:** 509.

Coping with Fatigue. The Arthritis Foundation. Free brochure available from local chapter, or call the national office. Also, if your client has arthritis, ask about an area Arthritis Self-Help Course.

Cromwell, F. (Ed.). (1986). *Occupational Therapy for the Energy Deficient Patient*. Binghamton, NY: Haworth. $19.95.

Digging for Clues to Fatigue. *Facts & Issues*. New York: National Multiple Sclerosis Society. Free reprint written for individuals with MS gives suggestions for managing fatigue.

Feiden, K. (1992). *Hope and Help for Chronic Fatigue Syndrome*. New York: Prentice Hall, Simon and Schuster. $11.

Fisher, G. C., & Strauss, S. (1989). *Chronic Fatigue Syndrome: A Victim's Guide to Understanding, Treating and Coping with This Debilitating Disease*. New York: Warner. $10.95.

Heloise. (1992). *Heloise from A to Z*. New York: PutnamBerkley. $10.95.

National Sleep Foundation. (1994). Publications include free pamphlet, *When You Can't Sleep: ABC's of ZZZ's*. Section II.

Solomon, N. & Lipton, M. (1991). *Chronic Fatigue and Other Ailments*. Tarrytown, NY: Wynwood Press, Gleneida Publishers. Check your local library.

Stevens, C. (1991). *Helpful Household Hints*. Northbrook, IL: SK Brown.

Young, G. (1991, November). Energy conservation for post-polio individuals. *Journal of Orthopedics*. Occupational therapist teaches methods to post-polio patients in the Kaiser-Permanente Health Plan.

20

The Client with Hearing Loss

The individual who is born deaf or, because of trauma or disease, acquires a loss of hearing early in life learns to adjust. Special schooling and a determination of the best way to communicate, whether by speech and/or signing, leads to a full life.

Our focus here is on the person developing a hearing loss, most frequently as a result of aging. Hearing loss is the third most prevalent chronic condition among older adults, after arthritis and hypertensive disease. It is estimated that hearing loss affects about 30% of adults aged 65 through 74; this rises to 50% for people 75 through 79. More than 10 million older people in the United States are hearing impaired.

Hearing loss is an invisible disability. Your client may not seem aware of a hearing loss. Other family members who are conscious of a lack of attention or apparent loss of memory put the changes down to senility, just getting "confused, being uncooperative, unresponsive, old."

A sense of isolation becomes an increasing problem for a client with a hearing loss. Parts of sentences are lost; conversations are difficult to hear, so the individual is just turned off. Social activities become limited as the person withdraws out of embarrassment and frustration. Stress within the family may rise. Members talk about, or seem to talk about, the individual as though he or she is not there or not capable. A feeling of insecurity or even paranoia may grow. This is where the health care professional can mediate and help find solutions.

ASSESSMENT

Make an informal assessment of your patient's hearing. Ask if:
- Words are more difficult to understand.
- Other people's speech sounds slurred or mumbled and seems worse when there is background noise.
- Family gatherings and those of friends, even television and concerts, are less enjoyable because of what goes unheard.
- Some speech is hard or impossible to understand, commonly the grandchildren's.
- Certain sounds seem annoying or overly loud.
- There is a ringing or hissing sound constantly or intermittently in the background.

If the patient appears to have a hearing loss, referral to a physician for a check-up is the initial step before seeing an otolaryngologist, or ear specialist. Hearing loss is sometimes due to a treatable disease, such as diabetes. Other causes range from injury due to prolonged noise (perhaps at work prior to retirement) viral infections, vascular disorders (such as a heart condition or stroke), head injury, tumors, heredity, some medications, and age-related changes in the ear. It is not even uncommon for the problem to be a build-up of wax of which the person is unaware. Once removed, hearing improves noticeably.

Types of hearing loss in older people include the following:
- Conductive—blocking of the sounds carried from the ear drums to the inner ear, which may be caused by ear wax, fluid in the middle ear, abnormal bone growth, or infection in the middle ear.
- Sensorineural hearing loss—damage to parts of the inner ear or auditory nerve. In older people, this impairment is called presbycusis. It leads to changes in delicate workings of the inner ear, which makes understanding speech difficult. The individual with presbycusis often says, "You don't have to shout. I'm not deaf."
- Central auditory dysfunction—a rare form of hearing loss, even in older people, caused by damage to nerve centers in the brain. Sound levels are not affected, but understanding speech is. Causes include high fever, head injury, tumors, or vascular problems. This type of loss is treated by training with an audiologist or speech pathologist.

When assessing a patient's hearing loss within the home or institution, balance should also be evaluated. An individual with a hearing loss sometimes has increased trouble with balance and ambulation. If there is a problem, evaluation includes the possibility of a walking aid and additional safety measures in the home, such as grab bars in the bathroom. Various kinds of help for hearing loss are available, including medication, special training, surgery, or an alternate listening device.

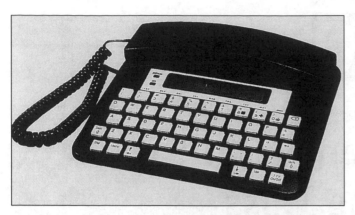

Figure 20-1. The telecommunication device for the deaf, or TDD, consists of a keyboard, display screen, and a modem on which a telephone receiver is placed. (Advanced TTY 8840 model. Photo courtesy of Lucent Technologies, Inc., Town and Country, MO.)

HEARING AIDS

An individual cannot go out and buy a hearing aid without a written statement from his or her physician that the individual needs one or has waived medical evaluation. As stated earlier, a hearing loss can mask another kind of treatable medical problem.

Many types of hearing aids are on the market; professional advice is important in finding the best one for your patient. The customer is buying not only a unit to increase sounds, but a product that includes services such as necessary adjustments, counseling in its use, and maintenance and repair through a warranty period. A larger unit that fits over the ear is sometimes easier to handle and provides added power. A unit with tiny adjustments is cosmetically more attractive but may be physically difficult for an older client to operate. A hearing aid is just that, an aid, not a replacement for natural hearing. The constant level of all noises, the occasional whine, and the inability to hear as clearly as the individual wishes might cause frustration. Training or help from the family will reduce these stressors. The AARP distributes a free report that describes the different kinds of hearing aids. See Resources.

Other types of help for hearing impairments do not depend on equipment. Speech reading, for example, teaches the client to learn visual cues from facial expressions, body posture, and gestures. Auditory training, which may include hearing aid orientation, is designed to help the hearing-impaired handle specific communication problems more easily. Counseling is also a possibility for the person who needs help understanding his or her limitations, especially if depression and isolation are part of the pattern.

AMPLIFIERS AND OTHER HOUSEHOLD AIDS

Several solutions exist for major tasks around the home requiring hearing, i.e., communicating by telephone, hearing when the doorbell rings, or hearing a regular timer on the oven or clock.

It is most important that people with hearing impairment be able to communicate on the telephone, not only for staying in touch and socially active but in case of emergency. The Accessible

Products Center, Lucent Technologies, distributes amplifier phones, flashing signals, and other aids for people with auditory loss. **Source: 335B**. Check with your local phone company. If your client wears a hearing aid, make sure that the telephone has a telephone pick-up switch that reduces background noise while the person is in conversation. The switch, usually indicated with a "T," has to be set before the individual wearing a hearing aid uses the phone, then is returned to its regular position when done. Some older telephone models are not compatible with this system, but the pick-up switch is now required by law on new phones. For noncompatible models, the user will need to carry a portable, battery-powered, adaptive coupler. Federal law requires that coin-operated phones be hearing-aid compatible.

The telecommunication device for the deaf or TDD consists of a keyboard, display screen, and a modem on which a telephone receiver is placed (Figure 20-1). The response may come in as a message on the screen or with an auxiliary written tape if desired. A TDD is available through Lucent Technologies (**Source: 335B**), Nationwide Flashing Signal (**Source: 375**), or your local phone company.

A portable device, the Tone Talker, enables a hearing impaired person with usable speech to see messages sent from any touch-tone phone and to respond by voice. The Tone Talker has a display and a microphone on a suction cup that attaches to the receiver. The person communicating with the hearing impaired person needs only the keys on a touch-tone phone to spell out words to the Tone Talker device used on the hearing impaired person's telephone receiver. Built-in words and phrases may be generated by a two-key code. Cost is about $300. **Source: 139**.

Electronic stores, such as Radio Shack®, carry a variety of aids. **Source: 430**. These include telephone amplifiers from built-in to portable, visual or flashing phone ringers, indoor and outdoor extension ringers, headset radios that allow listening at a preferred level, headphones for watching television with a louder volume, a personal listening-aid system (see *Mealtime Manual*, Chapter 11), and a piercing two-tone indoor siren for fire or intrusion.

Self-help firms carry a variety of listening devices. Nationwide Flashing Signals, Inc. (**Source: 375**) and Independent Living Aids, Inc. (**Source: 279**) sell telephone amplifiers, doorbell and phone signalers, baby cry signalers, auxiliary bellringers for placing in another room, personal listening devices, television decoders, and vibrating alarm clocks. Hello Direct® (**Source: 256**) carries a Phone Flasher and amplifying phones. If not near the door, a person with limited hearing may not hear a ring or a knock. A portable, two-part, electronic pager system lets an individual hear the doorbell. The transmitter plugs into any wall outlet near the front door; the remote receiver into a wall outlet near the individual. A ring at the front door can be heard in the kitchen, laundry, garage, or bedroom. Battery-operated. Cost is about $20 and up. **Sources: 159, 241, 295, 375, 476**.

An even less expensive unit consists of a wireless, battery-powered doorbell that attaches outside the door and a chime box that plugs into any outlet the user wishes. Extra chime boxes may be ordered. Cost is about $11 and up. **Sources: 109, 171**.

The Tele-Consumer Hotline provides fact sheets on telephone problems and distributes a resource directory of devices for the hearing, speech, or vision impaired. They will provide, for a fee, cost comparisons between different companies. To find out which services are available in your state, call 800-332-1124 (Voice/TDD) or 202-483-4100 (Voice/TDD) between 9 a.m. and 5 p.m. Monday through Friday.

One problem that may require a change in meal preparation patterns is a gas stove. New stoves have a soft pop that signifies when a burner is on. The flame is almost invisible. If your client has a hearing loss and any visual limitation that precludes seeing the flame, or any confusion, it would be wise to modify the kitchen so that cooking is done by a microwave oven or another electrical unit.

FAMILY, FRIENDS, AND CHANGES IN THE HOME

Instructing the patient and family in ways to maximize hearing ability is part of the treatment plan. Teach them to speak at the normal rate, but not too quickly. A common problem is overarticulating, which distorts speech sounds and makes visual clues more difficult. Shouting also distorts a message as well as its meaning. People should speak to the hearing-impaired individual from a distance of three to six feet. Explain to the speaker how to position oneself with good light on the face so that lip movements, gestures, and facial expressions are clearly seen.

Rearranging the living room to maximize position and light is a concrete step the family can take. No one speaking to an individual with a hearing loss should be more than six feet away. An individual should wait until he or she is visible to the hearing-impaired person before speaking. Visual clues are picked up from the lips so speakers should avoid chewing, eating, or covering their mouths while speaking. One should never speak directly into the person's ear, because this prevents utilizing visual cues. Reducing background noise in the home or in a gathering of people helps the listener to concentrate on conversation.

The client should be instructed to ask people to repeat if a point is missed and to tell others that there is a hearing problem so they will make communication easier. Talking with one person at a time is much easier than with a group. The person can ask or arrange to do this with practice. When background noises drown out the speaker even when the hearing-impaired person is wearing hearing aids, he or she might try an inexpensive hi-fi amplifier, which is hooked up to a microphone and pair of headphones. Pointing the microphone at the person who is talking picks up the conversation clearly. At large social gatherings, the person with a hearing impairment should be encouraged to request a seat near the speaker or know that asking for the public address system to be used is appropriate.

If your client with hearing impairment is going to be hospitalized, ask if there is a program that distributes hearing amplifiers at the institution. Many patients who are hearing impaired get overlooked and become confused in an unfamiliar environment. The AARP has started a volunteer program that might be picked up by others. When a patient has problems hearing, the loan of a portable amplifier is made while in the hospital. Another program in hospitals encourages putting a sticker on the patient's chart and bracelet to alert the staff. The program was developed in 1980 by the Suzanne Pathy Speak-up Institute, a New York-based, educational organization dedicated to assisting people with hearing loss.

HEARING LOSS AND DRIVING

An area of great concern regarding safety is that of hearing loss and driving. The older person who is beginning to experience hearing loss is more likely to be inattentive to or unaware of surroundings, such as the noise of oncoming vehicles, even horns. If you note a patient having difficulty, recommend that he or she see a doctor about wearing a hearing aid, especially when driving. In some states, the use of a hearing aid is required by law.

HEARING EAR DOGS

Hearing ear dogs assist the hearing impaired by increasing independence, mobility, and personal safety. They are trained to respond to and alert their owners to sounds, such as the telephone, a TTD, door bell, oven buzzer or timer, smoke detector, a problem with another member of the family, a baby's cry, and even cooking noises, such as the whistle of a teakettle or specific sounds a person may request. The cost of training a hearing ear dog for a four- to six-month period is about $3000 to $4000, but this is usually covered by donations from sponsors and various organizations. The dogs are available free of charge to qualified individuals who are asked for a donation if they can afford it. The person must be severely or totally deaf and show a need to qualify for the dog's services. The person must live alone or be in a position where there is no one on which to rely. Priority groups that have the greatest need for hearing ear dogs include young deaf adults leaving home to live independently, deaf couples with young children, and elderly deaf people who could previously hear. For information, contact Canine Companions for Independence, Inc., Dogs for the Deaf, International Hearing Dogs, Inc., or ask for a referral from an agency dealing with deafness. Addresses are in Appendix C.

There are about 2000 trained dogs who now serve as ears for deaf individuals in the U.S. (Figure 20-2).

ORGANIZATIONS

Several organizations are concerned with hearing problems. Addresses are given under Deafness and Hearing Loss in Appendix C.

- Alexander Graham Bell Association for the Deaf.
- American Deafness and Rehabilitation Association.
- American Association of the Deaf-Blind.
- American Speech-Language-Hearing Association—professional organization that answers questions and mails information on hearing aids, hearing loss, and communication problems. Provides list of certified audiologists and speech language pathologists. Section VI.
- Hearing Aid Helpline.
- Hear You Are, Inc.
- Helen Keller National Center for Deaf-Blind Youths and Adults.
- National Association for the Deaf.

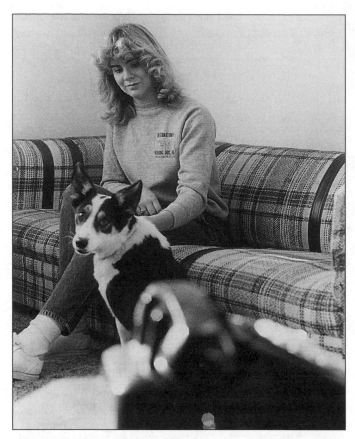

Figure 20-2. This hearing dog alerts his owner to the ringing telephone. (Photo courtesy of International Hearing Dogs, Inc., Henderson, CO.)

- National Hearing Aid Association.
- National Institute on Deafness and Other Communication Disorders, National Institutes of Health—distributes information on hearing, balance, and other related topics for both health care professionals and the public.
- Self-help for Hard of Hearing People, Inc.—national self-help group for the hard of hearing, provides information on coping with a hearing loss, new hearing aids, and technology. Publishes the bimonthly *SHHH Journal*.

RESOURCES

Addresses for publishers, periodicals, and organizations are given in Section Four.

Have You Heard? Hearing Loss and Aging. #D12219. Washington, DC: American Association of Retired Persons. Large print, free. Written for the person with a hearing loss. Explains how to recognize the problem and the reasons, where to go for assessment, gives tips for coping with a hearing loss by the individual, family, and friends, summarizes mechanical devices available, gives resources of organizations and publications.

Hearing Aids. #D13766. Washington, DC: American Association of Retired Persons. Free. Explains audiogram test and how to understand results; describes three most common types of hearing loss, and surveys types of hearing aids. Explains that cost must usually be borne by consumer.

Hearing Impaired/Visually Impaired: Resource Guide. (1991). Bethesda, MD: American Occupational Therapy Association. #4100, $10 AOTA members, $20 non-members. Bibliographies, audiovisuals, and resource personnel.

Now Hear This—A Consumer's Guide to Testing for Hearing Loss, and the Selection and Purchase of a Suitable Hearing Aid. (1992). King of Prussia, PA: Forum. $9.95 plus $3 handling.

SHHH Journal. See Periodicals.

So Now You Have a Telecommunications Device for the Deaf. National Association for Hearing and Speech Action. Guide for people with speech or hearing impairments to using a TDD to communicate effectively and efficiently on the telephone. Single copies free.

Trychin, S., & Wright, F. (1989). *Is That What You Think?* Washington, DC: Gallaudet University. $12, order through Self Help for Hard of Hearing People, Inc.

United States Government TDD Directory. Revised annually. Pueblo, CO: U.S. Consumer Information Center. Free.

PERIODICALS

Hearing Health.
SHHH Journal.

21

The Client with Developmental Delay

Learning to handle food preparation is an important step in attaining independence. Dependence on others for food is often considered the epitome of helplessness. The client with developmental delay, however, has many problems that affect the ability to handle the various facets of meal preparation. These include sensory, mental, and physical difficulties.

Sensory losses alter awareness of one's own body. The kinesthetic or space feedback is hard to gauge, such as when placing objects. Figure-ground perception is disturbed, making it difficult to combine movement and vision. Actions must be deliberately and slowly performed. Singling out an object is hard because of visual inefficiency.

The same skills that are used in activities of daily living and crafts are required for meal preparation. The occupational therapist and other health care professionals may assist the patient to greater skills in homemaking and independence while using other modalities.

There are losses in depth perception, perspective, and discrimination. Spatial constancy is disrupted, so that finding the edge of items when cutting is hard. A guide for cutting reduces this frustration. Aids designed for the blind may be adapted for use here. See the slicing aid in *Mealtime Manual*, Chapter 9.

Concepts like "how much is enough?" are foreign, so measurements must always be used. Color-coded measuring cups and spoons eliminate the need to read numbers. These may be adapted at home with mystic tape or purchased as a set. **Source:** 486. See Resources.

Time is not a concrete concept, so sequences rather than time frames must be used for doing tasks. A large numbered, color-marked timer helps prevent burning. The idea of setting the table while the meal is cooking makes sense to us timewise, but not to the client with developmental delay until sequenced into the schedule.

Disturbances extend to auditory functions. Poor listening skills become evident. When a client has to concentrate on the physical demands and skills, as when opening a can, there is inability to distinguish single sounds at the same time. New information passed on during a physical task interrupts the flow of past information, and action stops.

Physical problems interact with mental ones. Incoordination makes use of tools more difficult. There may be mild or severe unilateral neglect, or hemianopsia, when function on one side is affected.

Concepts are minimal and confined to one object and place. Since a concept taught for one task or place does not carry over or generate to other locations, working within the home or residence is necessary. Repetitions move the tasks from concept to reality. Posters, flip charts, photos, and drawings help the individual retain a sequence and follow it the next time and the next until it becomes habit. Polaroid photos help capture a sequence for more personal and understandable recognition by the client. Illustrated recipes must be used for even simple procedures, like heating soup.

Picture This: An Illustrated Guide to Complete Dinners is for the non-reading cook (Figure 21-1). The author, an occupational therapist, presents 12 main dishes with salads. The illustrations for each recipe, drawn by the creator of Joe Palooka, are divided into Food, Supplies (pans, kitchen utensils, appliances), and What To Do (including periods of time for making salad and setting the table). Handles of measuring cups and spoons are color coded. This book may also be used by patients with aphasia, limited vision, inability to read English, or children helping their parents. **Source:** 486. See Resources.

Life skill programs are designed for helping the person with developmental delay increase independent performance in everyday personal and household chores (Figure 21-2). The Keeping House section includes sheets for Progress Report, Activity Assessment, Routine Assessment, Picture Cards for tasks, and a video with interactive discussion questions on procedure, safety, and sharing jobs. As one example, Kitchen Introduction includes setting and clearing the table, doing dishes, cleaning up, and disposing of garbage. Other subjects focus on shopping, ordering a meal out, and getting involved in the community. Each includes a curriculum package, cue cards package, and teaching video. **Source:** 62. See Resources. *A Home Cooking Picture Cookbook*

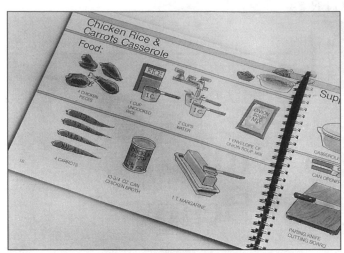

Figure 21-1. *Picture This: An Illustrated Guide to Complete Dinners* is for the non-reading cook. (Photo printed with permission from *Picture This: An Illustrated Guide to Complete Dinners* by Susan Bachner.)

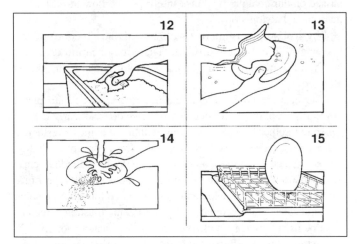

Figure 21-2. The Keeping House Picture Cards for tasks are shown here. (Reprinted with permission from Attainment Company, Inc., Verona, WI.)

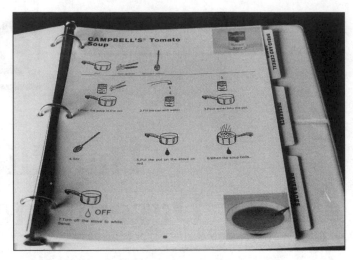

Figure 21-3. *Look 'n Cook* uses name brand products for people with developmental disabilities, non-readers, and beginning cooks. (Reprinted with permission from Attainment Company, Inc., Verona, WI.)

comes with an *Instructor's Guide*, a video, a menu maker for meal planning, and colored picture recipes. **Source:** 62.

Look 'n Cook, a color-coded cookbook, uses name brand products for people with developmental disabilities, non-readers, and beginning cooks (Figure 21-3). It is designed to be used with the total *Look 'n Cook* teaching program. Each recipe is divided into two parts: the items needed for the recipe and the procedure. Both pictures and written instructions are given. Name brand items include soup, baked beans, frozen dinners and pies, other frozen entrees, hamburgers, grilled cheese sandwiches, rice, potatoes, fruits and vegetables, desserts, and beverages. Described as a "survival" book, it gives the user a platform from which to launch into non-readymade food recipes. **Source:** 62.

Changing the order of doing a task confuses the client with developmental delay. Decision making is difficult, and spontaneity may be devastating. A person with developmental delay will do a task exactly the same way each time. Dishes are kept in the same order, food in the same place.

Safety awareness must be constantly reinforced. Planning ahead for contingencies requires the same structural outlines, whether understanding what to do in case of fire or if burned, or having designated emergency meals on hand if there is illness or bad weather.

Flip charts of job sequences help the non-reader learn a new task, such as dishwashing (Figure 21-4). The pictures are arranged in order, with words on the back for the reader. The materials come in book form and must be cut and assembled by the therapist or other health worker. **Source:** 132.

Illustrated cards for shopping and other activities are available for the client with developmental delay (Figure 21-5). **Source:** 62.

Another product, the Supermarket Shopping Passport®, includes 315 picture cards, a 20-compartment divider into which the cards of items needed can be put, a pen, and a storage box. Cost is about $55. The Crestwood Company also makes sets of cards for the drugstore, shopping center, personal needs, fast food and casual dining, and "table talk." Cards might also be used for encouraging planning by the client, increasing vocabulary, and meal planning by selecting foods desired. **Source:** 154.

It may take the client with developmental delay much longer to learn than the person with no learning problems. Once, however, he has learned the basics of food preparation, the level of independence and self-confidence increases. Creativity begins to grow. These skills may now be carried into and shared in the community. Both social activities involving food and a work situation, like salad preparation or dishwashing at a restaurant, become success stories.

Many programs serving a caseload of clients with developmental delay are short-staffed. Able-Net, Inc., has developed a staff training module that offers ways the direct-care staff can use "no-tech" or "low-tech" methods to foster active participation in activities ranging from meal preparation to communication and leisure. The modules include Partial Participation, Electrical Systems, Batter Systems, Output Communication, and Instructional Strategies. For example, an electric mixer attached to an adapted

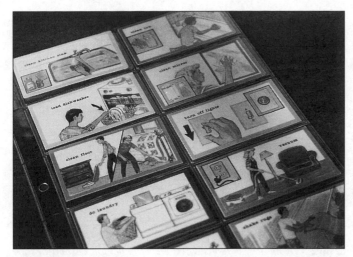

Figure 21-4. Flip charts of job sequences help the non-reader learn a new task, such as dishwashing. [From *Housework: Words and Chores for Daily Living Skills* (Books 1, 2, and 3] by Anita M. Riley and Paula A. Farmer Whitted, copyright 1990 by Communication Skill Builders, Inc., Div. of the Psychological Corporation, San Antonio, TX. Photo printed with permission.)

switch would allow the client to turn on a mixer, while the staff member moved the mixer around the bowl. For information, contact AbleNet, **source** 4.

RESOURCES

Addresses for publishers, periodicals, and organizations are given in Section Four.

PUBLICATIONS

Bachner, S., with illustrations by Tony DiPreta. (1984). *Picture This: An Illustrated Guide to Complete Dinners*. Lexington, KY: Special Additions. Twelve complete meals. $27.50 plus $1.50 postage and handling. Colors are used to match measuring utensils, no reading required. Other materials available from Special Additions include the Meal Preparation Kit containing *Picture This*, color-coded measuring cups and spoons, as well as a page-size magnifying sheet. Cost of measuring set is $17.50 plus $2.75 postage and handling; page magnifier is $5.00 plus $.70 postage per sheet. *Cooking-Up Learning*, how to integrate cognitive processes and goals into specific, food-related activities. Includes instructor's 3-ring manual, $50 plus $4.50 handling. The Shopper's Assistant for adolescents and adults is a set of laminated ingredient cards, instructor's guide, and recommended activities to simplify shopping and enhance skills in visual processing and academic functioning. Cost is $28 plus $2.25 postage and handling. *Effective Assessment and Programming for Kitchen Activities* is a manual to establish background and baseline information for kitchen programming. Cost: $28 plus $3.75 handling and postage. **Source:** 486.

Busselle, R. (1990). *An Exposure of the Heart*. New York: Penguin. $8.95. Author's account of her association with a center for people with developmental disabilities.

Caregiver Education Guide for Children with Developmental Disabilities. Frederick, MD: Aspen Reference Group, Aspen.

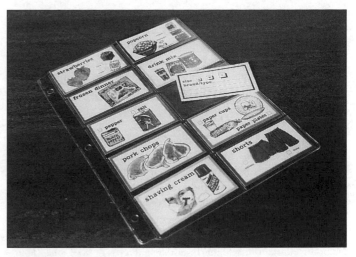

Figure 21-5. Illustrated cards for shopping and other activities are available for the client with developmental delay. (Reprinted with permission from Attainment Company, Inc., Verona, WI.)

$179. Ready-to-use caregiver education checklists, worksheets, forms, plans, and information sheets. Subjects cover common diagnoses, behavior management, psychosocial issues, physical management, home care, activities of daily living, nutrition and feeding, communication technology, care coordination with professionals and family. Annual updates sent on approval.

Developmental Disabilities Adults: Resource Guide. Bethesda, MD: American Occupational Therapy Association. #4240, $10 AOTA members, $20 non-members. Bibliographies, audiovisuals, resource personnel.

Facts About Adult Children with Developmental Disabilities and Their Families. Washington, DC: American Association of Retired Persons. #D15469, free. Discusses how parents, their adult children, service providers, and policy makers can plan together to ensure a secure future.

Gaule, K., Nietupski, J., & Certo, N. Teaching supermarket shopping skills using an adaptive shopping list. *Education and Training of the Mentally Retarded*, 20, 53-59.

Hannah, M. A., et al. (1977). *SCIL: Systemic Curriculum for Independent Living*. Novato, CA: Academic Therapy Publications. Four 3-ring binders, $165. Comprehensive life-skills training for adolescents and adults with learning disabilities. Covers independent skill areas such as money, time, measurement, telephone, home care, community living, and leisure time. Each topic is handled in small, sequential steps that pinpoint behavioral objectives, using checklists, and giving recommended lesson plans to help implement treatment.

Hayes, M. L. (1993). *You Don't Outgrow It: Living with Learning Disabilities*. Novato, CA: Academic Therapy Publications. $16. Problems faced by the person with learning disabilities do not vanish with the advent of maturity, though they do change in degree and emphasis. Subjects covered include family responsibilities, household management, employment, and higher education. Recommended resources.

Kaufman, S. Z. (1988). *Retarded Isn't Stupid, Mom!* Baltimore: Paul H. Brookes. $15. Family's story of their daughter's triumphs and sorrows, real-life events, and increasing independence as she moves toward adulthood.

Kurt, L., & Batshaw, M. (1996). *Handbook of Developmental Disabilities: Resources for Interdisciplinary Care*. Frederick, MD: Aspen. $59. Designed for pediatric services: covers interdisciplinary assessment, management/treatment approaches, orthotics/prosthetics, feeding/nutritional concerns, functional skills training, mobility/ambulation, assistive technology, and planning for adulthood. Includes resource directory.

Steed, F. R. (1977). *A Special Picture Cookbook*. Austin, TX: Pro-Ed Books. $18. Simple to more complex recipes including cake mix, cookies from scratch, green bean casserole, salads, pancakes, stew, and spaghetti. Individual must be able to match letters with can or box and read short phrases for some recipes.

Stumpf, S. H. (1990). *Pathways to Success: Training for Independent Living*. Washington, DC: American Association on Mental Retardation. $22.95. Examines effectiveness of small apartment settings as part of training program for independent living. Gives personal perspectives for program staff, family, and graduates.

Trainer, M. (1991). *Differences in Common: Straight Talk on Mental Retardation, Down Syndrome, and Life*. Bethesda, MD: Woodbine House. $14.95. Essays by a mother evoke the pleasures as well as challenges of raising her son who has Down's Syndrome and is now in his twenties.

PERIODICALS

American Journal on Mental Retardation. American Association on Mental Retardation.

Education and Training of the Mentally and Developmentally Disabled. For professionals.

Exceptional Children, and Exceptional Parents. Written for parents, caregivers, and professionals.

AUDIOVISUALS

See *Caring for Persons with Developmental Disabilities: A Training Program for Respite Care Providers* in Chapter 6.

22

The Client with Traumatic Brain Injury

Helping the individual with a traumatic brain injury (TBI) is an area of increasing concern for institutional and home health care professionals. There are more than 100,000 traumatic brain injuries per year in the United States. Of the 50% of the injured who survive, 9% remain in a coma indefinitely. Nineteen percent are inactive at home and require re-training in the basic activities of daily living, including feeding and self grooming. Seven percent return eventually to former activities but at less than their previous levels, and 15% have a full recovery.

Occupational, speech, and physical therapists, as well as other health care professionals treating TBI patients, must fully assess and then treat the cognitive losses and in some cases the physical limitations. Cognitive problems include short-term memory loss, inability to read or comprehend, inability to organize plans and carry them out, lack of awareness of errors or safety precautions, unrealistic goals, and not anticipating either the consequences or the effect of one's actions on others. Psychosocial problems include sudden emotional shifts in mood, periods of aggressiveness, depression, decreased self-esteem, paranoia, and high- or low-drive sexual issues. These deficits impact on all areas of daily living, including home management and meal preparation.

A significant number of traumatically brain injured clients live for extended periods of time, perhaps their whole lives, in transitional centers. Here they receive behavior management training, counseling, group socialization activities, and medication control. A group homemaking class for clients with traumatic brain injuries allows development of cognitive, physical, and behavioral skills (Figure 22-1). Others receive this training at home with the help of home health care workers and family.

Counseling with and educating the family plays a major role in recovery of both the patient and family. Cooperation, communication, and careful adherence to methods and objectives is necessary for success. Patience on the part of professionals and family is paramount, because rehabilitation can involve many specialties: physical, speech, and occupational therapists; social workers and psychologists; nurses; and physicians. Rehabilitation may last for

months, even years. Finding a support group for both the patient and the family allows sharing and venting of feelings as well as reinforcement of progress.

Cognitive activities within the area of homemaking involve repetition of basic tasks, such as simple food preparation, setting the table, washing dishes, and then a move to planning of meals and shopping. Safety awareness must be stressed and constantly reinforced. Microwave cooking may be indicated if handling burners and ovens appears dangerous or short-term memory is poor. Drawings, check-off lists, and simple charts help reinforcement and learning.

Visual reminders, such as large calendars, carry-along date-books, and specific locations for items like keys, help the individual with short-term memory loss keep better control of his or her immediate surroundings and learning (Figure 22-2). The key holder on the light switch shown is by Design Ideas. **Source:** 167.

Materials designed for people with developmental delay may be used in treating the client with traumatic brain injury. See Chapter 21. There is, however, a big difference when working with patients who have traumatic brain injury. Unlike many clients with developmental delay who have never had the skills for independence, individuals with traumatic brain injuries have lost these skills and grieve for these losses. Rather than being integrated into the community, they are being re-integrated, often at a level lower than when they left it. The depression and feeling of low esteem must be understood and dealt with in order to help the patient with traumatic brain injury recognize success in small or large steps.

A therapist's total skills in cognitive re-training will be called into play when working with individuals with traumatic brain injury. Continuing education courses are held by professional organizations and institutions. See Resources. However, to more fully understand the needs, frustrations, and problems faced by those with traumatic brain injury and their families and to appreciate resources available, one should participate in some of the conferences and organizations for TBI or head injury survivors and their families.

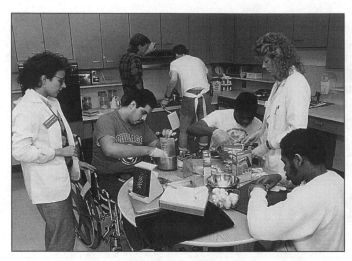

Figure 22-1. A group homemaking class for clients with traumatic brain injuries. (Photo courtesy of the O.T. Dept., Rehabilitation Institute of Chicago.)

Organizations that assist those with traumatic brain injury and their families include the following (addresses are in Appendix C):

- Coma Recovery Association. Provides information on treatment techniques and offers legal services.
- The Family Caregiver Alliance (FCA). Non-profit and advocacy organization assists families of adults with chronic or progressive brain disorders. Publications list on brain disorders and caregiving issues available.
- National Head Injury Foundation, Inc. (NHIF). Leading national support and advocacy group for individuals with head injuries and their families.
- The National Institute of Neurological Disorders and Stroke. Publications list available.
- The Perspectives Network (TPN). Non-profit, service group that organizes forums for people with brain injury where family members and professionals can share concerns. Also provides peer communication network for teens, families, and adults concerned with head injury. Publication list available.
- Research and Training Center on Rehabilitation and Childhood Trauma. Conducts research to increase knowledge of injuries among children. Emphasizes training programs and interventions that can be replicated nationally; produces audiovisuals, curricula/training materials, journal articles, newsletter, and other publications. Information and referral service. Also see Chapter 6 for additional organizations and referral sources.

RESOURCES

Addresses for publishers, periodicals, and organizations are given in Section Four.

PUBLICATIONS

Angle, D. K., & Buston, J. M. (1991). *Community Living Skills Workbook for the Head Injured Adult.* Frederick, MD: Aspen. $83. Treatment activities divided into eight modules: occupational therapy, family education, home management, money management,

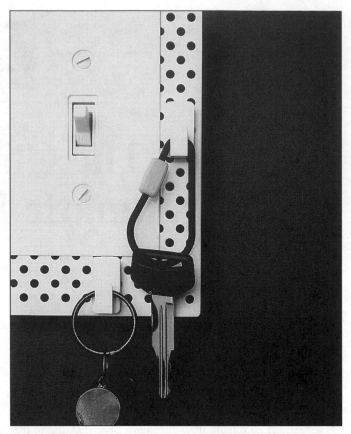

Figure 22-2. Here, an emergency whistle helps the individual with short-term memory loss keep better control of immediate surroundings and learning. (Photo courtesy of Design Ideas, Springfield, IL.)

interpersonal skills, leisure, transportation, and prevocational and vocational skills.

Brain Injury Survivor and Caregiver Education Manual. (1996). Frederick, MD: Aspen Reference Group, Aspen. $169. Comprehensive resource to help families respond to needs of individual with brain injury. Professional's tools include hand-outs, checklists, forms, questionnaires, and charts. Covers children and adults, types of disabilities, psychosocial and behavioral issues, meal planning, transitional living, driving techniques, and community re-integration. Annual supplements sent on 30-day approval.

Cera, R. M., et al. *Patients with Brain Injury.* Vero Beach, FL: The Speech Bin. $6. Guide for families outlines their role, defines eight levels of recovery (Rancho Los Amigos Cognitive Scale), and gives helpful activities. **Source:** 488.

De Boskey, D. S., Hecht, J. S., & Calub, C. (1991). *Educating Families of the Head Injured: Medical, Cognitive, and Social Issues.* Frederick, MD: Aspen. $70. In-depth information for families of severe head injury individuals. Loose-leaf manual allows assembling an individualized resource specific to the needs of the family and patient.

Giles, G. M. (1996). *Coping with Brain Injury: A Guide for Family and Friends.* Bethesda, MD: American Occupational Therapy Association. #1143, $4.50 AOTA members, $5.50 non-members. Defines mild to serious brain injury, prepares caregivers for challenge of helping injured family member get back to activities of daily living, gives realistic expectations for children and adults who have suffered TBI, coping with physical and emotional changes, discusses home, community mobility, and resumption of work.

Head Injury: A NARIC Resource Guide for People with Head Injuries and Their Families. (1994). Washington, DC: National Rehabilitation Information Center. 6-page listing of organizations, periodicals, books, and lists of articles. Free. Also will send listing of independent living centers.

Hoffman, M., et al. (1989). *Brain Injury Rehabilitation: A Manual for Families.* Houston, TX: The Institute for Rehabilitation and Research. $60 plus shipping and handling. Illustrated manual focuses on rehabilitation process (seizure management, sexuality, mobility, cognitive/perceptual, communication, independent living, educational/vocational, and therapeutic recreation/leisure skills). Aims to help family understand effects of TBI, participate in rehabilitation process, adjust to changes in role and relationship, and become aware of resources for assistance.

Hughes, B. K. (1990). *Parenting a Child with Traumatic Brain Injury.* Springfield, IL: Charles Thomas. $15.95.

The Institute for Rehabilitation and Research, Rehabilitation Interventions in TBI, TIRR-Department of Education, Houston, has a national database of educational resources on traumatic brain injury. Includes videos and non-published materials. Complete listing of all materials is $50. Printouts of two resources are available at no charge.

Kreutzer, J., & Wehrman, P. H. *Cognitive Rehabilitation for Persons with Traumatic Brain Injury.* Vero Beach, FL: The Speech Bin. $39.95. All phases of cognitive assessment and intervention; using games, computer treatment, re-training memory, community and workplace re-entry. Chart of mass-market games with suggestions for use.

Lazzari, A. *Help for Memory.* East Moline, IL: Lingui Systems. $34.95. For clients eight years old to adult with memory deficits or learning disabilities. Strategies for selecting, organizing, and retrieving information, coding and grouping, using aids, applying memory techniques. Exercises, tip sheets, and carry-over activities.

Mebane, W.M., Jr. (1991). *Getting Our Heads Together: A Helpful Handbook for Families of Head-Injured People* (rev. ed.). Asheville, NC: Thoms Rehabilitation Hospital, Inc. of W.N.C.

Miller, C., & Campbell, K. (1987). *From the Ashes: A Head Injury Self-Advocacy Guide.* Seattle, WA: Phoenix Project. $20 plus $5 shipping. Handbook written by two women with brain injuries. Addresses functional and psychological problems, finding treatment, psychic pain, and life changes. Bibliography and glossary.

National Head Injury Association. (1994). *National Directory of Head Injury Rehabilitation Services.* Washington, DC: NHIA. $40. Detailed list of thousands of services, including rehabilitation programs.

New York State Head Injury Association. (1991). *For Families from Families: What They Told Us About Having a Child with a Traumatic Brain Injury.* Albany, NY: New York State Head Injury Association. $3; and *Sisters and Brothers, Brothers and Sisters in the Family Affected by Traumatic Brain Injury,* $3.

Nightingale, N. R., & Jennifer L. (1992). *Step-by-Step Meals for People with Cognitive Challenges.* San Antonio, TX: Therapy Skill Builders. $66. Menus are designed to promote good nutrition, safety, reduce need for adaptive devices, and use easy-to-find ingredients. Each menu includes Meal Preparation Schedule, Kitchen Checklist, and Preparation Process.

Occupational Therapy Practice Guidelines for Adults with Traumatic Brain Injury. (1996). Bethesda, MD: American Occupational Therapy Association. $20 AOTA members, $25 non-members. 16-page reference tool for health care facility managers, managed care organizations, third-party payers, and occupational therapy practitioners. Defines evaluation, frequency, duration of treatment, explains patient care management, and gives billing codes.

O'Hara, C. C., & Harrell, M. (1990). *Rehabilitation with Brain Injury Survivors: An Empowerment Approach.* Frederick, MD: Aspen. $85. 110 specific evaluation and assessment checklist items; list for relatives to use in observing TBI survivor's memory, language, and other skills; 202-point checklist for assessing independent skills in personal health, safety, household management, consumer skills, and more. Covers physical, cognitive, behavioral.

Parrot Software has several computer programs for aiding in the rehabilitation of people with traumatic brain injury. Some that relate to homemaking include *Making Change for Money Plus,* Windows, $134.95; *Cooking Time Management Plus,* Windows, $79.95; *Compensatory Memory Strategies: Chunking Plus,* Windows, $134.95. A complete descriptive catalog is available.

Rosenthal, M., et al. (1989). *Rehabilitation of the Adult and Child with Traumatic Brain Injury* (2nd ed.). (1989). Philadelphia: F.A. Davis. $75. Nature of the problem from onset of injury into re-entry into the community: early assessment and evaluation, specific problems related to head injury, specialized assessments (psychiatric, OT, PT, ST, neuropsychological, treatment approaches, rehabilitation of the child with traumatic brain injury).

Senelick, R. C., & Ryan, C. (1991). *Living with Head Injury: A Guide for Families.* New York: Demos. $12.95. Step-by-step guide through process of rehabilitation.

Traumatic Brain Injury: Resource Guide. Bethesda, MD: American Occupational Therapy Association. #4130, $10 AOTA members, $20 non-members. Bibliographies, audiovisuals, resource personnel.

PERIODICALS

See Appendix D for addresses and rates.

Cognitive Rehabilitation. Bi-monthly, multidisciplinary journal.

Continuing Care.

Exceptional Children. For parents, caregivers, and professionals.

Exceptional Parent. Publication for parents of children with disabilities.

Journal of Cognitive Rehabilitation. Professional multidisciplinary publication.

Journal of Head Injury: A Search for Understanding. Articles by and for head-injury survivors and health care professionals on the recovery process.

The Journal of Head Trauma Rehabilitation. Clinical management and rehabilitation of people with head injuries.

L.I.N.K.S. (Living in New Kinds of Situations). Monthly, $45. For people with developmental disabilities. Order through the

National Association for Private Residential Resources.

National Head Injury Foundation Newsletter. Quarterly, for families and professionals.

This Brain Has a Mouth. Magazine by and for head injury survivors. Resources and experiences from survivor's perspective.

Update. San Francisco, CA: Family Survival Project. Articles for families with adults who have organic or traumatic brain injuries. Book reviews, resources.

AUDIOVISUALS

See Chapter 21.

Golfus, F., & Simpson, D. E. *When Billie Broke His Head...And Other Tales of Wonder*. 57-minute VHS video, Order No. CM-136, $245. Award-winning journalist, brain injured in an accident 10 years ago, meets people with disabilities around the country, as he searches for "intelligent life after brain damage." Available from Fanlight Productions. **Source:** 200.

CONTINUING EDUCATION

Courses on traumatic brain injury and re-training are held at several institutions around the country. These include the Howard A. Rusk Institute of Rehabilitation Medicine, New York University Medical Center, and the Rehabilitation Institute of Chicago.

23

The Client Who Has Cancer

Good nutrition is an important part of the medical program for an individual with cancer. The person who is properly nourished and has a diet high in protein and calories is better able to tolerate the stresses of cancer and treatment. The body's natural defenses against disease are stronger. Recovery from surgery is faster, because the nutrients help rebuild tissue.

Sometimes, the side effects of cancer treatment seem worse than the disease. Eating problems as a result of chemotherapy and radiation may be divided into five major categories: nausea and vomiting, loss of appetite, mouth soreness and dryness, fatigue, and intestinal upset. Other reactions include changes in taste and feelings of fullness. Patients who eat a good diet during treatment periods, however, have less severe side effects.

There are many ways that more than 80% of patients receiving treatment can reduce the effects of chemotherapy. Encourage your client to inform the oncologist about side effects, or speak with the doctor yourself. Nausea and vomiting affects between 40% and 80% of people undergoing chemotherapy. Counseling your patient in advance helps avoid a pre-determined response (known as the stomach flip-flop when entering the clinic). Encourage the client to eat foods that travel through the stomach quickly, including milk shakes, gelatin, ice cream, and puddings. Nibbling on starchy foods, such as crackers or toast, or sipping cool drinks like lemonade can also relieve nausea. Avoid fatty, fried foods, which take longer to digest. Schedule rests after a meal so that the food digests more quickly. Activity slows down digestion. The physician may also prescribe anti-emetic drugs.

Nutritionists recommend a diet high in protein and carbohydrates. The patient should eat small amounts of food frequently with plenty of fluids between meals. Part of your role as a health care professional includes finding a nutritional diet that meets the patient's needs.

You may also be concerned with reducing energy expenditure so the individual can perform as much of the meal preparation as he or she wants. Counsel with other members of the family, emphasizing the importance of good nutrition and showing ways they can prepare easy-to-swallow and digest, highly concentrated, nutritional foods.

Making a menu plan, even plotting the caloric intake with a calorie counter, helps the patient and family ensure that the patient is getting enough to eat. The dietitian will help make out a balanced daily menu plan. It should include the following:

- Dairy products: Two or more servings of milk or other dairy products.
- Meat, other proteins: Two or more four-ounce servings of meat, poultry, fish, or eggs. Alternate sources are peanut butter, dried beans, peas, or nuts.
- Vegetables: Two or more ½-cup servings, with one a dark green, leafy or yellow vegetable.
- Fruit: Two or more ½-cup servings, with one being citrus juice or fruit.
- Bread or cereals: Four or more servings. One serving is one slice of bread, one cup of cold cereal, or ½ cup of rice, pasta, or grits.

Most cancer patients lose weight because they do not take in as much food as their bodies need. Recipes for highly concentrated foods will maximize nutritional intake. Use whole milk, half-and-half cream, and evaporated milk rather than water when preparing cereals, soups, puddings, and cocoa. Double milk is another suggestion: add equivalent amounts of dry milk powder to regular milk for puddings, cheesecake, pasta sauces, and other foods. High-protein foods like cheese, rich ice cream, and eggs may be used. Other calorie enhancing tips include the following:

- Stirring a pat of butter or margarine into hot foods, including cereals, soups, rice, pasta, and eggs.
- Using cream as a topping for desserts, poured over cereal, and in sauces with meat and fish.
- Serving sour cream on potatoes and vegetables and in gravies and salad dressings, and mixing it into mashed potatoes or with brown sugar to top fruits.
- Adding ice cream to milkshakes, even those made with nutritional supplements.
- Mixing extra mayonnaise into salads and sandwich fillings.

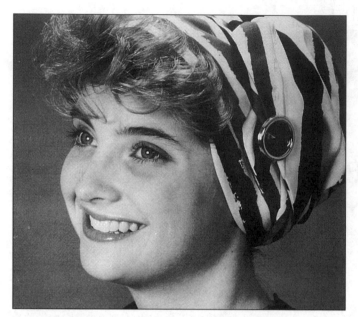

Figure 23-1. The Headliner is a fashionable, comfortable cover-up for women. (Photo courtesy of Designs for Comfort, Inc., Northfield, IL.)

- Spreading peanut butter on banana and apple slices, mixing it with sour cream if it is too dry.

Proper oral hygiene helps keep the mouth free of sores. Teach the client to rinse his or her mouth with a solution of warm water, salt, and baking soda and to use a soft toothbrush to keep gums and teeth clean. Avoid mouthwashes, foods, and beverages that contain alcohol.

Pureed and mashed foods are easiest to swallow. Mousses made with double milk, milkshakes, and yogurt are soothing. Highly spiced foods and those rough in texture should be avoided. A food processor or blender is an essential, energy-saving appliance for the preparation of easy-to-swallow food. See Resources for books with recipes. Commercial supplements may also be recommended to achieve the desired nutritional level. See Resources in Chapter 4.

Foods that are soft in texture and high in calories and protein include bread and rice pudding (made with extra liquid), chocolate milk and cocoa, cheesecake, cottage cheese (4% fat), cream soups, custards and puddings, eggnog, eggs soft-cooked, scrambled, made into an omelet, or chopped in salad, gelatin salads, hot cereals with milk or cream, ice cream, sherbet and frozen yogurt, malted milk, meat and fish salads, milkshakes, mousses, nutritional supplements (commercial), pureed and baby foods, and soufflés. See the *Non-Chew Cookbook* under Resources in Chapter 5.

When cramps and diarrhea are side effects, avoid chewing gum and foods that cause gas. Encourage your client to eat slowly and often, having small meals in a relaxed atmosphere. Reduce both roughage for a period of time and foods prepared with sugar. The physician may recommend that your patient eat foods high in potassium to replace what has been lost. Potassium-rich foods include bananas, red meat, potatoes, salt-water fish, and mushrooms.

Constipation is a common side effect of pain medication and some anti-cancer drugs. When this is the case, increase roughage—add prune juice as a beverage, cooked prunes stirred into cereal, or prune whip. Grating raw fruits and vegetables makes them easier to swallow. Encourage liquids and light exercise.

If possible, incorporate walks into your client's daily schedule, both to help the digestive process and to reduce stress. Relaxation techniques, such as imagery and meditation, often reduce stress that affects appetite.

Fatigue is a devastating, often unexpected, side effect. Teach the patient to pace activities and focus on priorities. During periods of chemotherapy or radiation treatment, set up transportation programs to reduce stress on the patient. If family or friends are not available, volunteers can often be found through a church or the local chapter of the American Cancer Society®. Emphasize the need to delegate household tasks that are tiring and not worth the effort. Find funding sources for aides or volunteers who will take over jobs like cleaning, shopping, and laundry. Set up a schedule that allows rest periods during the day and includes an appropriate level of physical exercise to reduce tension. Recommend respite times when friends or relatives can care for the children or for the patient, letting spouse and children get away.

The person who is receiving chemotherapy may have some loss of sensation and tingling in the hands and toes. When in the kitchen, make sure that oven mitts are worn when using the stove or oven. Feet should always be protected with shoes or slippers.

The woman who has had a mastectomy may require physical and occupational therapy to help reduce edema in the upper extremity, to strengthen affected muscles, to learn one-handed techniques, and to help adapt undergarments and other clothing. The Reach to Recovery program offers volunteer counseling through the American Cancer Society®.

Part of post-surgical and post-chemo or post-radiation therapy may include encouraging your client to face the days ahead with hope and confidence. Programs like Reach to Recovery with peer contact and books like *Cancervive* can help.

A patient who has suffered side effects of treatment, such as hair loss or radiation burns, may shy away from social contact, even sitting at the table with the family. As a health care worker, you can increase self-esteem by suggesting ways to improve appearance. Wigs, combination cap and hairpieces, and cosmetic programs all increase a sense of security and well-being.

The American Cancer Society® with the Cosmetic, Toiletry and Fragrance Association program Look Good...Feel Better helps the individual improve both appearance and self-image through devices such as cosmetics and wigs. For information, call the local chapter or 800-395-LOOK. TLC, a mail-order firm created by the American Cancer Society® for breast cancer survivors, sells items from headwraps to breast prostheses and lingerie. **Source:** 529. Special clothing for cancer patients is discussed in *Clothing for People With Special Needs*. See Appendix F.

The Headliner is a fashionable, comfortable cover-up for women who have alopecia (hair loss) from chemotherapy or have limited hand function that makes grooming difficult and fatiguing (Figure 23-1). The washable, adjustable cap creates an illusion of a full head of hair as well as providing warmth and comfort for sensitive scalps. It comes in a variety of fabrics and 14 hair colors. Cost is about $15 to $20 for scarves and turbans, $14 and up for the hairpiece. The Headliner is available through local wig, post-mastectomy, and home health care stores. Private insurance carriers usually accept Headliner as a reimbursable item when accompanied by a doctor's refillable prescription for a "medical hair prosthesis." **Manufacturer** and **source:** 166B.

See special eating utensils for sensitive mouths in Chapter 5.

Resources for information and support include the local chapter of the American Cancer Society®, the American Brain Tumor Association, Make Today Count, National Leukemia Association, National Lymphedema Network, the Cancer Information Service, National Institutes of Health, and Y-Me. See organizations listed in under Cancer in Appendix C. Local programs through hospitals and visiting nurse associations frequently present the "I Can Cope" course. This series of six sessions covers the disease process, daily health problems, nutrition, living with limitations, expressing feelings, and locating resources. Speakers vary but usually include physicians, physical and occupational therapists, a chaplain, social worker, and an attorney.

RESOURCES

Addresses for publishers, periodicals, and organizations are given in Section Four.

PUBLICATIONS

The American Brain Tumor Association provides patient services and educational materials plus funds research. Free publications include *Basic Series: AFBTR Dictionary, A Primer of Brain Tumors, Coping with a Brain Tumor, Living with a Brain Tumor—A Bibliography, When Your Child is Ready to Return to School,* plus a tumor series that covers various types of tumors and therapies. Additional publications cover Support Group Information, Treatment Facilities Listing, and Using a Medical Library. A newsletter, the *Message Line,* describes research advances and updates to their publications. There is no charge to patients for services.

Anderson, G. (1990). *The Cancer Conqueror: An Incredible Journey to Wellness.* New York: Andrews and McMeel. $7.95. Step-by-step transformation from despair to hope and a positive attitude by an individual with lung cancer.

Bloch, A. S. (1990). *Nutrition Management of the Cancer Patient: A Practical Guide for Professionals.* Frederick, MD: Aspen. $54.50. Nutritional problems and needs of cancer patients, dysphagia, cancers that affect swallowing or digestion, impact of therapies, home care, resources, and references.

Bloch, A., & Bloch, R. (1992). *Fighting Cancer: A Step-by-Step Guide to Helping Yourself Fight Cancer.* Bethesda, MD: National Cancer Institute. Free manual of inspiration and tips by a couple who successfully fought husband's disease.

Bruning, N. (1991). *Coping with Chemotherapy.* New York: Ballantine, Random House. $3.95. Author went through chemotherapy.

Cancer: Resource Guide. Bethesda, MD: American Occupational Therapy Association. #4210, $10 AOTA members, $20 non-members. Bibliographies, audiovisuals, resource personnel.

Chemotherapy and You. (1991). Washington, DC: National Cancer Institute. NIH Publication No. 92-1136. Free book for patients available from the Institute. Suggestions for patient to help self.

Cox, B. G., Carr, D. T., & Lee, R. E. (1987). *Living with Lung Cancer* (2nd ed.). Gainesville, FL: Triad. $7.95. Guide for patients and their families describes diagnostic tests, treatments, and side effects.

Drum, D. (1996). *Making the Chemotherapy Decision.* Los Angeles: Lowell House. $27. Part I—Medical aspects including drugs used and side effects, being an active patient; Part II—Nutrition, appearance, emotional support, stress-relieving techniques, when therapy doesn't work.

Eating Hints: Recipes and Tips for Better Nutrition During Cancer Treatment. (1987). Bethesda, MD: National Cancer Institute, U.S. Department of Health and Human Services, Public Health Service, National Institutes of Health. Publication No. 87-2079, free.

Edge, F. (1995). *Borrowed Time: Living with Cancer with Someone You Love.* Lantzville, BC: Oolichan Books. $14.95. Husband draws on his personal experience as a support person to provide insights into living with cancer. Gives resources.

Facing Forward: A Guide for Cancer Survivors. (1990, July). NIH Publications No. 90-2424. Free from the National Cancer Institute. Covers emotions, appearance, insurance, continued health care, employment.

Hart, J. (1993). *Love, Judy: Letters of Hope and Healing for Women with Breast Cancer.* Berkeley, CA: Conari. $10.95. Author has faced two bouts of breast cancer and shares her model of focusing on living during challenging life experiences such as cancer.

Kaura, S. K. (1991). *A Family Doctor's Guide to Understanding and Preventing Cancer: Environmental Risks and Solutions.* Santa Fe, NM: Health Press. $24.95.

Kohlenberg, S. (1993). *Sammy's Mommy Has Cancer.* New York: Magination Press, Brunner/Mazel. $9. Children learn that a person with serious illness has good days and bad days. Read together as a family, it offers a sense of safety and encouragement at a frightening time.

Love, S. (1991). *Dr. Susan Love's Breast Book.* Reading, MA: Addison-Wesley.

Management of Cancer Pain. Free booklet from the Agency for Health Care Policy and Research Publications Clearinghouse.

Nessim, S. (1991). *Cancervive: The Challenge of Life After Cancer.* Boston: Houghton Mifflin.

Oncology Patient Education Manual. Frederick, MD: Aspen Reference Group, Aspen. $210. For all practitioners working with oncology patients. Practical hand-outs, charts, diagrams, questionnaires, instruction sheets. Covers prevention, pre- and postoperative care, rehabilitation, pain management, palliative interventions, psychological issues, nutrition, and nutrition-related side effects. Annual supplements sent on 30-day approval.

Taking Time: Support for People with Cancer and the People Who Care About Them. Washington, DC: National Cancer Institute. Free.

When the Woman You Love Has Breast Cancer. Y-Me National Association for Cancer Information and Support, Inc. Free.

When Someone in Your Family Has Cancer and *Talking with Your Child About Cancer.* National Cancer Institute. Free.

When Your Brother or Sister Has Cancer. American Cancer Society. Free.

Zacharian, B. (1996). *The Activist Cancer Patient: How to Take Charge of Your Treatment.* New York: Wiley. $14.95.

Background of treatments and communicating with physician. How to find relevant information and support groups.

ORGANIZATIONS

Candlelighters—assists parents of young children with cancer, peer support.

Make-A-Wish Foundation—for children with terminal illness.

Make Today Count—for people with cancer and their families.

Reach to Recovery—for women who have had mastectomies, visitation by peers, through local cancer societies.

The Starlight Foundation—for children.

Y-Me National Breast Cancer Organization—has men's hotline to assist husbands of patient with cancer.

PERIODICALS

Cancer Smart. New York: Memorial Sloan-Kettering Cancer Center. See Periodicals.

COPING Magazine.

Premix Post, Baxter Healthcare Corporation. **Source:** 79. Quarterly newsletter informs customers of products and services from the company as well as recent developments and opportunities in cancer care.

AUDIOVISUALS

Surviving Cancer: The Road Ahead. VHS, 60 minutes. Aurora Publishing Co., $39.95. **Source:** 63. Men and women who survived cancer help newly diagnosed patients understand the confusing, intimidating world of treatment and recovery.

Also see Chapter 5

Fiore, N. A. (1984). *The Road Back to Health: Coping with the Emotional Side of Cancer.* New York: Bantam Doubleday Dell. $4.50.

Graham, J. (1982). *In the Company of Others: Understanding the Human Needs of Cancer Patients.* New York: Harcourt Brace Jovanovich.

Johnson, J., & Klein, L. *I Can Cope: Staying Healthy with Cancer.* Wayzata, MN: DCI Publications. $8.95. One of the authors is an oncology nurse who co-founded the American Cancer Society's "I Can Cope" program. Emphasizes need for good communications with specifics on clarifying feelings and enhancing self-esteem.

Kaufmann, D. (1987). *Surviving Cancer—A Practical Guide for Those Fighting to Win.* Washington, DC: Acropolis Books Ltd.

Margie, J. D., & Bloch, A. S. (1983). *Nutrition and the Cancer Patient.* Radnor, PA: Chilton. $11.95. Resources, references, and recipes for coping with cancer. Written for professional and lay people.

Mitchell, J. S. (1988). *Winning the Chemo Battle.* New York: Norton. $9.95.

Benjamin, H. H., with Turbo, R. (1987). *From Victim to Victor: The Wellness Community Guide to Fighting for Recovery for Cancer Patients and Their Families.* Los Angeles: Jeremy P. Tarcher. $15.95. Distributed by St. Martin's Press.

Dodd, M. J. (1987). *Managing the Side Effects of Chemotherapy and Radiation.* New York: Prentice Hall. $12.95. Consumer's guide to managing the side effects of treatment, nutritional advice, recipes, Self-Care Behavior Log with worksheets for communicating with health care workers.

Section Two

IN AND AROUND THE KITCHEN AND THE HOME

Safety in the Home

A safety assessment of the client's entire home should be part of every home management rehabilitation program. Involving the patient through use of a checklist is one way of noting problems and gives an outline for follow-up and changes. A detailed house tour checklist that can be used with your client to pinpoint hazards is available through Serif Press. Free brochures and booklets for making a house survey are available through other agencies as well. See Resources.

Neat housekeeping is essential to safety. Scatter rugs, loose papers, spills, clutter, and extension cords all can cause accidents. Falls and fires are two major causes of casualty and death among the elderly. Broken or faulty equipment that needs repair is a common problem, from loose handles, warped steps, and wobbly railings to frayed wires.

While the client is involved with meal preparation tasks, the therapist or other health care professional should continue the safety assessment through careful observation. This includes factors such as what the patient wears, i.e., loose long sleeves, floppy slippers, or long robes (older women who are losing height because of osteoporosis frequently have hems that need to be shortened for safety), the adequacy of lighting in the food preparation and cooking areas, the ability to carry or handle items within the house, and the way of handling the stove and appliances.

Is the area around the stove top free of flammable objects? Are burners turned off immediately? Are handles of pans kept to side or rear so they do not extend out from the cooktop? Are important controls located at the back of the stove, necessitating reaching over lit burners and hot pots? This is increasingly the case with better models of gas stoves. Modification with a properly designed cooktop or a change to microwave oven cooking are the best answers, but they are hard to make with an older homemaker who is reluctant to change or with an individual who has limited funds. Use of portable appliances can reduce reliance on a gas stove. A discussion with family members might help the transition.

Safety for Older Consumers: Home Safety Checklist asks questions and illustrates the dangers (Figure 24-1). In the photograph, the danger of wearing long sleeves while reaching over a burner

is paired with a question and the statistic that 70% of all people who die from clothing fires are older than 65 years of age. The suggestion is that long, loose sleeves should be rolled back and fastened with pins or elastic bands while working. Two other solutions are to eliminate the sleeves or use Velcro® bands to hold them while working. See Resources.

The National Burn Information Exchange found that two of every three burn cases are due to clothing ignition. Victims tend to be the very young, very old, and those with a disability. The health care professional can recommend changes in clothing selection to the patient and family. Cotton and linen burn quickly but can be made fire-retardant. Wool is safest and burns slowly, extinguishing itself. Some man-made materials burn quickly; others have melting and dripping properties that cause danger. Showing the consumer how to read labels, understand the properties of the fabric, and make sure a garment is treated is an additional facet of training. A brushed or piled surface, for example, which exposes tiny fiber ends, is highly conducive to flash burning. Garments for both the young and the elderly require careful selection.

SAFE FOOTING

Safety assessment involves checking for obstacles like furniture or wires, a telephone cord where people walk, poor lighting, uneven steps, loose rugs, or the lack of a rubber mat in the tub. Falls are one of the most common accidents, especially among the elderly. The second leading cause of accidental death in the United States, more than 12,000 in the home per year, falls are topped only by motor vehicle accidents. Older people with hip weakness, poor balance, and those using prescription medicines run the greatest risk of falling. See Chapter 1. Serious injuries result 10% to 25% of the time. A Personal Emergency Response System may be indicated for the person who is apt to fall and is alone much of the time. See Chapter 3.

Inattention is the major reason for falls. "Watch your step" should be the clarion cry. Lack of awareness of obstacles, such as

KITCHEN
CHECK THE RANGE AREA

Are towels, curtains, and other things that might catch fire located away from the range?

    yes   no

Do you avoid wearing clothing with long, loose sleeves while you are cooking?

    yes   no

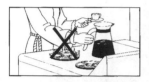

Do not wear clothing with long, loose sleeves while you are cooking.

Do you avoid using a gas range or oven to heat your home?

    yes   no

Are kitchen ventilation systems or range exhausts functioning properly and are they in use while you are cooking?

    yes   no

Placing or storing non-cooking equipment like pot holders, dish towels, or plastic utensils on or near the range may result in fires or burns.
• Store flammable and combustible items away from range and oven.
• Remove any towels hanging on oven handles. If towels hang close to a burner, change the location of the towel rack.
• Shorten or remove curtains which could brush against heat sources.

CPSC estimates that 70% of all people who die from clothing fires are over 65 years of age. Long, loose sleeves are more likely to catch fire than are short sleeves. Long, loose sleeves are also more apt to catch on pot handles, overturning pots and pans and causing scalds.
• Roll back long, loose sleeves or fasten them with pins or elastic bands while you are cooking.

When you use gas appliances to heat your home, they can produce deadly amounts of carbon monoxide.
• Never use your range or oven to heat your home.

Indoor air pollutants may accumulate to unhealthful levels in a kitchen where gas or kerosene-fired appliances are in use.
• Use ventilation systems or open windows to clear air of vapors and smoke.

Figure 24-1. The danger of wearing long sleeves while reaching over a burner. (U.S. Product Safety Commission, Washington, DC.)

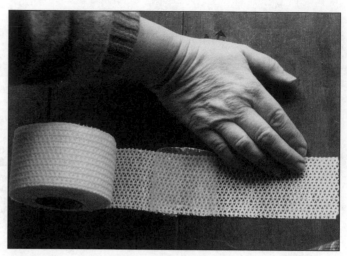

Figure 24-2. A double-adhesive strip, called "Lok-Lift," adheres to the rug and floor. (Photo by J.K.)

rug edges, toys, and items left on the stairs for carrying up or down; hurrying or thinking about something else; depression; peripheral neuropathies; poor eyesight; side effects of medication; and not looking where one is going are the main causes of an individual falling.

Cultivating safe practices reduces the chances of an accident. The first two basic steps are instilling the need to go slow and to clear all stairwells. Stairs should never be used for storage; yesterday's newspaper or a single garment can lead to a serious slip. Teach your client to keep a basket next to the steps for gathering items together into a reasonable load for him- or herself or the family.

The third step in evaluation is checking the construction of stair treads. In older homes, these may be warped or loose and need repair before causing an accident. Adding a second railing will increase safety going up and down, especially when the client is limited to use of one hand. If the person tends to walk at night or awaken confused, a gate at the top of the stairs, a remote or touch control light beside the bed, and night lights illuminating the way to the bathroom should be installed. Outside the home, steps may be given a non-slip surface with a combination of sand and paint.

Increasing visual discrimination on steps is helped by adding extra light that does not cause a glare or cast shadows. Switches at both ends of the stairs prevent groping in the dark. A wireless, wall switch may be installed at the most convenient place for turning on a lamp up to 50 feet away. Cost is about $35 from hardware stores and mail-order firms. **Source:** 262. Another answer is a sensor light that goes on automatically when there is movement within a certain radius, usually about 15 feet, and shuts off automatically after about four minutes. Cost of a sensor light is about $30 and up from hardware stores and mail-order firms. **Sources:** 96, 255.

Painting a white strip on the edge of each basement or other tread in a darkened staircase, or painting the top step and a space

at the bottom on the floor white increases contrast and safety. Where it is not possible to paint, fluorescent, light- or bright-colored tape can be put along the edge of each step.

Two-thirds of falls occur without changing levels in the home—the rug edge, the forgotten spill, wet leaves, ice, uneven pavement, even relatives of the banana peel. Proper footwear helps ensure against falls. Untied shoes are a ticket to misadventure; elastic laces or Velcro® closures are an insurance policy for those who cannot bend and tie. Crepe, rubber soles provide the greatest skid resistance; leather, the least; standard rubber and neoprene fall in between. Use of a tripod or quad cane helps provide extra security in both familiar and strange surroundings.

Removing small scatter rugs is a primary safety precaution (Figure 24-2). Securing rugs that the patient insists on keeping is the second step. A double-adhesive strip, called "Lok-Lift," adheres to the rug and floor. The knitted cellulose and plastic mesh, which is impregnated with acrylic adhesive, eliminates slipping of rugs but still lets them be lifted for cleaning. **Manufacturer:** 391. Cost is about $12 and up per roll from hardware stores and mail-order firms. **Sources:** 239, 262, 476. Also see carpet tapes and mats in *Mealtime Manual* under Safety in your Kitchen and Around Your Home.

Teaching a client how to fall safely is usually done by a physical therapist. Principles include the following:
• Stay relaxed and do not stiffen; crumple like a sack, rolling onto padded or fleshy parts of the body.
• Turn the body to one side while falling to land on a well-padded area—the thigh or side of the buttocks.
• Keep the fingers relaxed and spread wide apart with arms outstretched, but not locked.

Reaching to change light bulbs or to get a seldom used dish from a top shelf can lead to falls. Temporary or makeshift supports result in permanent injuries. A client should be taught to ask others to get items needed or change bulbs.

On infrequent occasions, an ambulatory patient who is steady on his or her feet needs to reach items stored in upper cabinets. Although step stools are usually not recommended, it is better to teach the correct way and use the right stool than to ignore the problem. The stool should be stable and have a handle to hold onto while standing on the top step. Any loose screws or braces must be tightened.

The step stool shown in Figure 24-3 has a rubber-covered base and a high handle for holding while reaching. It is available through hospital supply firms. Cost is about $84. **Sources:** 90, 105, 198, 461, 580.

FIRE SAFETY

Many potential causes of fire may be prevented with simple modifications to the home. This includes electrical units, such as lights and appliances, as well as storage around the stove and actual use of the range. When a client insists on smoking, use of cigarettes in bed must be banned; ashtrays should be deep and non-tippable; and the patient taught to snuff out cigarettes completely. The Fire Safety Check by the National Association of Home Builders includes a safety checklist designed to aid older people in reducing the risk and incidence of fire in their homes. See Resources.

In older homes, electrical safety is often a concern with overloaded outlets and frayed wires. Extension cords should not be run under rugs, through holes in the wall or floors, or strung through doorways. Constant wear rubs off the insulated covering and may start a fire. Appliances must be unplugged before cleaning, even with a damp sponge or cloth; few appliances are immersible. If a patient is forgetful, a timer is a good insurance aid while cooking. As part of planning for home assessments, call or write the U.S. Consumer Product Safety Commission (CPSC) to obtain an free home audit checklist and guide. See Resources.

In an older home, your client may be depending on extension cords to provide power for lights and other appliances. Be sure that the cord being used is rated to handle the demands of the appliances plugged into it. Check the wattage rating on the label, then add the wattage of the appliances plugged into it. If amperage is listed instead of wattage, multiply the amp rating by 110 to obtain the allowed wattage. Electrical products are rated by independent testing organizations such as Underwriters Laboratories. If the power requirements are more than the cord's rating, your client needs to get another cord. Do not let the individual client use an extension cord with any heating appliance or with a vacuum cleaner, unless it is a heavy-duty cord designed for use with powerful machines. If any extension cord or outlet feels warm to the touch or if appliances plugged into an extension cord cause a fuse to blow or circuit breaker to trip, the cord should be immediately replaced.

When too many electrical wires are a problem, a Velcro® kit organizes and separates wires. Kits are available through hardware and office supply stores. **Manufacturer:** 557.

Discuss handling of a stove or kitchen fire with the client. Then have the instructions repeated back to you. Install missing safety aids. Rules for preparing for and handling a fire are given in a reproducible form in Appendix G.

Smoke detectors and power failure lights should be part of every person's home but are especially important for the person who is immobilized or has difficulty seeing or hearing. Smoke detector batteries should be changed every six months: "Change your watch, change your battery" is an easy slogan to remember. One type of smoke detector screws into the light fixture. The bat-

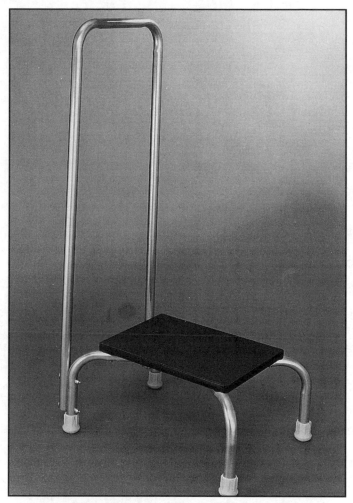

Figure 24-3. This step stool has a rubber-covered base and a high handle for holding while reaching. (Photo courtesy of Winco, Inc., Ocala, FL.)

tery is constantly recharged. Cost is about $35 from mail-order firms. **Sources:** 482, 508.

Power-failure lights should be placed in areas of the house where the client would be walking in the event of a power failure, i.e., bedroom, bathroom, hallways, and kitchen (Figure 24-4). The unit stores up power while the electricity is on, then comes on immediately when power is cut. The one shown costs about $15 from housewares, hardware, and variety stores, or through mail-order firms. It also serves as a flashlight and may be carried around the house if required. **Manufacturers** include 87, 221, 463. **Sources:** 96, 159, 255, 262.

Some patients, such as those with multiple sclerosis or peripheral neuropathies, while ambulatory, cannot function without seeing where their feet are. For them, having a security light that goes on when power fails can mean the difference between being independent and having an accident.

Portable appliances should always be unplugged when not in use. This includes units with on-off switches and toasters or toaster ovens. Fires have erupted from the new thermoplastic appliances like coffeemakers and toasters even when off, but plugged in and hit by an electrical short or other disturbance. Thermoplastic is highly combustible, and the fire spreads quickly.

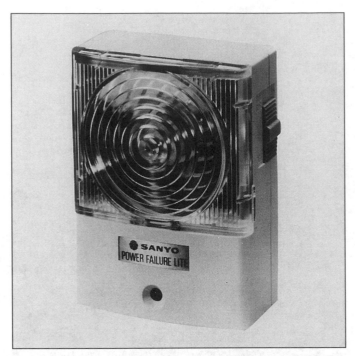

Figure 24-4. This unit stores up power while electricity is on, then comes on immediately when power is cut. (Photo courtesy of Sanyo Electric, Inc., Little Ferry, NJ.)

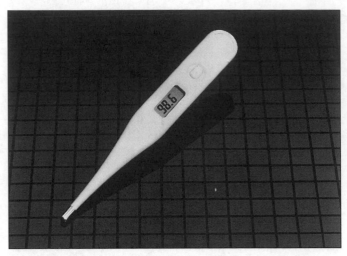

Figure 24-5. This unbreakable digital fever thermometer has a large, easy-to-read display that holds current reading until turned off. (Photo courtesy of The Lumiscope Co., Inc., Edison, NJ.)

Although not limited to the kitchen, space heater safety should be stressed. This problem is especially prevalent among the elderly who feel the cold more and seek added warmth. The National Fire Protection Association says that a heater should be at least 36 inches away from combustibles. This includes wallpaper, furniture, bedding, clothing, curtains, papers, pets, and people. It should never be left on when the client is not home or is sleeping. Check the wires for fraying, splitting, or overheating. Explain the danger of water and electricity, and remove heaters from any bathroom not large enough to have the heater completely away from the tub and sink. Suggest alternate ways to handle the problem, such as turning up the thermostat 20 minutes before a bath or shower, putting warm water in the tub and letting bathroom heat up with the door closed, getting occupational or physical therapy training to speed the bathing process, hiring an aide for the shower or bath, or purchasing a heating unit that plugs directly into the socket so that it is not on the floor. Cost is about $40 from department stores and mail-order firms. **Sources** include 578. Any of these expenses is minuscule compared to the tragedy of fire and the costs of burn rehabilitation.

GLASS DOORS

If there are glass patio doors or glass shower doors located in the home, the health care professional should make sure that they are safety glass. If the patient is forgetful or has limited vision, decals or pressure tape should be added at several heights to any glass door so that the person will see them and not have an accident caused by thinking the door is open when it is not.

BEING PREPARED FOR AN EMERGENCY

Organizing an emergency center and emergency pantry with your patient and his or her family helps them be prepared. The center should include a flashlight, extra batteries, dry-powder fire extinguisher, first-aid kit, aerosol spray for burns; optional items are candles, safety matches, and a poison antidote kit (if children in the home). Power failure lights may be installed in several places in the home, such as the bedroom, bathroom, kitchen, and hallways.

When medical emergencies arise, a regular glass thermometer may be difficult to handle and read for the person with weak hands, incoordination, or visual limitations (Figure 24-5). **Manufacturers** include 338. Cost is about $15 and up from pharmacies and hospital equipment firms.

An emergency pantry is essential for the person who lives alone, is elderly, or is unable to get out in inclement weather. A well-organized stockpile of canned and packaged non-perishable foods minimizes discomfort and helps maintain good nutrition. It is sometimes lifesaving—the person with diabetes should always keep some orange juice and other accepted food items on hand in case of a medical crisis. The supplies should be carefully labeled with dates of purchase and should be kept readily accessible and periodically rotated with new items added.

When the power is out, fruit and vegetable juices provide nutrition without cooking. Crackers, canned bread, dry cereals, dry milk, and non-refrigerated cheese also require no cooking. More often, it is inclement weather rather than loss of power that keeps the elderly or a person with a disability indoors. Prepared foods that take no refrigeration include canned or dried soups, meats and stews, tuna, salmon, beans (plain, baked, or as salads), noodle and rice mixes, canned fruits and vegetables, spaghetti, rice, instant potatoes, staples, and condiments. Adequate food for the person on a therapeutic diet and baby food are additional essentials where indicated.

HOME SECURITY

Home security is another area for assessment. Residential burglary affects one out of 12 homes in the United States. Not only is there loss of property, there may be damage, and the invasion often has a negative psychological impact on the victim.

Leaving doors unlocked while home or away on grocery or other errands and letting deliveries such as mail pile up are clues that attract robbers. Help your patient find someone to bring items in daily if he or she is not up to the task. Check window and door locks. If the person cannot handle the key or lock, make adaptations such as push-button locks and built-up or extended handles. Encourage keeping the door locked at all times. The key may be hidden in a special place for health care workers and other responsible helpers. Teach the individual about property identification, Neighborhood Watch programs, and use of local law enforcement personnel. The National Burglar and Fire Alarm Association will send information on setting up a security system. Security systems are available through local firms or by mail order, with costs ranging from about $300 and up. **Manufacturers** of security systems include 263, 387. Units include door-answering intercoms with optional door release, door surveillance options that work during daylight and at night, window lock sensors, and video cameras attached to a VCR system. **Sources:** 255, 468. Also see Personal Emergency Response Systems in Chapter 3.

Security lighting illuminates danger spots and helps keep intruders away. To find out how well-lighted a patient's home is, ask a relative or friend to walk around the outside after dark. Is there a clear path from the street to the door? Is the door lighted so the keyhole is easy to find? Are there dark areas where someone could hide? Various types of lights may be added, including a timing device, a motion sensor light that goes on when someone crosses the detector's path, or a photocell that goes on at dusk and off at dawn. A chore service or other volunteer group can install these for clients who do not have family or others to assist.

RESOURCES

Addresses for publishers, periodicals, and organizations are given in Section Four.

PUBLICATIONS

Burn Prevention Tips. Tampa, FL: Shriners Burns Institutes. Free, illustrated booklet covers kitchen, microwave oven, hot water, gasoline, surviving a home fire, matches, emergency treatment of burns, camping equipment.

CPSC Guide to Electrical Safety with home audit checklist. Washington, DC: U.S. Consumers Products Safety Commission. Free.

Fire Safety and Older People. Marlboro, MD: National Association of Home Builders Research Center. $6 plus $2 handling. Safety checklist and outline of a model public education program.

Fire Safety Tips for Older Adults. Large-print brochure. And *Learn Not to Burn* for home health workers who assist the homebound or elderly. Both from the National Fire Protection Association. Write for current catalog with additional materials on kitchen fire safety, electrical fire safety, portable fire extinguishers, smoke detectors, fire prevention around the house, heating without getting burned, preventing burns at home, and fire safety for people with disabilities.

King, M. P., & Deily, J. (1987). *Coping and Home Safety Tips for Caregivers of the Elderly.* Charlottesville, VA: Jefferson Area Board for Aging and Northwestern Virginia Health Systems Agency. Write for current cost and availability of companion video.

The National Burglar Alarm and Fire Alarm Association. Information on setting up a security system, $2.

The Perfect Fit: Creative Ideas for a Safe and Livable Home. Washington, DC: American Association of Retired Persons. Free, request No. D14823. Well-illustrated booklet covers whole house.

Perkins-Carpenter, B. (1993). *How to Prevent Falls.* New York: St. Martin's. 97-page large print, self-help book.

Preparing for Emergencies: A Checklist for People with Mobility Problems. (1992). Washington, DC: American Red Cross. Free in packages of 25. May be used with clients to make home surveys and set up emergency plans. Includes questions, creating a plan, including drawing floor plan, preparing a disaster supplies kit, and emergency plan with names and phone numbers of contacts.

Pynoos, J., & Gohen, E. (1990). *Home Safety Guide for Older People: Check It Out, Fix It Up.* Washington, DC: Serif Press. $12.95. Checklist of hazards and listing of solutions for common problems. Excellent safety assessment guide to follow and use in teaching clients.

Safety for Older Consumers: Home Safety Checklist. (1986). Washington, DC: U.S. Consumer Product Safety Commission. Free, illustrated, large-print checklist covering the whole house. Photocopying and reprinting of information is encouraged.

Weinruch, R., Hadley, E. C., & Ory, M. G. (1991). *Reducing Frailty and Falls in Older Persons.* Springfield, IL: Charles C. Thomas. $85.

Local utility companies also can provide safety checklists and brochures for home owners, with many of the materials geared toward the elderly or parents with young children.

AUDIOVISUALS

Beating the Burglar. Washington, DC: Criminal Justice Service, Program Department of the American Association of Retired Persons VHS program, 8:43 minutes. How to protect yourself at home or when away. Free loan with hand-outs, request 90 days in advance.

Kitchen Planning, Storage, and Home Modifications

Being able to function safely and efficiently within one's home is a prerequisite for independent living. Although this guide focuses on meal preparation and home management, evaluation and planning for modifications must include the whole residence. Entranceways allow coming and going not only for shopping, but for medical or social engagements and emergencies as well. If a patient cannot use the bathroom by him- or herself, it is difficult to consider being independent for an extended period of time. A comfortable, barrier-free living room and bedroom, again, are part of daily needs. References are given for information in all of these areas.

KITCHEN PLANNING

The kitchen is a work room. Planning an efficient workplace for meal preparation is part of any home management rehabilitation program. If your client is hospitalized, considerations of needed modifications should be started then. More often, however, the planning is done on-site, because the hospital stay was too short or non-existent. Home health care professionals, usually an occupational therapist, physical therapist, or home economist, with a primary care nurse, work with the patient and family.

The extent of remodeling depends on the physical needs of the patient and available funding. If the problem is loss of vision, relearning to use the kitchen by feel, re-doing storage for easier retrieval, and teaching safety precautions may be all that is necessary. If using one hand, adding stabilizing aids, reorganizing storage to reduce lifting, and ensuring safety awareness may be adequate. On the other hand, if the patient was severely affected by a stroke, is non-ambulatory, or has loss of vision on one side, many changes will have to be made. For the person confined to a wheelchair, work surfaces must be lowered or an alternate preparation area set up. See chapters on kitchen planning and kitchen storage in *Mealtime Manual*.

PRINCIPLES

When beginning any alterations or modifications in a kitchen, careful measurement is crucial. If the homemaker is in a wheelchair, the counters should be set so that the undersurface just clears the arms of the chair. Wheelchair measurement, trunk balance, dimensions of comfortable safe reach, and ability to bend are considered in the evaluation.

The process of evaluating barriers and planning changes is done with the patient and, when possible, the family (Figure 25-1). Although much of the work is done within the office, one or more home visits are recommended.

If a wheelchair is used in the kitchen, at least one counter should be open underneath so the chair occupant can roll under and work efficiently (Figure 25-2). Having an open area next to the oven makes handling hot foods safer and easier.

A few basic rules apply to every kitchen plan:

- The work area is free of traffic. Family members have a way around the main preparation space.
- The plan allows efficient movement between centers, i.e., sink, stove, refrigerator, food storage, and eating place.
- The work surface is unbroken, if possible, allowing movement from refrigerator to counter to sink to counter to stove, in a straight line or L or U shape.
- A sit-down place to eat within the kitchen is preferred.
- Eating area or dining room for full family meals is easily accessible, with door removed if necessary for efficient passage.
- Lighting fully illuminates work areas, and controls are within reach.

Have your client mentally or physically move through the steps taken to prepare a single dish. If his or her energy were high-priced fuel, there would be ways found to cut down steps. Relocating the sink, stove, and/or range can cut miles off meal preparation over the course of time. The well-known triangle is still the best solution.

A portable work center adds additional counter space without extensive remodeling. In a large kitchen, it is a step saver

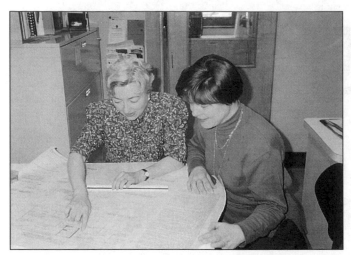

Figure 25-1. Although much of the work is done within the office, as here, one or more home visits are recommended. (Photo courtesy of Barrier-Free Design, O.T. Dept., Howard A. Rusk Institute of Rehabilitation Medicine.)

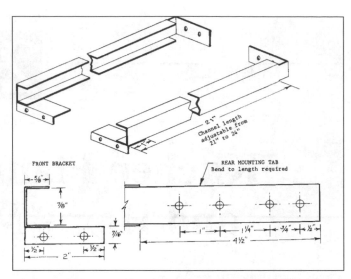

Figure 25-3. The slides on this unit are formed from heavy, zinc-plated steel and adjust for 21- to 24-inch cabinet depths. (Photo courtesy of Washington Products, Inc., Massillon, OH.)

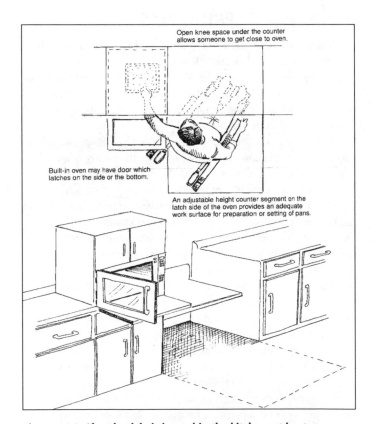

Figure 25-2. If a wheelchair is used in the kitchen, at least one counter should be open underneath so the chair occupant can roll under and work efficiently. Having an open area next to the oven makes handling hot foods safer and easier. (Illustration by G.K.)

when in a central position. Wood- or formica-topped units are commercially available from kitchenware stores and mail-order firms. Heavier units on wheels are not recommended, because they take too much energy to move.

When counter top area is limited, a breadboard slide provides extra working space (Figure 25-3). Check with your local build-

ing supply firm. **Source:** 563.

A wooden work center provides additional space (30 by 48 inches) and has an overlapping surface so that the homemaker may sit on a stool or chair (Figure 25-4). Unit also serves as a sit-to-eat place in the kitchen. In selecting a work island, make sure there is adequate leg room for your client to sit while preparing foods. If trunk balance is unsteady, a chair with arms should be used and the feet supported on a footstool. Cost of this and similar units is about $200 and up. **Source:** 510.

When an additional control panel is needed within reach of food preparation area but electrical remodeling is not possible, an extension cord and reel is one answer (Figure 25-5). Patient must be taught that only one heating unit, such as the microwave or electric kettle, can be used at a time. Cost is about $20 and up from hardware stores and mail-order firms. **Source:** 239.

Portable power strips are another solution. See Electricity in *Mealtime Manual.*

Modifying current electrical outlets so they are accessible to the person in a wheelchair or limited in ability to bend may be done with an upright outlet (Figure 25-6). Cost is about $30, and installation can be done in minutes. **Source:** 13.

Some kitchens have features for added convenience and easier functioning when a family member is older or has a physical disability. The counters are standard height but pull-out surfaces and open vertical storage installed at varied levels allow use from a seated or standing position (Figure 25-7A). The open kitchen allows the cook to be part of family activity while working. The 30-inch high counter serves as both a dining table and a sit-down work surface for meal preparation, kitchen chores, and folding laundry. The Whirlpool® appliances have front- or side-mounted controls. The refrigerator has pull-out shelves and baskets and through-the-door dispensers for ice and water (Figure 25-7B). The cooktop is installed in a counter that is open below, giving closer access in a wheelchair or for the worker who is ambulating but must sit to work (Figure 25-7C). A mirror above the cooktop lets the seated cook see into pots and pans. The vent control has been modified and placed

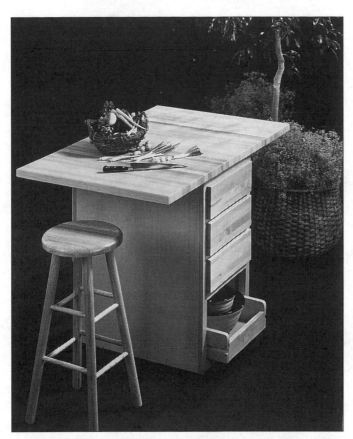

Figure 25-4. This wooden work center provides additional space and has an overlapping surface so that the homemaker may sit on a stool or chair. (Photo courtesy of Taylor Woodcraft, Malta, OH.)

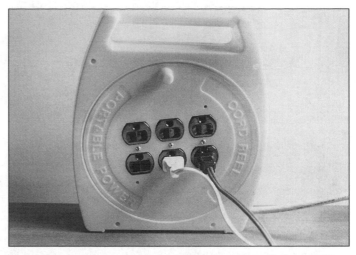

Figure 25-5. This portable unit has a 25-foot line, six grounded outlets, and a circuit-breaker button. (Photo by J.K.)

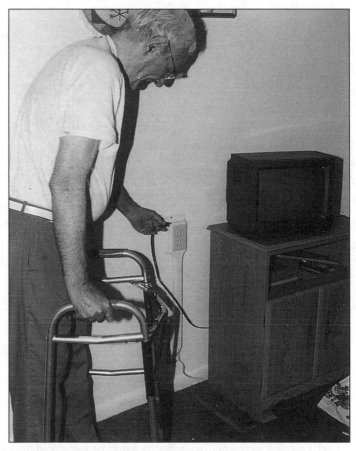

Figure 25-6. Modifying current electrical outlets so they are accessible to the person in a wheelchair or limited in ability to bend may be done with an upright outlet. (Photo courtesy of Accessible Work Systems, Inc., Bellevue, OH.)

along the front edge of the cooktop counter. The mid-storage space is open for a quick reach to condiments and frequently used utensils. The Whirlpool® self-cleaning oven is at an intermediate height for use by seated or standing individuals.

A cooking island allows use from a wheelchair and has an extra shelf on which to set pans while stirring or adding foods (Figure 25-8A,B). The microwave oven is set into the island with a pull-out shelf just below. Open floor space permits unhampered propelling of the wheelchair. Another pull-out board next to the wall oven lets the cook immediately set down hot pans. The inexpensive, mid-range storage units hold a variety of foods quickly accessible.

A galley-style kitchen can be lowered for use from a sitting position (Figure 25-9). In the photo, the long counter on the right serves as a preparation as well as an eating place and has a pass-through to the next room. The narrow electric scooter moves easily in the corridor and has a swivel seat to allow close approach to the cooktop and oven, set on the counter. **Source** for scooter: 47.

A small, wheelchair-height kitchen concentrates the work area in one corner (Figure 25-10). The pipes under the sink are set back to avoid contact with the lower extremities. The cooktop has controls on the side for easier access with weak upper extremities. Pans can be slid to and from the sink or filled with the spray hose.

A larger wheelchair kitchen requires extensive remodeling (Figure 25-11A,B,C,D). The sink was lowered for use from the wheelchair. Cabinet doors were removed as well as the baseboard

so the wheelchair could roll under. This made it possible to reach and use large drawers for storage. The drawers are on ball-bearing slides so they roll with less effort. Not shown are the cooktop controls located at the front and a pull-out board that allows sliding pans from the stove top. A mirror above the cooktop reveals contents of pans to the seated cook. A pull-out board next to the wall

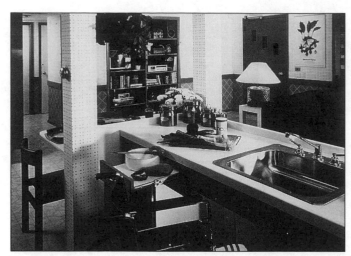

Figure 25-7A. This Horizon House kitchen has features for added convenience and easier functioning when a family member is older or has a physical disability.

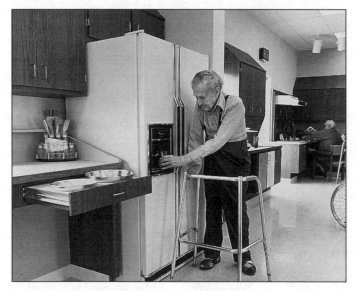

Figure 25-7B. The refrigerator has pull-out shelves and baskets and through-the-door dispensers for ice and water.

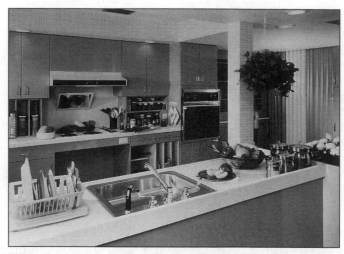

Figure 25-7C. The cooktop is installed in a counter that is open below, giving closer access in a wheelchair or for the worker who is ambulating but must sit to work. (Horizon House, Howard A. Rusk Institute of Rehabilitation Medicine. Photos 25-7A,B,C courtesy of Whirlpool® Corp., Benton Harbor, MI.)

for easier reach and increased light: drawers and pull-out shelving that bring products closer to the user; height reduction of cabinets with adjustable shelves to eliminate the need to climb; and a corner pantry unit with adjustable shelving holding more square feet of storage than a lazy susan. A work area at the sink may incorporate a seat and offers easy access to storage, cooking, work surface, and dishwasher. Recessed work areas do not interfere with kitchen traffic, and wasted space in corners is eliminated with almost eight square feet of floor space returned to kitchen, making it seem larger. Price is competitive with traditional cabinets and is frequently less. Design services to builders, developers, and home owners are free. For descriptions and prices, write **source** 321.

Full kitchen packages have been developed for apartments in adapted and senior housing centers. Each kitchen has an under-counter refrigerator and a cooktop and sink with open knee space for a wheelchair to roll under. **Source:** 177. Additional adaptations for efficient and increased use of lower and mid-storage space is required in most cases.

MAJOR APPLIANCES

Reaching to a standard height stove is fatiguing and dangerous for the person who is working from a wheelchair or must sit to work. Most controls are at the back of the stove, which requires reaching over hot, often lit, burners. One of the first appliance changes that might be recommended for safety and efficiency is the installation of an accessible cooktop. The client can then roll under it in a wheelchair or sit next to it in a chair. The controls may be located on the front, middle, or side. A counter space to slide pans as they come off cooktop burners minimizes the need to lift.

Some electric cooktops have two burners and a grill with large, easy-to-turn knobs located at the front (Figure 25-13). **Manufacturers** of cooktops include Amana (37); Dacor (157); Gaggenau (216); General Electric (221); Jenn-Air (293B); Thermador (523).

oven allows the resting of items as they are removed. A slide-out unit next to the dishwasher stores items on two shelves.

Drop-down or pop-up work centers may be incorporated into a kitchen or other part of the house. With open space underneath, the optimal height can be constructed for the person in a wheelchair, the individual who sits to work, or the ambulatory person who needs more surface. When not in use, the unit may be folded away. Project plans for foldaway units are regularly featured in magazines such as *Better Homes & Gardens*, *Family Circle,* and *Woman's Day.*

A modular system of cabinets may be mounted at various heights (Figure 25-12). They are hung on a single rail. The electrically adjustable height counter top accommodates a sink and cooktop. A modular base system is also available. **Source:** 228.

LifeSpec cabinet systems are designed for the changing abilities of the aging. Design elements include shallow depth shelving

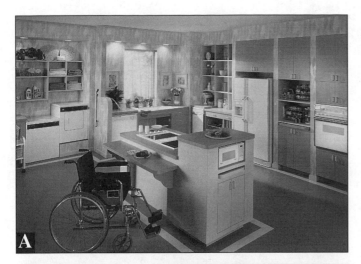

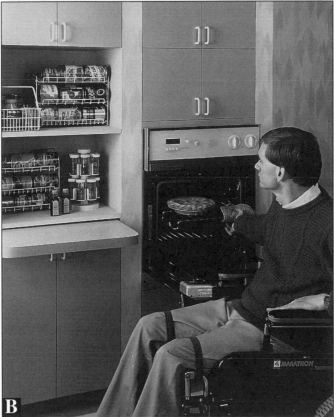

Figure 25-8A,B. The cooking island in this kitchen allows use from a wheelchair and has an extra shelf on which to set pans while stirring or adding foods. The microwave oven is set into the island with a pull-out shelf just below. Another pull-out board next to the wall oven lets the cook immediately set down hot pans. (Photos courtesy of Whirlpool® Corp., Benton Harbor, MI.)

Refrigerators are available in a wide range of designs. Some homemakers who use wheelchairs prefer a swing-out or pull-out lower freezer; others choose a two-door model with the freezer on one side and refrigerator on the other. People with limited reach appreciate pull-out shelves (Figure 25-14, Figure 25-15).

Some flexible refrigerator units come with five different configurations, including top cabinets and lower pull-out drawers that

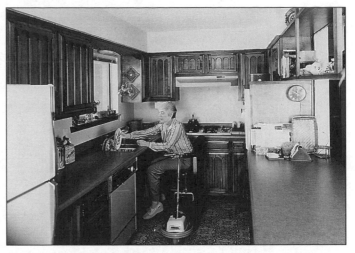

Figure 25-9. This galley-style kitchen has been lowered for use from a sitting position. (Photo courtesy of Amigo® Mobility International Inc., Bridgeport, MI.)

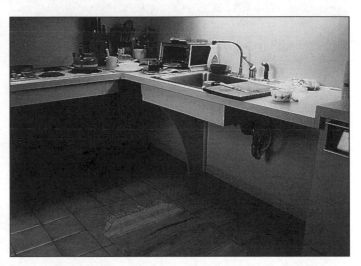

Figure 25-10. This small, wheelchair-height kitchen concentrates the work area in one corner. (Photo courtesy of Barrier-Free Design Service, O.T. Dept., Howard A. Rusk Institute of Rehabilitation Medicine.)

may be placed wherever desired, such as under a cooking island or next to the sink (Figure 25-16). The drawers slide easily enough that they have been used by a client with complete loss of function in her upper extremities so that she uses her feet as hands when cooking. **Source:** 497B.

Electronic, push-button dishwashers require light touch rather than turning of a knob to operate (Figure 25-17). Look for interior storage that pulls out for easier access for the person with limited reach or who is using a wheelchair.

A portable dishwasher that may be placed on a counter for the person who cannot bend is **manufactured** by 566.

Plumbing for the kitchen is discussed in *Mealtime Manual*, Chapter 13. Whether in the kitchen or bathroom, easy-to-handle faucet controls permit more independence and safer use of hot water. An E-Z Flo automatic faucet control allows turning on of the water with pressure on a wand by the slide of the hand; water

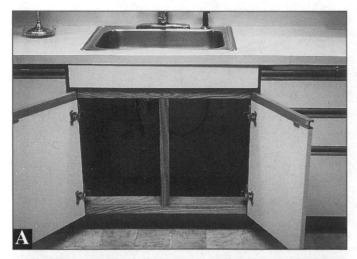

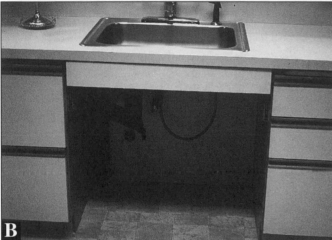

Figure 25-11A,B. This larger wheelchair kitchen required extensive remodeling. The sink was lowered for use from the wheelchair. Cabinet doors were removed as well as the baseboard so the wheelchair could roll under.

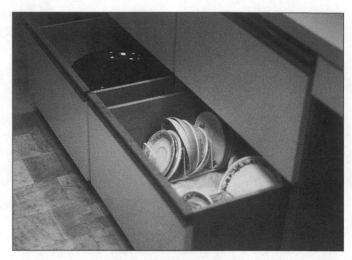

Figure 25-11C. The drawers are on ball-bearing slides so they roll with less effort.

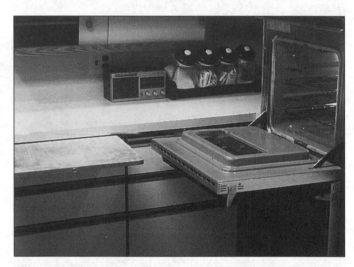

Figure 25-11D. A pull-out board next to the wall oven allows resting of items as they are removed. (Photos 25-11A,B,C,D courtesy of the Barrier-Free Design Service, O.T. Dept., Howard A. Rusk Institute of Rehabilitation Medicine.)

flow ceases when the wand is released. It fits all faucets and costs about $29 from plumbing suppliers. **Manufacturer: 207B.** When making major changes, an instant hot water heater or push-button controls may be installed at the side of the sink. Plumbing suppliers carry units that maintain temperature of water at a safe level and automatic faucets that turn on when a hand or object is placed underneath the spout. **Manufacturers** include 307. See *Mealtime Manual*, Chapter 13, under Plumbing. When not making major changes, a tap turner may be devised or purchased, or a single-handle faucet control installed.

Several styles of single-handle faucet controls are on the market. Make sure that your client can adjust water flow without touching the spigot. **Manufacturers: 163B, 184, 242, 307.**

Planning a kitchen with an adjoining laundry center increases efficiency (Figure 25-18A,B). Designed for use from a wheelchair, a dryer may be raised on a box-like platform for easier loading and unloading. Both the washer and dryer should have front-mounted controls. Low design of a washer allows handling from a wheelchair. The laundry center may be closed off from the kitchen by drawing a vertical blind from its storage slot between the dish stor-

age cabinet and laundry center wall.

When space is at a premium or the washer and dryer are out of range on another floor, a full-sized, stacked laundry center may be installed in a small area such as the bathroom, a hall closet, or the kitchen (Figure 25-19). The user must, however, be able to stand to reach the dryer or have a long reach. **Manufacturers** include 221, 348.

Some washing machines and dryers may be placed beside each other at an optimum height for the user or stacked (Figure 25-20). Push-button controls are mounted at the front. **Manufacturer: 60.**

STORAGE

Efficient kitchen organization includes the ability to retrieve and replace items quickly and easily. Chapter 14 in *Mealtime Manual*

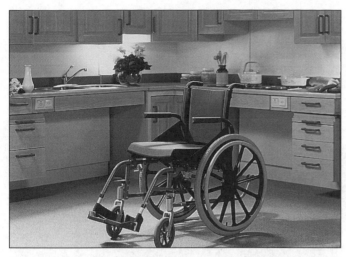

Figure 25-12. This modular system of cabinets may be mounted at various heights. (Photo courtesy of Grandberg Superior Systems, Saskatoon, SK, Canada.)

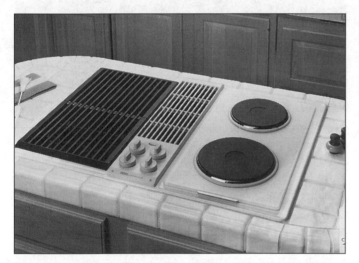

Figure 25-13. This electric cooktop has two burners and a grill with large, easy-to-turn knobs located at the front. (Photo courtesy of Jenn-Air® Co., Indianapolis, IN.)

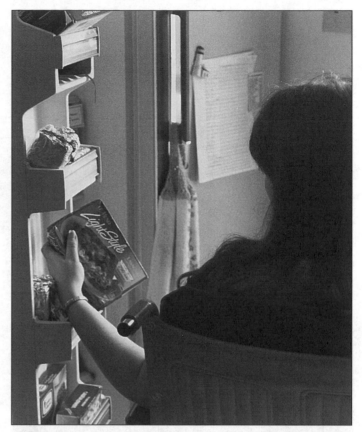

Figure 25-14. This homemaker who uses a wheelchair and has marked weakness in her upper extremities prefers a two-door refrigerator with convenient shelves on the door. (Ballard Green, Ridgefield, CT. Photo by J.K.)

outlines principles and gives commercial solutions. Maximizing storage in an already built kitchen may be done with commercial cabinet inserts, such as made by Clairson International. **Source:** 123. Individuals with strength in their upper extremities might consider pot racks that hang above meal preparation areas. Cost is about $100 and up from kitchen supply and mail-order firms. **Manufacturer:** 137. **Sources:** 128, 306, 482, 490.

If handling knobs on cabinet doors is difficult because of hand limitations, adjustments can be made (Figure 25-21). The knobs shown are constructed of a large electrical ring tongue, plastic wire, or plastic-coated steel cable (small aircraft size), and a short section of rubber tubing or soft rubber hose. Remove the knob from the cabinet door, hook the ring tongue on the bolt and replace. Length may be altered to fit need but should allow a hand to slip completely through the loop.

Oversized, plastic-covered foam knobs for cabinets and drawers are available from **source** 161.

Spacewall is a new concept in storage (Figure 25-22A,B). Wood boards with grooves between them are used for a section of wall. Special hardware may be hung at the desired height and location to create a storage wall. Kitchen adaptable accessories include metal wire flat and angled shelves, plate supports, tool/wooden spoon holders, utility baskets, square storage holders, single and double hooks, towel and bottle racks, and acrylic shelves. **Source:** 485.

The mid-range between the upper cabinets and the back of the counter surface is often neglected when considering storage. Seldom used for meal preparation tasks, the back of the counter allows for accessible storage of frequently used items.

An over-the-sink shelf provides extra mid-storage space and frees the counter for heavier appliances (Figure 25-23). Of handcrafted pine, it fits over the back of sinks up to 33 inches wide, is 38 inches long by 9 inches high by 4½ inches deep, and does not interfere with faucets. Cost is about $15 and up from mail-order firms. **Manufacturer:** 203. **Sources:** 328, 361.

Desk toppers may be adapted for kitchen use and add two shelves of space on the counter (Figure 25-24). They are available from office supply and mail-order firms. Cost in wood or metal is about $20 and up. **Sources:** 109, 211, 225, 219, 258.

The spice cabinet shown in Figure 25-25 attaches under the upper cabinet, then pulls down when in use. It may be installed with screws or adhesive tape. **Manufacturer:** 297. Cost is about $16 from housewares stores and mail-order firms.

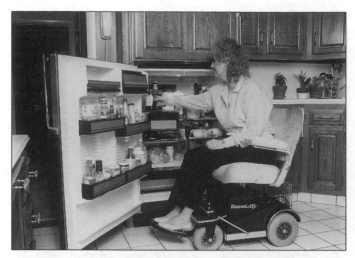

Figure 25-15. This woman works from an electric scooter and finds that a low refrigerator with wide doors provides more accessibility. (Photo courtesy of Electric Mobility, Inc., Sewell, NJ.)

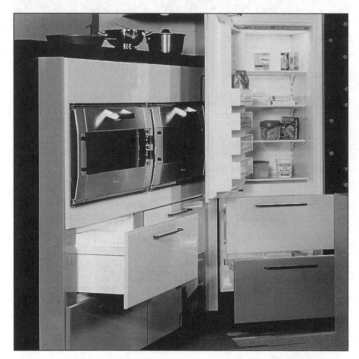

Figure 25-16. These flexible refrigerator units come with five different configurations. (Photos courtesy of the Sub-Zero Freezer Co., Inc., Madison, WI.)

Adding extra lights under the cabinets to illuminate the counter work surface increases safety and ease when preparing foods. A single fluorescent tube light is made by 221. Cost is about $15 and up from hardware stores. Slim-line halogen light bars are available from lighting and mail-order firms. **Source:** 482.

Lifting objects up off the floor and replacing bulky chests with open shelves reduces bending and leaves more floor space for the person in a wheelchair. This may be done with adjustable shelf brackets available from building suppliers. Shelves of inexpensive wood may even be finished by the patient as part of therapy. **Manufacturer** of brackets: 494. Shelf systems that may be added

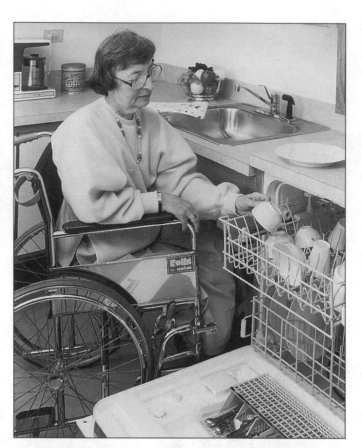

Figure 25-17. Electronic, push-button dishwashers require light touch rather than turning of a knob to operate. Photo courtesy of Whirlpool® Corp., Benton Harbor, MI.)

to existing wall areas are available in styles that lean against the wall or use suction cups and do not have to be attached by screws or nails. Cost for a four-shelf unit is about $135 from housewares firms. **Sources:** 274, 468, 490.

Designed for use as work stations, adjustable-height units may be used in the kitchen, living room, study, or bedroom (Figure 25-26). For people who use wheelchairs, the open space underneath allows a close approach to work and turning in a limited area. The same unit may be installed higher for the individual who wishes to stand while working. **Source:** 12.

DOORS AND WINDOWS

Adapting door knobs with slip-on handles and friction materials assists people with weak grasp or arthritis.

Commercially available lever handles may also replace round knobs so doors can be operated with the arm or palm of the hand (Figure 25-27). **Sources:** 23, 312.

The off-set door hinge is a handy solution-maker in a home where doors are too narrow for a wheelchair to pass through easily. The set of hinges adds about 1½ inches of extra clearance. Cost is about $20 a pair from self-help firms. **Distributors:** 23, 176. **Sources:** 23, 198, 383, 461, 468. See Chapter 13 in *Mealtime Manual*.

An automatic door opener assists not only the person who uses

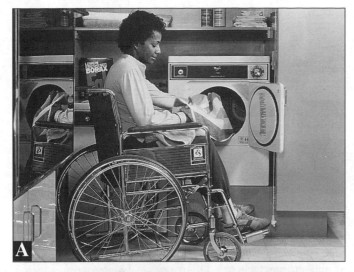

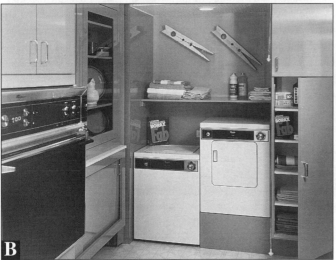

Figure 25-18A,B. Designed for use from a wheelchair, the dryer has been raised on a box-like platform for easier loading and unloading. The adjacent closet stores supplies. (Photos courtesy of Whirlpool® Corp., at Horizon House, Howard A. Rusk Institute of Rehabilitation Medicine.)

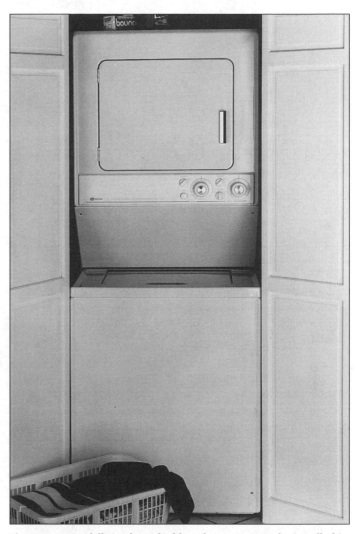

Figure 25-19. A full-sized, stacked laundry center may be installed in a small area. (Photo courtesy of the Maytag® Co., Newton, IA.)

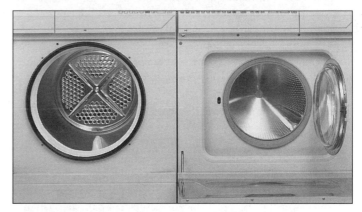

Figure 25-20. This washing machine and dryer may be placed beside each other at an optimum height for the user or stacked. (Photo courtesy of Asko, Inc., Richardson, TX.)

a wheelchair but anyone who has difficulty ambulating, use of only one hand, back pain, or general weakness (Figure 25-28). **Manufacturers** include 23, 390, 414.

Handling doors when carrying items and when in a wheelchair is easier with a door closer (Figure 25-29). A "door butler" closes the door every time and installs with two screws for indoor or outdoors, even gates. In white for indoors or UV- protected black for indoors or outdoors, cost is about $18 from hardware stores and mail-order firms. **Source:** 482.

Low windows and sliding doors give the person in a wheelchair a full view. Gliding patio doors also eliminate barriers to the outside. **Sources** include 48, 345, 406. Handling a sliding door, however, takes moderate to good strength. This is often not possible for the person with weakness, arthritis, or back pain to manage without stress. A push-button patio door opener electrically opens the sliding door. A timed delay allows the person in a wheelchair or ambulating slowly to walk through before it automatically closes. It

installs on existing or newly constructed sliding glass doors and is available with an optional locking device and selection of three push-button controls. **Sources:** 23, 264.

An automatic remote control for roof and awning windows

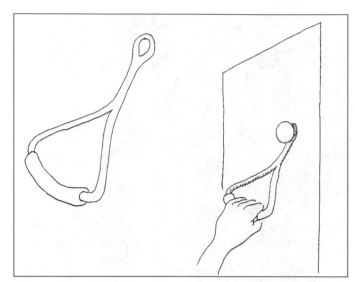

Figure 25-21. If handling knobs on cabinet doors is difficult because of hand limitations, this type of cabinet door handle helps. (Original design by Fred Carroll, the Independence Factory. Illustrated by G.K.)

operates up to four windows. The operator is installed in place of the window handle. Then, an electrical cord is run to a command nodule plugged into an outlet. Pressing a button on the command nodule opens or closes the window. If it should start raining, a sensor strip on the sash of the window tells the unit to close the window automatically. Cost is about $230. **Source:** 48.

ENTRANCES AND EXITS

Comings and goings from one's home may require modification (Figure 25-30). Ramps allow a person with limited mobility or using a wheelchair to get in and out of the house. Another answer is a porch lift. The vehicle may require its own modifications, such as a van lift for a wheelchair, a lift or a carrier to allow a caregiver to get the chair or scooter in and out of the car.

A durable medical equipment supplier will have samples of items. Study periodicals written for the consumer with a disability, such as *Accent on Living*, *Mainstream*, *Spinal Network*, *Team Rehab*, and *Rehabilitation Gazette*. See Resources on where to obtain additional information. **Sources** for ramps include 36, 238, 260, 412, 415, 431, 437 (rubber). Also see Chapter 25 in *Mealtime Manual*.

When pain or limited range in lower extremities makes regular stair risers impossible, a portable half-step may be used when not at home.

An answer for one's residence is permanent half-steps (Figure 25-31). The existing stoop may be divided in half and one side extended to allow construction of the steps. Railings to provide security are always recommended and eliminate the need for a cane while going up or down. Because this project is expensive, check local resources for physical or financial help if needed.

Indoor stair lifts adapt two-story homes for people who cannot manage stairs, whether because of poor ambulation or in a wheelchair (Figure 25-32). Use of the lift requires training in operation and safety awareness, especially for the patient with poor trunk balance or vision. If medically prescribed, the cost of rental is tax-deductible. Purchase of a lift is not always tax-deductible, because it is considered to raise the value of the home. The unit may, however, be removed when no longer needed. Ask a local representative to come for an on-site visit to assess all details. The width and design of the stairs, physical ability and weight of the patient, style of seat, and location of control are all considerations. **Manufacturers** include 9, 44, 100, 117, 572.

A wheelchair lift, designed for private residences or public buildings, carries a person in a wheelchair from one floor to another (Figure 25-33). The three basic components are the rail system, the driving machine, and the platform. Doors on each end protect the user while in transit. Controls are located within the lift enclosure. Platform may be folded up against the wall when not in use. **Manufacturers** include 9, 117. A vertical wheelchair lift, which is available through the same manufacturers, may also be used where space is minimal and stairs must be kept free. For major modifications in a home, residential elevators allow the person in a wheelchair to use all levels of the home. **Manufacturers** of elevators include 9, 564, 572.

For an individual to remain at home alone for the day, responsible for home management or just caring for him- or herself, independence is necessary in many areas. Handling toileting activities is one task that may call for modifications, such as safety bars, raised seats, even widened bathroom doors. When self-cleansing is not possible because of weak upper extremities, limited reach, or poor trunk balance, a bidet toilet attachment may be the answer. All components are activated by push-button controls; water and air temperature are adjustable. The unit, which installs on existing toilet, combines a toilet seat, spray nozzle, and blow dryer. Cost is about $300. See Chapter 6.

WORKING WITH A CONTRACTOR

Learning to work with a contractor is a talent the health care professional must develop when making home adaptations. Knowing how the contracting process works smoothes the process for the patient, the firm doing the work, and you. Family service magazines often have articles on working with contractors, and there are books available through local libraries. See Resources at the end of this chapter.

Finding the right contractor takes research and patience. Firms specializing in barrier-free design may be located in your area. Ads may be found in area or state publications for people with disabilities, or one can request information through a computerized search service, listed in Appendix C. The patient and family may have sources. Co-workers may offer suggestions. Recommendations might also come from local real estate agents, architects, building inspectors, bank mortgage officers, regional rehabilitation facilities, and agencies for the aging or people with disabilities. Always ask for and check references. Homeowners with whom the contractor has dealt may let you see completed work. You may contact the Better Business Bureau or government consumer affairs office for added information. Check credit standing. Find out if the contractor belongs

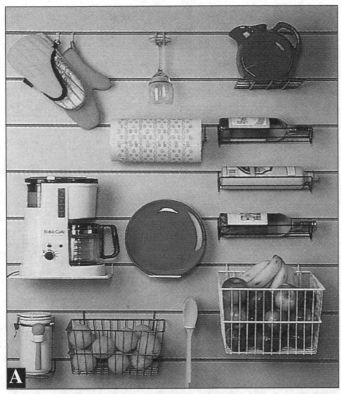
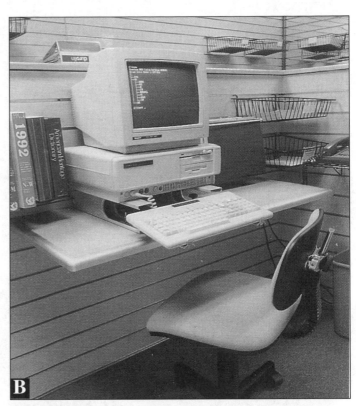

Figure 25-22A,B. Spacewall is a new concept in storage. Special hardware may be hung at the desired height and location. The desk and computer as well as the storage baskets are also hung on Spacewall. (Photos printed with permission of Spacewall Northeast, Inc., Waterbury, CT.)

to the National Association of the Remodeling Industry or the National Association of Home Builders.

The contractor will meet with you and the family. Interviewing and negotiation are two skills needed during this process. Preliminary plans to present to the contractor and a basic budget should be set before the first meeting. Ask that the firm submit proposals. If it is a large job, talk with at least three contractors, and give the family a chance to negotiate. Listen to ideas the contractor has. These may save money in the long run. The contractor will often have a book of work already done.

The family is responsible for studying and approving the contract. Make sure that they check financial details: total price, payment schedule, payment penalties, and that every part of the job is described, the dates to start and complete the job, product specifications, warranties, and workmanship. Post-construction responsibilities should be written into the contract. The contractor is responsible for obtaining all building permits, meeting all building codes and ordinances, and arranging for periodic inspections by the building inspectors. Depending on location, separate contracts may be required for electrical and plumbing work. Before signing, the patient and family must understand that the contract legally binds both parties.

In larger remodeling jobs, the patient and family must also be aware that normal routine may be upset for a while. You can help smooth this path, i.e., preparing them by organizing advance meal preparation and setting up an alternate working area before the work begins.

The ideal is, of course, that all the work be done while the

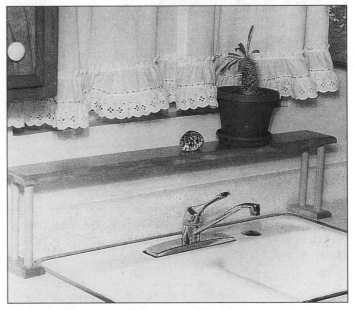

Figure 25-23. An over-the-sink shelf provides extra mid-storage space and frees the counter for heavier appliances. (Shelf by Fernanda Manufacturing Co., Hauppauge, NY.)

patient is still in hospital or rehabilitation center. On the other hand, that reduces the patient's involvement in the planning. It may even increase the cost, because simpler ideas often solve the problems once the patient is on the scene. Sometimes the most helpful

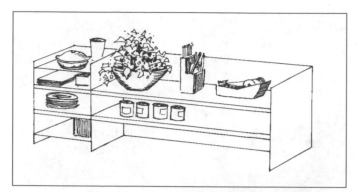

Figure 25-24. Desk toppers may be adapted for kitchen use and add two shelves of space on the counter. (Illustration by G.K.)

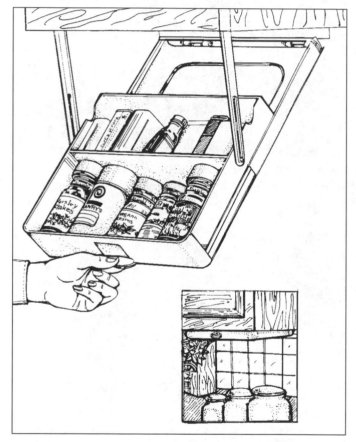

Figure 25-25. This spice cabinet attaches under the upper cabinet, then pulls down when in use. (Photo courtesy of Jokari U.S., Inc., Dallas, TX.)

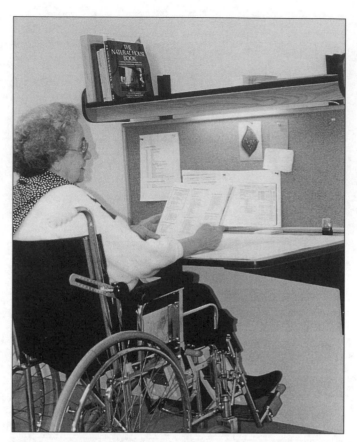

Figure 25-26. Designed for use as work stations, these adjustable-height units may be used in the kitchen, living room, study, or bedroom. (Photo courtesy of Accessible Designs Adjustable Systems, Inc., Athens, OH.)

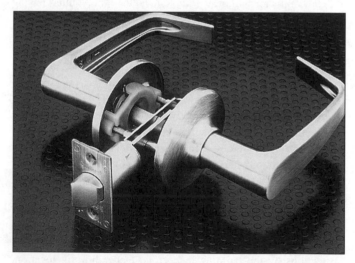

Figure 25-27. Commercially available lever handles may replace round knobs so doors can be operated with the arm or palm of the hand. (Photo by J.K.)

thing you can do is emphasize the length of the process to keep the family from rushing into construction in the mistaken belief that it can be finished before the client is discharged.

If your client lives in a rented home or apartment, you must also work with the owner from the beginning. Present the plan and reasons for the changes. Find out if present appliances can be stored and replaced if the patient moves. Landlords can be helpful. Sharing the remodeling plan with local newspapers and publications allows the owner to share positively in the event.

FUNDING

Discuss the role of your client as well as financial circumstances with the family. What do they feel they can afford? In matters of simple reorganizing and purchasing small, portable appliances, they may be able to fund the entire amount.

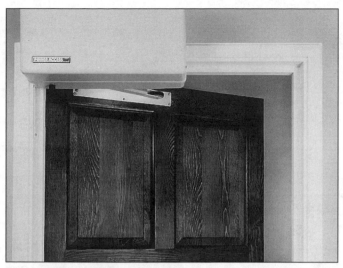

Figure 25-28. This automatic door unit is designed for use on apartment and other heavier doors. (Photo courtesy of Power Access Corp., Collinsville, CT.)

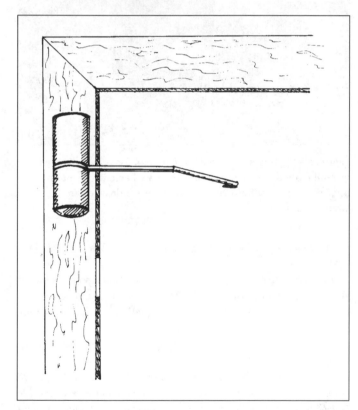

Figure 25-29. A "door butler" closes the door every time and installs with two screws for indoor or outdoors, even for gates. (Illustration by G.K.)

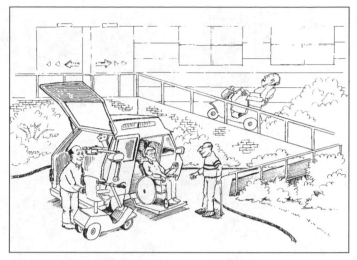

Figure 25-30. Comings and goings from one's home may require modification. (Illustration by G.K.)

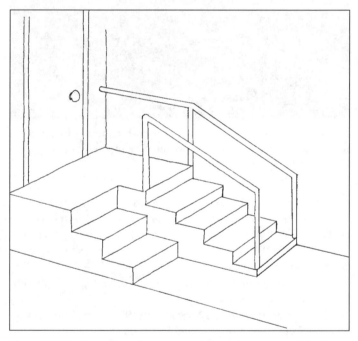

Figure 25-31. An answer for one's residence is permanent half-steps. (Illustration by G.K.)

Homemaking is considered an occupation. As such, funds for remodeling and equipment may be available through the State Vocational Rehabilitation agency in your area. This depends on the extent of your patient's role within the home, the diagnosis, and the current state budget. When the remodeling job is large, find out about the family's involvement with local organizations that might be willing to help. Check the *National Directory of* *Home Modification/Repair Programs*, which is listed at end of this chapter, for state programs. Contact agencies and groups affiliated with the disability your patient has. See Appendix A. Talk with Family Services who have programs to help families stay together and consider housing essential to this process.

RESOURCES

Addresses for publishers, periodicals, and organizations are given in Section Four.

PUBLICATIONS

A Place to Live: Independent Living. (1988). Bloomington, IL:

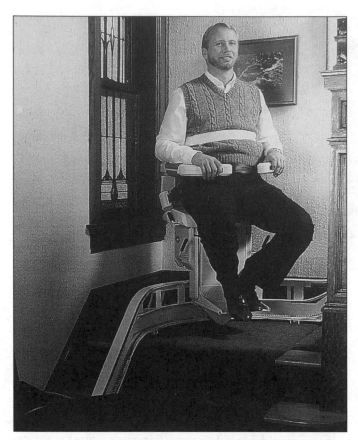

Figure 25-32. Indoor stair lifts adapt two-story homes for people who cannot manage stairs. (Photo courtesy of The Cheney® Company, New Berlin, WI.)

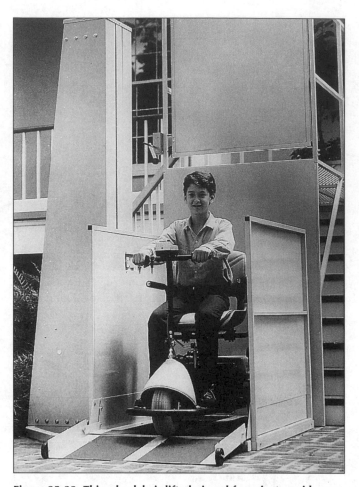

Figure 25-33. This wheelchair lift, designed for private residences or public buildings, carries a person in a wheelchair from one floor to another. (Photo courtesy of Access Industries, Inc., Grandview, MO.)

Accent Special Publications. $4.95. **Source:** 8.

Accessibility/Architectural Modifications: Resource Guide. Bethesda, MD: American Occupational Therapy Association. #4000, $10 AOTA members, $20 non-members. Bibliographies, audiovisuals, resource personnel.

Accessible Building Plans. Jackson Heights, NY: Eastern Paralyzed Veterans Association.

The Accessible Housing Design File. (1991). New York: Barrier Free Environments, Van Nostrand Reinhold.

The Accommodating Kitchen: Accessibility with Substance. Newton, IA: Maytag Consumer Center. Free from **source** 348.

ADA Compliance Guidebook. (1991). New York: Building Owners and Managers Association. 79 pages with grids, $30 association members, $40 non-members. Cites section of the law and describes its requirements.

The American Occupational Therapy Association has several publications to assist in barrier-free assessment and planning: *Readily Available Checklist: A Survey for Accessibility.* (1993). Produced by the Adaptive Environment Center, #1988, $25 AOTA members, $32.50 non-members; *Achieving Physical and Communication Accessibility.* (1991) Produced by the National Center for Access Unlimited. $25 AOTA members, $32.50 non-members; and *A Consumers Guide to Home Adaptation.* (1989). Produced by the Adaptive Environment Center (also available from the Center, $9.50 AOTA members, $12.50 non-members.

American Association of Retired Persons. (1992).

Understanding Senior Housing for the 1990's. Washington, DC: AARP.

Barrier-Free Product Catalog (2nd ed.). Minneapolis: National Handicap Housing Institute. $20. More than 500 manufacturers of hardware and appliances, product evaluations, model numbers, photos, and prices of each product.

Basic Kitchen Planning for the Physically Impaired (1989). Brochure from GE Consumer Affairs. Free.

Bostrom, J. A., Mace, R. L., & Long, M. (1987). *Adaptable Housing: A Technical Manual for Implementing Adaptable Dwelling Unit Specifications.* U.S. Department of Housing and Urban Development, Office of Policy Development and Research. Publication No. HUD-1124-PDR(1). Raleigh, NC: Barrier Free Environments, Inc. Free from HUD User, P.O. Box 6091, Rockville, MD 20850.

Branson, G. D. (1991). *The Complete Guide to Barrier-Free Housing: Convenient Living for the Elderly and the Physically Handicapped.* Croset, VA: Betterway Publications.

Building Design Requirements for the Physically Handicapped. Jackson Heights, NY: Eastern Paralyzed Veterans Association.

Cheever, E. (1992). *Beyond the Basics: Advanced Kitchen Design* (3rd printing). Hackettstown, NJ: National Kitchen and

Bath Association. Written for professional designers, includes section on wheelchair kitchens. Extensive background and resources.

Cheever, R., & Garee, B. (Eds.). *An Accessible Home of Your Own*. Bloomington, IL: Accent. $4.50. **Source:** 8.

Christiansen, C., & Baum, C. (Eds.). (1991). *Occupational Therapy: Overcoming Human Deficits*. Thorofare, NJ: SLACK Inc. Davidson, H. Assessing environmental factors. pp. 427 to 454. Broad scope to environmental factors that affect patients, includes a home evaluation form as well as neighborhood assessment. Barnes, K. Modification of the physical environment. Covers measurements, architectural barriers and solutions, discusses kitchen arrangement, safety factors in selection of appliances.

Christianson, M. A. (Principle author), & Taira, E. D., (Ed.). (1990). *Aging in the Designed Environment*. New York: Haworth.

A Comprehensive Approach to Retrofitting Homes for a Lifetime. Marlboro, MD: National Association of Home Builders Research Center. $10 plus $2 handling. Outlines process for remodelers and older homeowners to work effectively with each other. Helps assess client needs, identify appropriate financing arrangements. Audit form to complete as home is surveyed for modifications and design solutions. *Directory of Accessible Building Products* included.

A Consumer's Guide to Home Adaptation (rev. ed.) (1995). Boston: The Adaptive Environments Center. $12 including postage and handling. Well-illustrated, in large-print. Also available on audiotape.

Daniels, M. (Ed.). (1988). *The Inner & Outer Art & Practice of Making Your Home Accessible*. Berkeley, CA: Center for Independent Living. $30 donation.

Designs for Independent Living: Kitchen and Laundry Designs for Disabled Persons and Aids to Independent Living. Free from Appliance Information Service, Whirlpool® Corp. **Source:** 571.

Directory of Accessible Building Products. Marlboro, MD: National Association of Home Builders Research Center. $.50 postage. Descriptions of more than 60 commercially available products designed for use by people with disabilities and age-related limitations.

Hashagen, W. R. (1990). *How to Get It Built Better—Faster—For Less*. $22 from author, **Source:** 246. All phases of building from planning, financing, and permits through construction; checklists help guide user.

Housing Accessibility Information System (HAIS). Marlboro, MD: National Association of Home Builders Research Center. Available in hardcopy and FoxBASE software versions. $20 for either version. References currently available publications that address housing accessibility; hardcopy version includes full text of articles and brochures.

Housing for People with Disabilities: Development Process and Financing Mechanisms. Marlboro, MD: National Association of Home Builders Research Center. $5 plus $2 handling. Volume I focuses on organizing and planning; Volume II lists federal, state, local, and private resources available for housing development for people with disabilities.

Independent Living Home Appraisal. $15 from Consumer Care Products, Inc. Guide to making full home assessment for safety or remodeling. **Source:** 140.

Kitchen Planning for the Physically Impaired. General Electric Consumer Affairs, General Electric Company. Free brochure. **Source:** 221.

Kitchen Planning Standards, Circular Series C5.32, Council Notes, Building Research Council (1991). Vol. 12, No. 1. Urbana-Champaign, IL: University of Illinois at Urbana-Champaign. 16 pages. Clearly presented rules and specifications for planning any kitchen.

Petersen, M. J. (1995). *Universal Kitchen Planning: Design That Adapts to People*. Hackettstown, NJ: National Kitchen and Bath Association. $30 members, $50 non-members. Allows the health care professional to consider how the client with a disability might function in a kitchen, modifications that could be made, and how team of designer, therapist, and rehab engineer might work together. Case studies on accessible design well-illustrated. Large-print, resources.

Pynoos, J., et al. (1991, June). *National Directory of Home Modification/Repair Programs*. Los Angeles: Long Term Care National Resource Center at UCLA/USC. Free.

Rand, E., & Perchuk, F., with the Editors of Consumers Reports® Books. (1991). *The Complete Book of Kitchen Design*. Yonkers, NY: Consumers Reports® Books. $16.95. Planning, designing, selecting appliances and cabinetry, working with professionals.

Salmen, J. P. S. (1988). *The DoAble ReNewable Home*. #D12470. Washington, DC: American Association of Retired Persons. Free from AARP.

Securing Independent Housing with Accessible and Universal Design. (1995). Rosenhayn, NJ: Design Communications. $45. Process to purchase housing, potential home modifications, funding support, directory of modification suggestions. **Source:** 166.

Uniform Federal Accessibility Standards. (1988). Washington, DC: The General Services Administration, Department of Defense, Department of Housing and Urban Development, U.S. Postal Service, FED-STD- 795. Presents uniform standards for design, construction, and modification of buildings so that individuals with physical disabilities will have ready access to and use of them. In accordance with the Architectural Barriers Act, 42 U.S.C. 4151-4157. Free.

Universal Design: Housing for a Lifespan of All People. (1988). Washington, DC: U.S. Department of Housing and Urban Development. Concept is design that simplifies life for everyone by making more housing usable by more people at little or no cost. Free.

Wheelchair House Designs. Jackson Heights, NY: Eastern Paralyzed Veterans Association, Architecture Department. Illustrated house plans designed for its members.

Wylde, M. (1995). *Enabling Products Sourcebook 2*. National Kitchen and Bath Association.

Wylde, M., Barron-Robbins, A., & Clark, S. (1994). *Building for a Lifetime*. Newtown, CT: Taunton.

AUDIOVISUALS

The Adaptable Fire-Safe House. Marlboro, MD: National Association of Home Builders. $25 plus $2 handling. VHS video tour and information packet includes rendering, floor plan, product descriptions of adaptable features and fire safety system.

Adapting the Home for the Physically Disabled. 30-minute

VHS video, #1101, $89.95 from A/V Health Services, Inc. Helps people using wheelchairs or walkers modify their homes into functional living domains. Includes all rooms plus ramp construction. **Sources:** 1, 11, 65.

Changing Needs, Changing Homes: Adapting Your Home to Fit You. (1996). Bethesda, MD: American Occupational Therapy Foundation with funding from the Retirement Research Foundation. Available from the American Occupational Therapy Association. Videotape package designed to clarify the role of the occupational therapist, Specialized remodeler, and client in the process of home modification.

Hartford Insurance Company (Producer). *For the Rest of Your Life.* 45-minute VHS video. Stresses universal design and aging in the environment. $25 or free loan. **Source:** 367.

Vogt, P. and Associates (Director). *Toward Universal Design.* Washington, DC: Peter Vogt and Associates. Captioned VHS 15-minute color/sound video. Defines universal design in terms of what will it allow an individual to do over a long period of time; considers that only the built environment is that which handicaps and the ranges of people that we are designing for. Thought-stimulating introduction to field of universal design. $15 from Design Initiative, P.O. Box 222514, Chantilly, VA 22022-2514. (709) 378-5079.

Universal Design Kitchen, 5 minute VHS video, and *It's All in the Planning*, 10-minute VHS video. Free loan from Whirlpool Corp. **Source:** 571.

CONTINUING EDUCATION

Courses on environmental accessibility, universal design, and barrier-free assessment and planning are frequently offered through the American Occupational Therapy Association and through courses listed in publications for occupational therapists and other health care professionals.

Transporting Food and Equipment

Moving items around the house may be a major activity for your client. Teaching how to protect hands and arms from stress and reduce wear on legs and hips, especially if they are weak or affected by arthritis or incoordination, requires actually doing the steps of several activities. Teach your client how to reduce carrying and mileage by rolling loads, using big pockets, a basket, or a lapboard if he or she is a wheelchair user. Wheeling items allows doubling up on loads.

Carts, wheeled tables, trays, and lapboards all are discussed in *Mealtime Manual*, Chapter 16. These additional suggestions include ones that you can build or adapt for your client.

A purchased or simple home-constructed dolly reduces lifting and carries everything from groceries to laundry (Figure 26-1). It may be used for small items, such as laundry baskets, grocery bags in a container, or pails. Select units with four casters, because units with three casters tend to tip if unbalanced. You may still want to secure the carrying container to the dolly. A cord or handle allows pulling and eliminates bending. The wooden dolly shown is about $8 from mail-order firms. **Sources:** 241, 361, 508, 561B.

A double pail brackets together to carry both wash and rinse water or dark and light laundry at the same time (Figure 26-2). Attached to a dolly, it reduces both steps and lifting. **Manufacturer:** 452. About $9 from housewares stores.

A walker with a tray allows the person who requires support while walking to move items from place to place with more stability (Figure 26-3A,B). Some rolling walkers have hand brakes to control forward motion, a necessary feature for the person with Parkinson's or marked incoordination affecting gait. The tray on the unit shown is removable, leaving the seat and basket in place for use when shopping or doing other household tasks such as laundry. **Manufacturer:** 379. Cost is about $300.

Additional rolling walkers are shown in Chapter 13 and Chapter 30.

When helping a client select a cart for transporting items at home, options extend beyond carts designed for kitchen use. Those manufactured for kitchen use are often constructed for appearance, not design, especially units that fold, and do not offer adequate stability when one propels them.

Sturdy utility carts with large casters are available from office, hospital, and commercial restaurant supply firms. A raised handle lets the client maintain good posture while rolling the cart. **Manufacturers:** 90, 453. Cost of a well-constructed cart is about $45 and up. **Sources:** 58, 219, 225, 258. Carts of structural plastic will not mar walls, should they be hit while moving items. Cost is about $95 and up. **Manufacturers:** 258, 453.

Mail carts, designed for interoffice use, have deep carrying baskets. Housekeeping carts, as used in motels and hotels, are taller in height and may also be adapted to home activities, like carrying laundry, collecting wastebasket trash, and housecleaning. Both come with extra large casters that making propelling easier. **Manufacturers** include 453. Cost is about $99 and up. **Sources:** 58, 258. A portable working island/cart might be adapted from a "trade cart" that has drawers, two shelves, and two locking casters. **Manufacturer:** 453. Cost is about $195 from office supply firms. **Source:** 258.

A wheeled table modified with an attached ramp allows the sliding of items to and from the stove or counter (Figure 26-4). The ramp may be hinged to a commercial cart of the correct height. It should have strip of rubber under the distal edge of the ramp to provide friction and prevent sliding.

The AmbulMate™ caddy attaches to a quad cane, walker, crutch, or wheelchair, allowing the user to carry a few items (Figure 26-5). When used on a walker, it is attached on the inside, so the individual has a clear view. The space is designed to let one organize daily needed items, including eyeglasses, in a padded compartment. The solid base does not allow small articles to fall through. A beverage holder secures a 16-ounce container so it will not spill. Carrier is large enough to hold a half-gallon carton. Top closes to provide a smooth writing surface and to conceal contents if desired. It may be transferred from appliance to appliance, and it is dishwasher safe. **Manufacturer:** 336. Cost is about $35 for all Lumex walkers; $8 for adapter to other walkers. Available from rehabilitation supply firms including **source** 383.

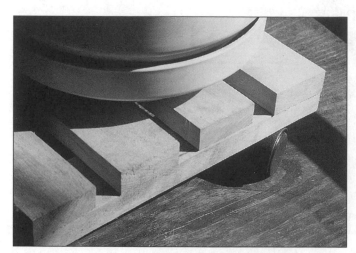

Figure 26-1. A purchased or simple home-constructed dolly reduces lifting and carries everything from groceries to laundry. (Photo by J.K.)

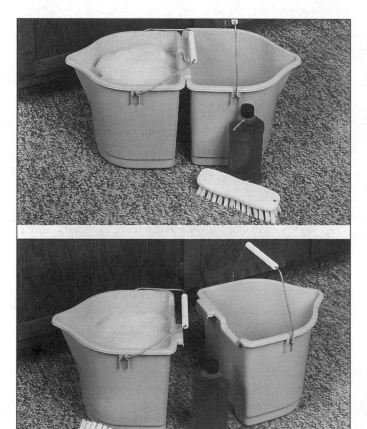

Figure 26-2. This double pail brackets together to carry both wash and rinse water or dark and light laundry at the same time. (Photo courtesy of Rubbermaid®, Inc., Wooster, OH.)

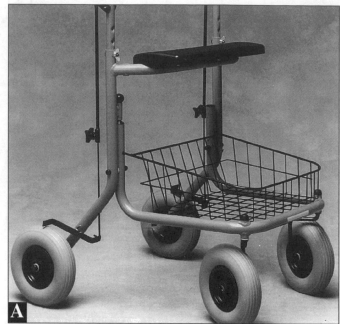

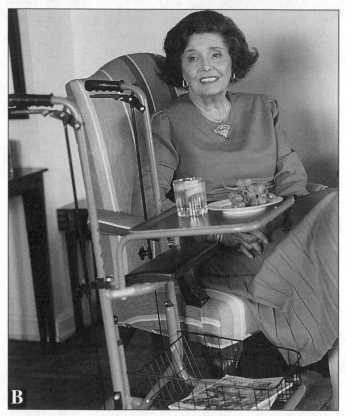

Figure 26-3A,B. This rolling walker has hand brakes to control forward motion, a necessary feature for the person with Parkinson's or marked incoordination affecting gait. (Photos courtesy of Noble Motion, Inc., Pittsburgh, PA.)

For a homemaker who has marked weakness in both upper and lower extremities, a special high cart with an adapted cutting board, a bracket for the mixer, and a ramp for sliding pots to and from the stove allow independent functioning (Figure 26-6A,B,C,D).

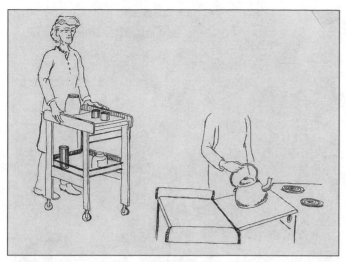

Figure 26-4. This wheeled table modified with an attached ramp allows the sliding of items to and from the stove or counter. (Illustration by G.K.)

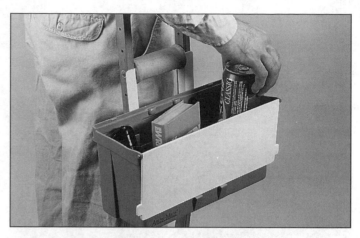

Figure 26-5. The AmbulMate™ caddy attaches to a quad cane, walker, crutch, or wheelchair, allowing the user to carry a few items. (Photo courtesy of Lumex®, Inc., Bay Shore, NY.)

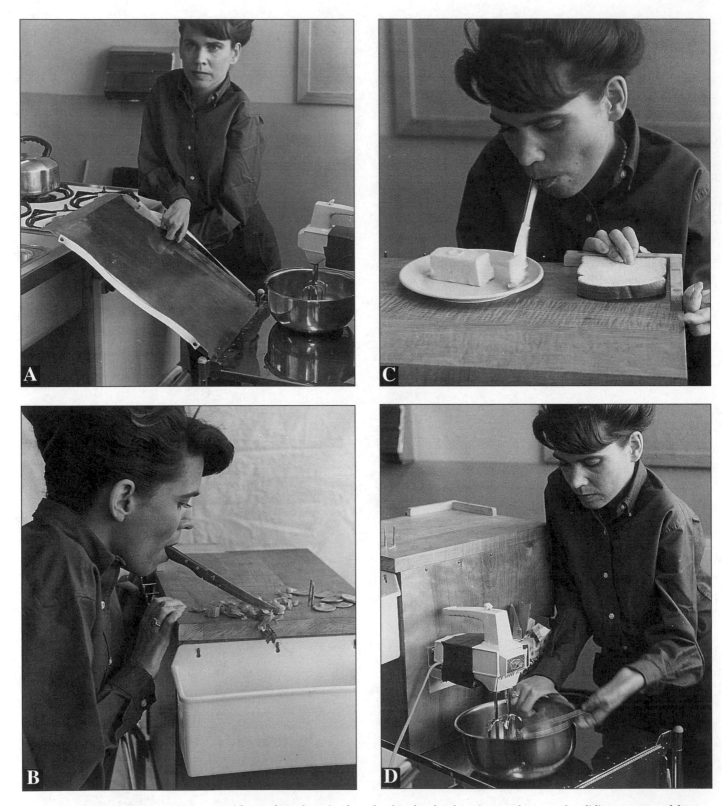

Figure 26-6A,B,C,D. A special high cart with an adapted cutting board, a bracket for the mixer, and a ramp for sliding pots to and from the stove allows her to function independently. (Photos courtesy of the O.T. Dept., Howard A. Rusk Institute of Rehabilitation Medicine.)

Section Three

KITCHEN TOOLS, APPLIANCES, AND TECHNIQUES

27

Selecting Equipment and Appliances

Kitchen equipment and tools are illustrated and discussed in detail in *Mealtime Manual for People with Disabilities and the Aging*. See the manual's index for aids to help with specific tasks: can opening, container opening, cutting, mixing, oven cooking, range top cooking, selection of tools and utensils, transporting items, vegetable and fruit or meat preparation. Also see devices that aid when there are specific disabilities.

The health care professional working in home management rehabilitation can constantly find new techniques and equipment that streamline meal preparation by reading newspaper articles and ads, and looking through catalogs. Developments include Teflon® liners for baking pans, lightweight electric kettles, non-breakable coffee carafes, adjustable-height electric can openers, storage canisters with snap-open tops (**Manufacturer:** 207B, **Sources:** 383, 482), versatile toaster/convection oven combinations (**Manufacturers** include 566), and the widely available Good Grips® utensils by Oxo® International, Div. of General Housewares, which made the jump from a specialized rehabilitation market into the general consumer's product line. **Manufacturer:** 397. See *Mealtime Manual* under peeling and cutting aids.

Creative use of new and traditional equipment will conserve energy, improve nutrition, and increase safety. Sometimes, a tool designed for another purpose, such as pliers or a woodbench vise, may be adapted for use in the kitchen.

When adapting kitchen tools, two features are required for built-up handles. First, they must be lightweight; second, they must be washable. Any tool that will be used at the stove or with hot appliances must have a heatproof handle. Quick solutions for tools not used with heat are foam rubber or pipe insulation, both of which are inexpensive and easily replaced. Pipe insulation is high density, so it is firmer. More permanent solutions are wooden file and garden tool handles or cut off and bored lengths of broom handles. Hollow aluminum tubes, as from discarded aluminum lawn furniture, are lightweight and dishwasher safe. A one-inch furniture cap slipped over the end covers sharp edges and keeps water out.

CUTTING AIDS

For the person with incoordination or limited vision, a funnel board helps transfer food (Figure 27-1). A handle at one end allows secure holding; the other end has two raised side panels to form the funnel. Rubber feet attached under each corner keep the board from sliding. A similar, commercially available model, constructed of polypropylene is shown in *Mealtime Manual*.

A cutting board with a concave surface helps keep food from scattering when chopping and moving it into a pan or bowl (Figure 27-2). It comes with a curved chopping knife. Cost is about $8 from kitchenware and mail-order firms. **Source:** 328.

Adapted cutting boards may be constructed with commercially available polypropylene or wooden boards. Smaller boards with a handle, often called paddle boards, are easier to lift and maneuver. **Manufacturers** of boards include 20, 210. Hardware for making a board is available locally or in sets from self-help firms **source** 518. Make sure to use stainless steel if two stabilizing nails are incorporated into the design.

A raised cutting board simplifies the task of picking up food pieces when hands are weak, incoordinated, affected by arthritis, or there is loss of vision (Figure 27-3). Foods are simply slid into a bowl or pan. A standard, wooden cutting board may be used, with a semi-circle cut out of one end, then sanded well. Wooden legs, about three inches long, or just high enough to fit over a low bowl or skillet, are attached at each corner at a 20° angle if possible. If a saw to cut slots for the legs is not available, you may attach them with deep-set screws through the top. Rubber tips on the legs prevent sliding. Finish board with a coating of salad oil. Note: This board works well for the person who is standing but may be too high for the individual who is sitting and has upper extremity weakness.

A small "top chop block" that has an undercut edge for slipping a plate under to catch cut up foods is **manufactured** by 20. Request catalog.

Spring-opening shears halve the amount of work needed when cutting (Figure 27-4). Loop-handled scissors and others

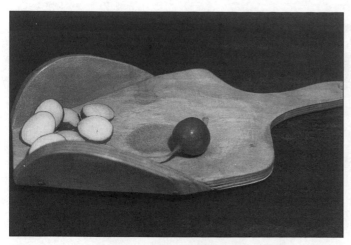

Figure 27-1. For the person with incoordination or limited vision, a funnel board helps transfer food. (Wood funnel board was designed by Francis Leserer. Photo by J.K.)

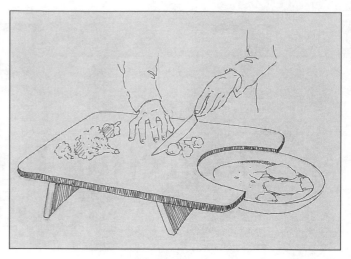

Figure 27-3. A raised cutting board simplifies the task of picking up food pieces. (Illustration by G.K.)

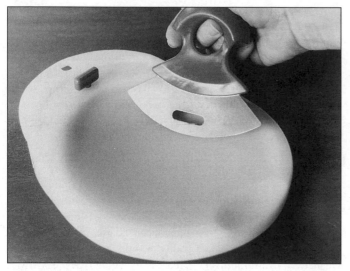

Figure 27-2. This cutting board with a concave surface helps keep food from scattering when chopping and moving it into a pan or bowl. (Photo by J.K.)

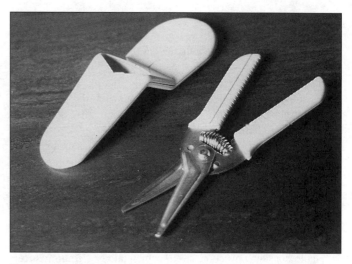

Figure 27-4. These heavier duty shears have rounded points for safety and will cut poultry, packages, and some foods. (Shears from Lillian® Vernon Corp., Virginia Beach, VA. Photo by J.K.)

that are spring-loaded are shown in *Mealtime Manual*. The heavier duty shears shown have rounded points for safety and will cut poultry, packages, and some foods. They store in a wall-mounted holder. Cost of these and similar shears is about $10 and up from housewares stores and mail-order firms. **Source:** 328.

Simplifying a task when a patient has marked involvement of the upper extremities can be accomplished by using the easiest, most efficient motions (Figure 27-5). The person with weakness in both hands, use of only one hand, or marked incoordination places the cheese in position, then pushes down on the bar. Cost is about $15 from housewares stores. **Manufacturer:** 422.

CONTAINER OPENING, MIXING, AND COOKING

A wedge that has been cut into the removable section of an adjustable-height, pull-out work surface stabilizes boxes, jars,

and other containers while opening with one hand or with weak hands (Figure 27-6). Cut-out is lined with rubber. When the rectangle is turned over, the base is solid, so there is a flat food-preparation surface.

Spring-opening pliers quickly release the foil tab on cans and work well with other tabbed containers (Figure 27-7). **Manufacturer:** 191. Cost is about $10 from rehabilitation suppliers. Other types of pliers may also be used in the kitchen.

A client with marked weakness and limited reach of the upper extremities may lift a food processor to a lower working surface while using it, then slide it back on the higher counter when not in use (Figure 27-8). The lowered surface is made from a cutting board cut to the width of the drawer with edges added on each side to stabilize it.

Selection of even small items makes a difference in handling meal preparation (Figure 27-9). Although many kitchen shakers are breakable, the salt and pepper shakers shown are made of lightweight plastic and are easy to grasp. They may also be used for

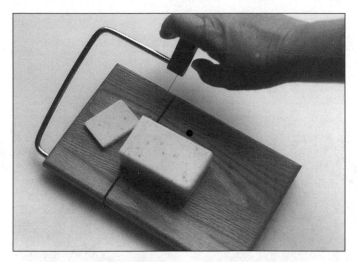

Figure 27-5. This cheese slicer cuts with a wire, so it requires no knife. (Slicer by Prodyne Enterprises, Montclair, CA. Photo by J.K.)

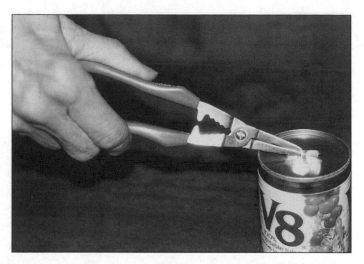

Figure 27-7. Spring-opening pliers quickly release the foil tab on this can and work well with other tabbed containers. (Photo by J.K.)

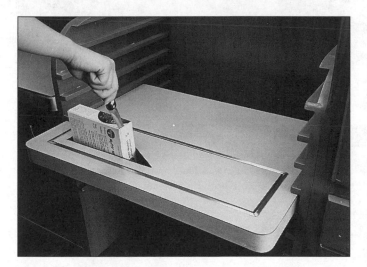

Figure 27-6. The wedge stabilizes boxes, jars, and other containers while opening with one hand or with weak hands. (Photo courtesy of the O.T. Dept., Howard A. Rusk Institute of Rehabilitation Medicine.)

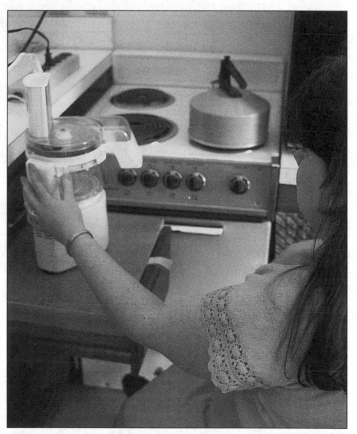

Figure 27-8. This woman lifts her food processor to a lower working surface while using it. (Ballard Green Housing, Ridgefield, CT. Photo by J.K.)

ground spices and herbs. **Source:** 538. Tupperware® also makes a set of salt and pepper shakers with pronged tops that automatically clean the holes when shut, a help for people with poor hand function or limited vision. **Manufacturer:** 538.

A pitcher with a built-in stirrer makes mixing juice concentrates or dry milk and other beverages easier when working with one hand or incoordination (Figure 27-10). Cost is about $12 from housewares stores and mail-order firms. **Sources:** 461, 476.

A metal bowl holder is designed for a person who has use of one hand and is also helpful when there is upper extremity weakness or incoordination (Figure 27-11). Cost is about $40 from rehabilitation supply firms. **Sources:** 11, 461, 553. The metal bowl with a loop handle is also sold separately by housewares stores. Cost is about $20. **Manufacturer:** 201.

The Remarkable bowl allows the cook to insert a portable electric mixer through the hole in the cover, avoiding splatters (Figure 27-12). The removable center may be easily replaced for storing food in bowl. **Manufacturer:** 538.

Another quick tip for reducing splatters is to slip a lightweight paper plate onto the mixer. Before assembling the beaters, mark where they insert, then punch a hole in those two places, and slip beaters in with plate at the top. Mix as usual, keeping the plate even with the top of the bowl. Food will be caught by plate and

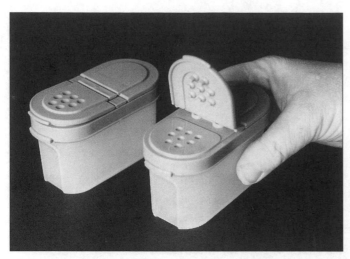

Figure 27-9. These salt and pepper shakers are made of light-weight plastic and are easy to grasp. (Shakers by Tupperware® Inc., Orlando, FL. Photo by J.K.)

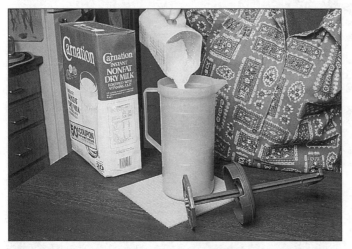

Figure 27-10. A pitcher with a built-in stirrer makes mixing juice concentrates or dry milk and other beverages easier. (Photo courtesy of the O.T. Dept., Howard A. Rusk Institute of Rehabilitation Medicine.)

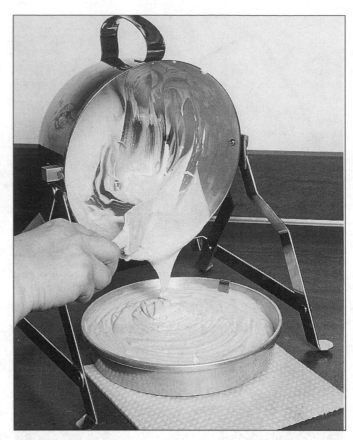

Figure 27-11. This metal bowl holder is designed for a person who has use of one hand and is also helpful when there is upper extremity weakness or incoordination. (Photo courtesy of the O.T. Dept., Howard A. Rusk Institute of Rehabilitation Medicine.)

with a bulb control, the other with a syringe mechanism, are shown in Chapter 2.

APPLIANCES

Major and home appliances are discussed and illustrated in *Mealtime Manual*. Please see the manual's index. Ensuring that a patient uses safety precautions with appliances is part of home management training. Reading over the instruction book of any new appliance should be mandatory, with emphasis placed on safe handling of the appliance, and caution emphasized about contact with water, heat, electricity, or gas.

One caveat: When selecting kitchen appliances, many popular units are constructed of heatproof thermoplastics. A new safety requirement is that the user always unplug the unit when not in use. This includes cool-sided toasters and toaster ovens. There have been a number of fire disasters where a plugged-in but turned-off unit has started a fire while the owner was not present.

Safe installation of a major home appliance is a first step when remodeling or making modifications. For example, a washing machine should not be located where the temperature falls below freezing. A trash compactor should be placed in an area free from spray paints or insect sprays that could emit explosive fumes; i.e., it should not be in the garage or near a workbench area. A brochure

drop back into bowl; plate may be torn off and discarded when mixing is done.

When two handles are needed for safe lifting of a one-handled saucepan, a second handle may be constructed with an aluminum tube and two hose clamps riveted to the tube (Figure 27-13). Check the circumference of the pan, allowing an extra inch, and buy two hose clamps of the size equal to that measurement.

A measuring spoon designed originally for use with medications may be supported in a cup or other container, or held by a small homemade stand so that the person with use of one hand or poor coordination can measure liquid ingredients (Figure 27-14A,B). Called a dosage spoon, it is graduated by quarter teaspoons and holds up to two teaspoons. Cost is about $2 from pharmacies. **Manufacturer:** 250.

Other oral medicine holders for giving liquid medication to children may be adopted for use in the kitchen. Two types, one

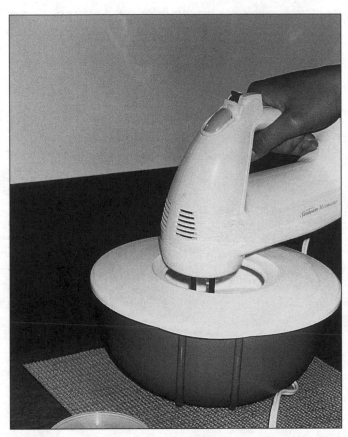

Figure 27-12. The Remarkable bowl allows the cook to insert a portable, electric mixer through the hole in the top, avoiding splatters. (Bowl by Tupperware®, Inc., Orlando, FL. Photo by J.K.)

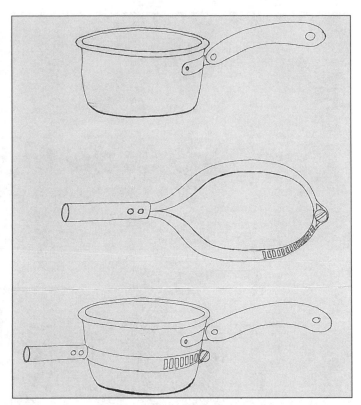

Figure 27-13. A second handle may be constructed with an aluminum tube and two hose clamps riveted to the tube. (Original idea from Fred Carroll, the Independence Factory. Illustration by G.K.)

giving guidelines is available from Whirlpool® Corporation. See Resources.

Controls and switches may be adapted for safer and easier use by clients with severe incoordination or weakness. Adapted switches are available through companies carrying therapeutic supplies, including AbleNet (4), Jesana Ltd. (294), Prentke-Romich (418), TASH (506), TFH Achievement and Special Needs (516), and Toys for Special Children (532). A local electronics or electrical engineer can also offer suggestions and may help build a needed prototype.

When portable appliances are difficult or unsafe to set because the hands come in contact with the hot metal, a dowel or spoked handle may be screwed onto the control so that it may be turned with the side of the hand (Figure 27-15A).

Counter-top appliances permit working at a safe, convenient level and reduce bending to an oven or broiler (Figure 27-15B). A compact grilling machine is designed so that meat or poultry does not have to be turned during cooking, splatters and smoke are eliminated, and fat runs off into a catching drip tray under the front of the unit. The lid has an extended handle that may be lifted with a potholder. Non-stick surface requires use of plastic or wooden tools for removing food; one comes with unit. UL listed. **Manufacturer:** 460. Cost is about $80 from housewares stores and kitchen mail-order firms. **Source:** 306.

A child or adult with severe disabilities can share in a kitchen activity by pressing on the jellybean switch on a lapboard to activate a food processor or other appliance (Figure 27-16A,B). The switch may be connected to a combination of controls to operate various electrical units. **Source:** 4. See Resources.

Commercial aids, such as the universal turner for stove and other knobs, are shown in Chapter 20 in *Mealtime Manual*. Turners for small knobs like timers may be made easily and inexpensively. Look for L-shaped or lever knobs at local hardware stores. To make sure that the diameter is the same, take a knob from the appliance you are modifying.

An inexpensive solution for knob turning may be made with a large crutch tip. The cavity of the rubber tip is filled with a hardening compound. Before it dries, the tip is fitted over the knob to be turned. If it is still difficult to turn the knob, then a hole may be drilled through the tip and a wooden dowel inserted to give greater leverage. (Original design by Fred Carroll, the Independence Factory.)

Safety is a major consideration when working with any appliance. Patients with developmental delay, traumatic brain injury, aphasia, or other difficulties that make reading and sequencing difficult may use a flip-chart or drawings to learn correct procedures in using an appliance. See Chapter 21. For teaching safety, *The Safety Guide for Older Consumers* gives a room-by-room checklist with large print and easy-to-follow illustrations. One on avoiding fires warns against long or loose sleeves when reaching over a range. See sample page in Appendix G and Resources at the end of Chapter 1.

For the client who depends on a toaster oven or convection oven for most of the cooking, toaster-oven sized pans by Nordicware® are available from housewares stores and through mail-order firms.

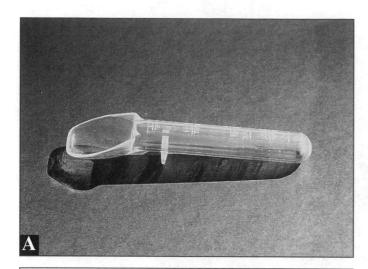

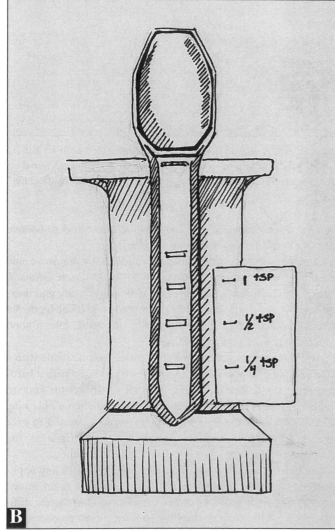

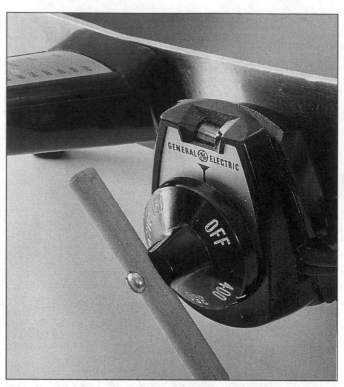

Figure 27-15A. This design was developed as part of the Institute project sponsored by the Campbell Soup fund. (Photo courtesy of the O.T. Dept., Howard A. Rusk Institute of Rehabilitation Medicine.)

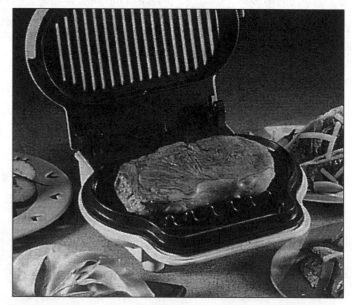

Figure 27-15B. This compact grilling machine permits working at a safe, convenient level and reduces bending to an oven or broiler. (George Foreman's Lean Mean Fat Reducing Grilling Machine. Photo courtesy of Salton/Maxim® Housewares, Inc., Mount Prospect, IL.)

Figure 27-14A,B. This measuring spoon, called a dosage spoon, is graduated by quarter teaspoons and holds up to two teaspoons. (Illustration by G.K.)

Manufacturer: 380.

When there is a performance or mechanical question, or a problem with an appliance, most major manufacturers have hot-lines to call. These include the following:

- General Electric—800-626-2000.
- Salton/Maxim—800-221-8794; 312-578-1111 (in IL.).

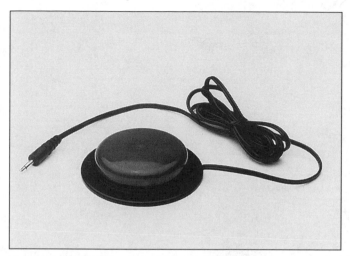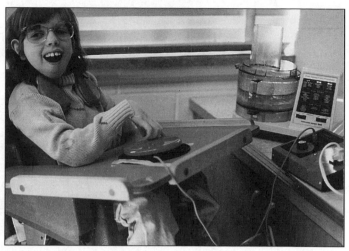

Figure 27-16A,B. This child with cerebral palsy is able to share in a kitchen activity. She presses on the jellybean switch on her lapboard to activate a food processor or other appliance. (Photos courtesy of AbleNet®, Inc., Minneapolis, MN.)

- Whirlpool® Cool Line—800-253-1301; 800-632-2243 (in Mich.); 800-253-1121 (Alaska and Hawaii).

RESOURCES

Addresses for publishers, periodicals, and organizations are given in Section Four.

PUBLICATIONS

Better Homes & Gardens Crockery Cook Book. (1994). Des Moines, IA. Meredith. $14.95. Easy recipes allow cook to begin main dishes early in the day while energy is highest and be relaxed when mealtime arrives.

Bridge, F., & Tibbetts, J. (1991). *The Well-Tooled Kitchen.* New York: William Morrow. $24.95. Guide to kitchenware with illustrations, addresses.

Consumer Reports®. Source for checking safety evaluations and costs of current appliances and home products. See Periodicals, *Mealtime Manual.*

Good Housekeeping. Frequent articles on selection of kitchen equipment and testing results on portable appliances. See Periodicals, *Mealtime Manual.*

Hoffman, M., & Hoffman, G. (1993). *Mabel Hoffman's All-*

New Crockery Favorites. New York: Bantam Doubleday Dell. $5.99. For crockpot or slow cooker.

Is That Newfangled Cookware Safe? (1991). Food and Drug Administration. #531Y, free from the Consumer Information Center. Advantages and safety concerns of seven popular types of cookware from aluminum and non-stick coating to cast iron.

Katona, C., & Katona, T. (1993). *Convection Oven Cookery.* San Leandro, CA: Nitty Gritty, Bristol. Gives range of possibilities, but not low-fat.

Levin, J., & Scherfenberg, L. (1991). *Breaking Barriers.* Minneapolis: AbleNet. $15. Use of simple technology to increase independence and participation. **Source:** 4. Also see Resources in Chapter 11 and assistive technology resources in Appendix F.

Nice Things to Know About Safety with Major Home Appliances. Appliance Information Service, Dept. CT, Whirlpool® Corporation. Single leaflet free. **Source:** 571.

Time Smart Guide. Free from Whirlpool® Corporation. Suggestions on managing home, cutting time in the kitchen and laundry, making the most of appliances, shopping, and cooking shortcuts. **Source:** 571.

The U.S. Product Safety Commission has many free publications that may be reproduced without permission for distribution to clients. Write for current list.

Teaching About Microwave Cooking

The microwave oven offers many advantages to the person with a disability. It may be put at the most convenient height and in the safest place. A side-opening door allows sliding of items to and from the oven to the counter top. Lightweight containers instead of heavy metal or glass pans may be used. Cleanup is easier. Meals may be prepared ahead of time for the person with severe disabilities, then heated when needed. Timing is remembered by the microwave oven so the person with short-term memory or cognitive loss does not have to worry about turning it off. Other features include speed of cooking and energy saving for the person who can cook and serve or eat from the same container. For the client with chronic obstructive pulmonary disease, it will not heat up the kitchen, and there is no danger when using oxygen. The person who lives alone can enjoy re-heated foods without losing taste. Tests have shown there is little loss of nutritional value from re-heating leftovers.

The older homemaker is, however, often not familiar with microwave ovens or with digital controls. In such cases, a single- or double-dial control with a customized heating chart is the best selection. Several companies still make a single dial, often for auxiliary kitchens of nursing homes and other institutions. Although one is sometimes difficult to find, **manufacturers** include General Electric, 221; Kenmore from Sears Roebuck, 468; Panasonic, 399; Sharp, 473.

If your client is unfamiliar with microwave cooking, a careful discussion of the parts, how to care for the oven, precautions, and its uses should be part of training. See Chapter 20 in *Mealtime Manual* for microwave ovens. Containers for microwave cooking should be selected for the type and amount of cooking the individual is going to be doing and with concern for any hand or upper extremity problems. Glass is heavy and breakable. Microwave-safe plastic is lightweight and unbreakable. A specific place should be set up for all microwave-safe containers. This is especially important if the patient forgets or has a family not familiar with microwave cooking.

For the person with loss of vision, the microwave oven offers safety and ease (Figure 28-1). A small shelf just below the oven will provide a place for setting pans when removing them from the oven.

A wheelchair-height, pull-out workplace directly in front of the microwave oven can be designed for a homemaker with limited endurance and weak upper extremities (Figure 28-2).

A microwave fish cooker consists of three parts: a cover, removable slotted tray, and pan (Figure 28-3). The lightweight plastic set may be used for steaming, poaching, or serving. The built-in rack keeps the tray above water and juices. It may also be used for vegetables and re-heating. It comes with directions for cooking and defrosting in the microwave, plus recipes. It is not designed for bacon and foods with high fat content. Top-shelf is dishwasher safe. Cost is about $8 from housewares stores and mail-order firms. **Manufacturer: 189.**

The stack cookware system by Tupperware® Inc. is a different concept in microwave cooking (Figure 28-4). Each recipe is prepared for a stacked, cooked meal, such as peas and mushrooms, meat loaves with sauce, and fruit compote. Then, the casseroles are stacked one on top of the other and cooked on high power for 25 to 30 minutes. There is no stirring or turning. This allows the homemaker or caregiver to prepare everything ahead of time. A *Cookware System Cookbook* gives more than 25,000 menu combinations. For more information, contact **manufacturer 538.**

Special microwave-safe tools have no metal parts, so they may be left in the microwave oven while cooking (Figure 28-5). The unique patent allows no toxins to transmit into foods. A dishwasher- and freezer-safe set of spoon, whisk, spatula or food slicer, and tongs is about $12 per set from gourmet kitchen firms. **Manufacturer: 429.**

New products have increased the versatility of a microwave oven (Figure 28-6A,B). A microwave roaster cooks and browns meats in a microwave. The meat is set on a rack so that fat drips away; vegetables can be added for a fast, one-step, one-pan meal. Four-piece set includes basting tray, roast rack, Flavor-Lock™ self-basting dome, and a carving knife. It will cook a whole chicken or up to a four-pound roast in 15 to 20 minutes. Cost is about $20 and up from variety stores. **Manufacturer: 310.**

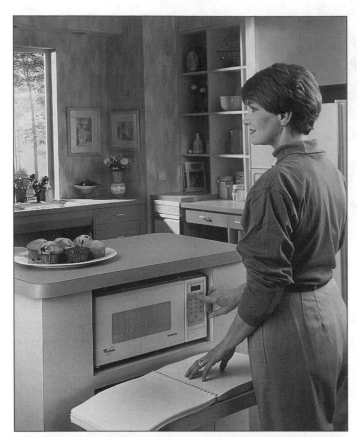

Figure 28-1. This woman sets the timer while checking her Braille cookbook. (Whirlpool® Kitchen. Photo courtesy of Whirlpool® Corp., Benton Harbor, MI.)

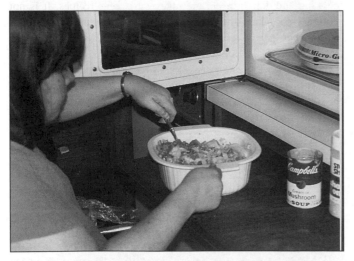

Figure 28-2. This woman is able to lift a lightweight container from the oven down to the pull-out board. (Ballard Green Housing, Ridgefield, CT. Photo by J.K.)

A microwave pouch holder protects the fingers when heating foods that are sealed in a pouch (Figure 28-7). When the food is cooked, the cook snips off one corner and pours food into a dish. Dishwasher safe. Cost is about $4 from mail-order firms. **Distributor:** 71.

See additional tools and containers in *Mealtime Manual,*

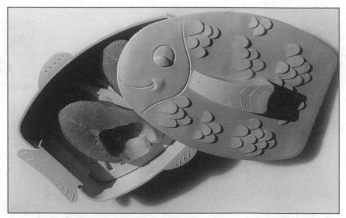

Figure 28-3. This microwave fish cooker consists of three parts: a cover, removable slotted tray, and pan. (Cooker by Ensar Corp. Photo by J.K.)

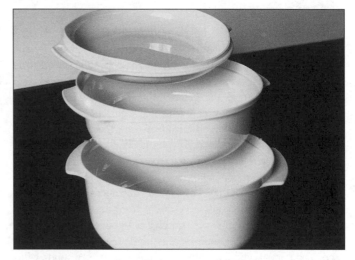

Figure 28-4. The stack cookware system by Tupperware® Inc. is a different concept in microwave cooking. (Unit by Tupperware®, Inc., Orlando, FL. Photo by J.K.)

Chapter 20, under Microwave Ovens and Accessories and in this guide in Chapter 9.

The following safety rules should be stressed to your patient:

- Potholders should always be used. Although only the food heats, the warmth transfers to the container and can cause burning if hands are not protected.
- To test if a dish is microwave safe, place a glass measuring cup filled with ½ cup water into the microwave oven. Then put the dish you wish to test near but not touching it. Microwave on high for 1 minute. If the water is hot but the dish is cool, it is microwave safe. If it is warm or has hot spots, it is not.
- Since microwaves may cook unevenly, foods should be cooked in small, uniform pieces and stirred, or the dish turned frequently. Let food stand for several minutes after removing it from the microwave so the heating process can continue. This avoids any cold spots that harbor bacteria. This is especially important when cooking chicken or pork. Cover meats tightly, rotate while cooking, and on removal check internal temperature with a meat thermometer (the correct reading for pork is 170°; for chicken,

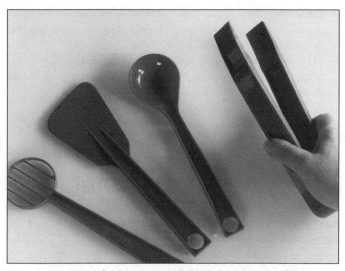

Figure 28-5. Special microwave-safe tools have no metal parts, so they may be left in the microwave oven while cooking. (Tools by R.A.S. International. Photo by J.K.)

it is 185°).

- Cooking longer at a lower temperature lets food heat more evenly.
- Round containers cook more evenly than square or oblong.
- Metal, aluminum foil, or twist ties should never be put in the oven.
- Dishes with metal trims or rims are not microwave safe.
- Packaging on prepared foods should be used once and discarded. Instructions for heating differ with foods and brands so directions must be carefully read and followed.
- Plastic bowls and plastic food storage containers should not be used in the microwave unless the label says microwave safe. Food inside containers such as margarine tubs might get hot enough for harmful chemicals to leach out of the plastic.
- Frozen foods and those with fillings may heat unevenly and be cool on the outside but very hot on the inside. When it is not possible to stir the dish, cut the item open before taking a bite.
- Foods should never be left in the microwave, but refrigerated if appropriate.
- The oven should be periodically cleaned with a soft cloth or sponge and warm water. Cleaning up spills immediately eliminates hardening of foods.
- If foods do harden, put a damp sponge or cloth on the spill until softened, then wipe up.
- Serious cleaning of the microwave may be accomplished by putting two tablespoons of baking soda or lemon juice in one cup of water in a microwave-safe, four-cup bowl. Place the bowl in the oven, and let it boil for about five minutes until the steam condenses on the inside walls of the microwave. Then wipe off the walls, the inside of the door, and the door seals.
- Odors in the microwave may be eliminated by combining ½ cup lemon juice and one cup of water in a large measuring cup. Microwave on high for three minutes. Let cool before removing.
- Vents should always be clear of objects so oven heats and cools correctly.

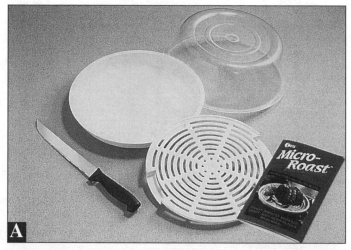

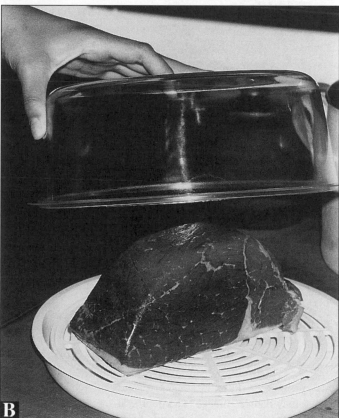

Figure 28-6A,B. This microwave roaster cooks and browns meats in a microwave. (Micro-Roast™ by K-Tel International, Inc., Minneapolis, MN. Photo by J.K.)

- Paper products like paper towels, plates, and napkins can be used to contain or cover foods for a short time, not longer than four minutes, in a microwave oven. Use sturdy paper plates or place the proper plate on a regular one for stability.
- Frozen entrees may be cooked right in their paper containers. Follow package directions.
- Covering food with waxed paper prevents splatters, because waxed surfaces stay moist but do not get soggy. Paper towels and napkins tend to get soggy when heating moist foods and overheated when covering dry foods.
- Wax-coated containers are not for heating, because the wax

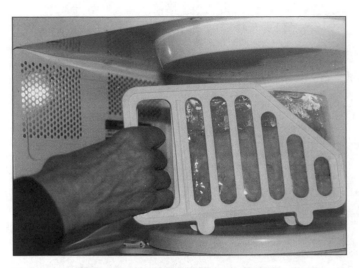

Figure 28-7. This microwave pouch holder protects the fingers when heating foods sealed in a pouch. (Photo by J.K.)

melts into the food.

- If using plastic wrap, it should be labeled microwave safe on the box. Use a container large enough that the plastic does not touch the food. Puncture the plastic wrap before and after heating to avoid scalding.
- The cover on any container with heated food should always be opened away from you. Use a long fork or other utensil to lift cover and protect hands and face from steam burns.
- Casseroles that have lids with handles in the middle allow safer handling. If you have weak hands, it is better to avoid covers. Continue to use waxed paper or plastic wrap, letting food cool a few minutes before removing the cover.
- For heavier foods, microwave-safe baking dishes and casseroles are best.
- Baby bottles should never be heated in a microwave, because they heat unevenly. Infants have been scalded.
- The oven should never be turned on without anything in it.
- If a fire occurs, do not open the door; immediately turn off the power and cover the vent with a towel to cut off oxygen.
- Never operate a microwave oven with a damaged door. If it has a swing-down door, do not use it as a shelf for food, because that may damage hinges. The door seal should always be tight and hinges in proper working condition.

If your patient is depending on a microwave for all cooking, here are some additional tips:

- A roll or sandwich may be heated without becoming soggy if placed on a paper towel-lined plate. Microwave only until warm, about 15 seconds, or bread will become tough and dry.
- Meat may be cooked in a microwave. To brown it, sprinkle with paprika or Worcestershire sauce.
- Poultry does not brown, but sauces, glazes, and crumbs added to the dish give a nice appearance to the poultry. Do not use egg or sour cream sauces, because they tend to curdle.
- Fish cooks very well in a microwave. Steam or "bake" it. Fish cooked in sauce dilutes the sauce.

- Casseroles should have ingredients such as pasta or rice pre-cooked before adding to the casserole. These ingredients may be cooked separately in the microwave.
- Fruit-based desserts and puddings cook well in a microwave. Most others do not, with the exception of recipes and mixes designed for microwave baking.
- Waxed paper is the ideal material for loosely covering foods in the microwave, like chicken and crumb-topped casseroles that splatter. Use it to line microwave-safe dishes and cake pans.

CHILDREN AND MICROWAVE USE

When parents are disabled, young children often take on home management and other responsibilities much earlier. Use of the microwave, however, is not as safe as it seems at first glance, or even when watching advertisements.

Children should use a microwave only under supervision until they are old enough (about seven years old) to know how to use a conventional stove. A child should be able to think out consequences, like the inner filling of foods becoming very hot so the food must sit and cool for a few minutes. He or she must be able to read instructions. The Shriners Burns Institute has documented a rise in the number of scaldings and burns to children by microwave foods. Some of these are to the esophagus by foods cool on the outside but scalding on the inside.

The child should also be tall enough to lift something carefully out of the microwave with both hands while standing on the floor. He or she should not have to stand on a chair. A child who is too short may spill the hot food down on his or her face and body.

For more discussion on microwave ovens, equipment, and references, see Chapter 20 in *Mealtime Manual*.

RESOURCES

Addresses for publishers, periodicals, and organizations are given in Section Four.

PUBLICATIONS

Keeping Up with the Microwave Revolution. (1990). Food and Drug Administration. 5 pages, #532Y, free from the Consumer Information Center. Examines FDA research on food packaging designed for use in microwave ovens. Also explains how microwaves work and gives cooking tips.

Anderson, J., & Hanna, E. (1997). *Microways: Every Cook's Guide to Successful Microwaving*. New York: Putnam-Berkley.

Dwyer, K. K. (1990). *Easy Living, Low-Calorie Microwave Cooking*. New York: St. Martin's Press. $14.95.

Keanneally, J. A., (Ed.). (1990). *Good Housekeeping's Illustrated Microwave Cookbook*. New York: Hearst, William Morrow. $25.

Better Homes & Gardens®. Meredith Corporation. Because microwave design changes rapidly, check for current cook book titles.

Teaching About Nutrition and Meal Planning

Achieving good nutrition is a primary goal when working with clients in the area of meal preparation and eating. Just because a person has a sudden or chronic disability does not mean that he or she will automatically change food habits.

There are areas where nutrition teaching is always imperative to the good health and rehabilitation of clients. These include eating for a healthy heart, healthy bones, and prevention of cancer. If you are a dietitian, a nutritionist, or have one as part of your multidisciplinary team, you have the basis on which to plan a nutritionally sound program with your patient. If not, consult with a Cooperative Extension Service Home Economist. Check in the telephone directory under County Government, Cooperative Extension Service.

Other resources for dietary consultation and information include the Food and Drug Administration Consumer Office, the Public Health Office, the nutrition or home economics department of a local college or university, and the dietitian or nutritionist of a local school, senior center, or hospital. Some organizations that provide help are the American Cancer Society®, the American Heart Association, the American Dietetic Association, and the American Diabetes Association. Materials abound that you may use in your treatment program. Some recommended guides are listed at the end of this chapter.

What are other local possibilities for improving nutrition for your clients? If finances are a major problem, your client may be eligible for the Federal Food Stamp Program, listed under the State Department of Human Resources, Family and Children Services, Food Stamp Program. Meals-on-Wheels programs bring prepared foods directly to patients for a nominal fee. Ascertain availability through local Senior Centers, Office for the Aging, or State and County Family and Children Services. Many senior centers provide noontime meal programs, which allow a chance for better nutrition as well as socialization.

THE FOOD PYRAMID

The Food Guide Pyramid is a nutrition tool that graphically shows the amounts of various foods a person should eat each day.

See diagram in *Mealtime Manual*. The pyramid has five major food groups replacing "the basic four." It focuses on limiting fat, particularly saturated fat, as well as limiting sweets in the diet. The pyramid is a simple guide that will help your client choose what and how much to eat from each of the five food groups to get the needed nutrients. The pyramid calls for eating a variety of foods and, at the same time, the right amount of calories to maintain a healthy weight. A range of servings is given for each group, because individual needs vary with age, sex, and activity level.

The five major food groups are represented in the major portion of the pyramid. The Bread, Cereal, Rice, and Pasta Group occupies the largest space at the base of the pyramid. The most servings of food each day should come from this group. The other food groups are represented above the base in progressively smaller sections. The smallest portion at the top of the pyramid is reserved for the Fats, Oils, and Sweets Group—foods that should be eaten sparingly.

WEIGHT AND NUTRITION

Maintaining an ideal weight is important for overall health. When a client's weight problem affects performance of daily living skills, he or she should be under a physician's care and should be referred to a dietitian or nutritionist. Certain conditions, such as vascular diseases, diabetes, or arthritis, require strict weight control. The person with arthritis affecting the lower extremities puts added stress on weight-bearing joints when overweight.

New studies, however, state that "normal weight" may be slightly higher than previously determined. The older person who has added five to 10 pounds over the years seems to improve chances for longevity. For women, this added protection also helps prevent fractures of osteoporotic bones.

Obesity is, however, a major health problem in America. More than 50% of the U.S. population is now overweight. Thirty-four million people are more than 20% over their desired body weight. Studies show that men and women with added weight around their waists—apple-shaped—are more likely to succumb to diabetes and heart disease than those who are pear-shaped, or with the weight around the hips. These people and those with health conditions aggravated by extra pounds should reduce. Naturally lean individuals should not try, however, to lose additional pounds, because they may end up with nutritionally inadequate diets.

To help teach the size of an average serving, you might use an electronic scale to visually reinforce the allowed amount of a particular food. An electronic scale weighs in $1/8$ pound or 5-gram increments with the touch of a switch and includes a standby mode battery saver. **Manufacturers** include 156, 498. **Sources:** 33, 98, 234. See an example in *Mealtime Manual*, Chapter 24.

Exercise is as important as calories in controlling weight. The individual with limited mobility may find that lack of exercise severely affects weight. Planning a daily time for exercise should be part of a multidisciplinary program, including home management training. The patient should always start with the physician's recommendation and increase exercises slowly. Flexibility and stretching exercises prevent aging joints from stiffening. Walking is an excellent activity for increasing cardiovascular health, muscle tone, and strength. It can be graded within almost any setting. Teach the patient to move around more at home and to use stairs if stable on his or her feet. Exercise programs for the sitting patient are available in audio- and videocassette forms as well as books. See Resources.

OSTEOPOROSIS

Osteoporosis is a major problem, most severely afflicting post-menopausal women, although men may also be affected. Ensuring adequate amounts of calcium and engaging in weight-bearing exercises throughout life are the two best steps to prevention. However, by the time an older patient is seen, there is often a marked loss of bone mass. This occurs especially in the spine, hips, and wrists. The weakened bones result in more frequent fractures, even potentially fatal broken hips. As health care professionals, we have a threefold responsibility: encourage the patient to get adequate calcium in the diet, through menu planning and checklists if necessary; engage in weight-bearing exercises on a daily basis; teach adequate safety precautions and training to prevent falls and possible fractures. Post-menopausal women should also be encouraged to discuss with their physicians the benefits and risks of estrogen and other medications as a deterrent to osteoporosis.

There is a major research focus on osteoporosis at this time. The fact that calcium-fortified orange juice has calcium carbonate, which is absorbed by the body, and that weight-bearing exercise does increase bone density are just two findings. Nutrition newsletters and health-oriented magazines are good sources for updating. See Resources.

If your patient is lactose-intolerant, tablets may be taken before a meal, or added to treat milk, or lactose-treated milk may be purchased. Recommend that your client speak with the physician. Other forms of milk may be more acceptable, including yogurt and kefir. See Resources for publications on lactose-free foods.

THE ELDERLY AND NUTRITION

Lack of good nutrition is a common problem among the elderly. Social isolation for those who live alone reduces their desire to cook or eat. Physical limitations make fixing food more difficult. The ability to taste and to smell decline in acuity, while poor-fitting dentures lessen eating enjoyment. Fixed income diminishes the buying power of the budget.

Some specific steps that can be taken include the following:
- Teach about convenience foods that are healthy and quick to fix.
- Set up a menu plan that provides for the whole week.
- Prepare foods ahead.
- Go on a supermarket tour to help rekindle the interest in eating. Many older consumers do not know about new products because poor eyesight, old habits, and reduced mobility make shopping a chore if not an ordeal.

The elderly also tend to overlook their fluid needs. Simple dehydration is a common problem. Eight glasses of fluid a day is required, even more so when older, for optimal kidney function and health. Water is the best liquid, although skim milk and fruit juices may account for part of the total. Make sure that there is an easy-to-handle mug or a pitcher from which the individual can pour water or another beverage. This may sound simplistic but helps solve a common problem. See Chapter 30 in *Mealtime Manual* for handling of beverages, Chapter 22 in *Mealtime Manual*, and Chapter 4 in this guide.

TEACHING ABOUT LOW CHOLESTEROL/LOW FAT

Changing food habits is the hardest barrier to overcome when guiding a client to better nutrition. More than one in four Americans, or more than 68 million people, have some form of cardiovascular disease (CVD). CVD annually kills about 175,000 Americans younger than 65.

The wealth of foods on shelves, the ambiguity of food labels, and the conflicting information that comes through the media leave the consumer in a quandary. Knowing the difference between cholesterol-free and low-fat, light and lite, and what is "fresh," almost takes a scientist to untangle. Rules regarding labeling have undergone changes for easier understanding. Legal definitions for cholesterol and fat now include the following:
- Cholesterol-free: Contains less than 2 milligrams of cholesterol per serving and 2 grams or less of saturated fat per serving. This means that products that contain vegetable oil, margarine, and peanut butter but no cholesterol cannot be labeled cholesterol-free. The reason is that fat, especially saturated, raises blood cholesterol. Products that never contained cholesterol, such as canned peaches, cannot be labeled cholesterol-free, because it never contained any. Instead, it may say "a cholesterol-free product."
- Low in cholesterol: Contains 20 milligrams or less of cholesterol per serving and per 100 grams of food, also two grams or less of saturated fat per serving.
- Reduced cholesterol: Contains 50% or less cholesterol per serving than the "regular" or original versions of the same product.

- Low-fat: Contains 3 grams or less of fat per serving and per 100 grams of food.
- Reduced fat: Contains less than 0.5 grams of fat per serving, provided that it has no added ingredient that is fat. A cake or biscuit mix that requires added oil would not qualify.
- (%) Fat-free: May be claimed only if the product meets the "low-fat" definition.
- Low in saturated fat: Contains one gram or less of saturated fat per serving and not more than 15% of calories from saturated fat.
- Reduced saturated fat: Contains 50% or less saturated fat than the "regular" or original version of the same product.

Understanding labels lets your patient buy more wisely. A label diagram is given in Appendix G. The page may be copied and enlarged as a teaching tool. Review the ingredients and explain that the largest amount of an ingredient by weight must come first. Read the ingredients, the number of calories, the various forms of sodium (salt, onion and other flavored salts, monosodium glutamate, baking powder, baking soda, meat tenderizer, bouillon, sodium-benzoate, -caseinate, -citrate, -nitrate, -phosphate, -propionate), and sugars in various forms (sucrose, glucose, dextrose, fructose, maltose, lactose, sorbitol, mannitol, honey, corn syrup, corn syrup solids, molasses, and maple syrup). With continued changes in labeling laws, review current articles. If possible, go on a supermarket trip with the client or use some of the Resources, especially the shopper's guide in Appendix G and also Chapter 30.

ALTERING EATING PATTERNS

The Food Guide Pyramid recommends limiting fats, oils, and sweets because they supply calories but little or no vitamins or minerals. The 1990 Dietary Guidelines for Americans recommends limiting fat to 30% or less of total calories. (Some medical researchers in heart disease feel this should be closer to 20%.) The guidelines recommend a daily maximum of approximately 53 grams of fat in a 1600-calorie diet, 73 grams in a 2200-calorie diet, and 93 in a 2800-calorie diet. Reduce the fat grams by one-third to meet heart researchers' recommendations.

To figure the number of grams of fat that provide 30%, or 20%, of the calories in a daily diet, multiply the total calories for the day by .30, or .20 (Example: 1800 calories x .30=540 calories from fat; or at the 20% rate, 360 calories). Then, divide the calories from fat by 9 (each gram of fat has 9 calories) to get the suggested maximum grams of fat per day. (Example: 540 calories from fat divided by 9=60 grams; or 360 calories from fat divided by 9=40 grams of fat.)

Cutting down is hardest to teach anyone when it comes to the questions of cholesterol and fat. The first guideline is to reduce any fat. This slashes calories and helps control weight. Second, reduce animal and saturated fats. Most patients think they are limiting the amount of animal fat they eat, but do not even know what is a normal portion size. Draw a diagram showing normal size portions of meat of approximately 3 ounces. Reproduce it in the actual size to let your client carry home a visual aid to realistically reduce the amount put on one's plate. A second homework

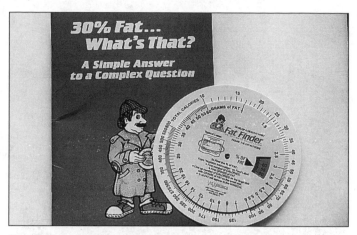

Figure 29-1. The Fat Finder helps determine the percentage of fat in a specific food or food combination. (Photo printed with permission from Vitaerobics, Encinitas, CA. Photo by J.K.)

sheet, in Appendix G, lets you encourage your patient to list each day's food intake for review during therapy sessions.

The CSPI cholesterol scoreboard helps the patient or group of clients understand the amounts of fat and cholesterol in various types of foods. This is one of many nutrition posters available from the Center for Science in the Public Interest. **Source:** 112. See Resources.

A reusable planning guide from Wellness Reproductions teaches about food groups and helps build a healthy menu. Overhead markers are used to fill in specific foods. Cost is about $12. **Source:** 567.

The Fat Finder helps determine the percentage of fat in a specific food or food combination (Figure 29-1). The American Heart Association recommends no more than 30% of calories come from fat; other researchers have suggested even less. With this dial, one takes the number of grams of fat in an amount of a given food, lines this up with the number of calories in the same amount of food, and is immediately given the percentage of fat. Cost is about $7 with an explanatory book about cholesterol. **Source:** 560.

A fat skimmer separates fat from liquids, returning only the broth for soups or broths (Figure 29-2). To use, dip the Lexan ladle in liquid, lift it out, and let fat rise to the top. Then, pull the small lever on the handle and broth pours back into the pan, leaving the fat in the ladle to be tossed away. It may be used with one hand but does take moderate coordination and vision to note where fat and liquid separate. Dishwasher safe. This unit is about $13 plus $4 postage and handling. **Source:** 255B.

The Skim-It fat separator may be easier for some clients to handle than a ladle, because it can be used with one or two hands (Figure 29-3). The scoop is dipped into the soup or stock up to the level of the slots; fat on the surface flows through the slots and collects in the bottom of the cup. It is then lifted out, disposed of, and the process repeated. Cost is about $5 from housewares stores. **Manufacturer:** 181.

To reduce the amount of salad dressing used, suggest that your clients purchase an adjustable spray bottle from the pharmacy. Pour dressing into it, then shake and spray. This will mist the salad with dressing at less than a quarter of what they might pour on.

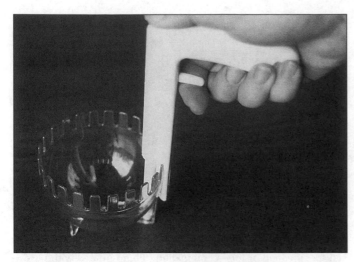

Figure 29-2. A fat skimmer separates fat from liquids, returning only the broth for soups or broths. (Fat skimmer by Heartwatch II, Wichita, KS. Photo by J.K.)

Teach your client to change the types of fats eaten in small amounts. Canola oil, vegetable oils rather than soft or hard margarine, and soft margarine rather than hard margarine are easy early steps. Switch to skim or 1% milk. Finally, teach alternatives to meat and higher fat dairy foods.

The only way for someone to change is to try new foods. Doing this as part of home management training raises the success rate. Find a good recipe using low-fat yogurt. Teach about low-fat cheeses, and use with a bean recipe. Stir-fry a little tofu with vegetables as a lunch. Add grains like oatmeal, wheat germ, and cooked barley to meat mixtures to extend the recipe and increase the carbohydrates and fiber. For those under budget restrictions, the double lesson is that it also stretches the dollar. Products are on the market that provide the taste of meat with low-calorie substitutes. One company, Dixie USA, Inc., distributes mixes of meat substitutes, including Beef (Not!)™ meatloaf, chili, taco fillings, burgers, and Chicken (Not!)™ mixes. Complete catalog is available from **source** 170B.

Holding monthly or periodic seminars on how to attain good nutrition is an excellent way to emphasize guidelines to a wider audience of clients. Tasting sessions and free hand-outs carry the lessons home. Local merchants may even be willing to donate low-salt and low-fat products as part of the tasting session, knowing that they will gain new customers for these products.

A program on low-fat cheeses, for example, might include a listing of accepted cheeses along with tips and recipes. Some starting tips include the following:
- A cheese slicer makes thinner slices for sandwiches.
- Shredded cheeses go further than sliced when used in casseroles and as toppings.
- Sharp cheeses require less, because the taste is stronger.
- Dry-curd or low-fat cottage cheese can replace ricotta in lasagna or manicotti.
- A blender turns cottage cheese into a smooth dip with herbs and garlic. This avoids the sour cream or cream cheese base.
- Lower fat, hard cheeses may be used in baked dishes.
- Homemade, low-fat yogurt cheese, made from drained yogurt, is a versatile snack and cooking base.

Organizations and groups involved with the promotion of foods are usually happy to provide materials for teaching about nutrition. Several of these are listed in Appendix C including the following:
- American Dairy Association.
- American Seafood Institute's Fish and Seafood Hotline.
- Canned Food Information Council.
- Fish and Seafood Consumer Information Center.
- Lactaid, Inc.
- National Dairy Council.
- National Fish and Seafood Promotional Council.

CONTROLLING SODIUM INTAKE

Conservative measures are the preferred course when a person suffers from mild high blood pressure or hypertension. Rather than start a patient on a lifelong course of medicine, physicians usually prefer to try non-drug therapy. Patients should be taught to lose weight—as little as 5% will help (unless the patient is already underweight), reduce salt intake (discussed here), exercise daily, and stop smoking.

Whether or not a patient suffers from hypertension or heart or kidney problems, it is wise to limit sodium intake. Table salt, which is 60% sodium and 40% chloride, is the major source of sodium in a normal diet.

But how much is in a glass of milk, in a baked potato, or in a ½ cup of canned beans? Purchasing or making up a chart and actually developing a before-the-chart and after-the-chart quiz for clients is one way of teaching. A Sodium Scoreboard poster is available from the Center for Science in the Public Interest. **Source:** 112.

An electronic salt checker immediately measures the salt level or salinity in a food or dish (Figure 29-4). Many medical studies recommend limiting salt intake from 1100 mg to 3000 mg per day. When there is high blood pressure, salt may be strictly limited. The unit shown helps a patient see what is being eaten while learning about salt content or when eating away from home. Food should be thoroughly stirred, then the clean tip inserted in the moist food or beverage. There is a gauge for hot and cold foods. An LED light indicates the salinity level. To find the milligrams of salt or sodium, the individual must multiply the answer times the number of grams of food (28 grams per ounce) in the serving. Five ounces or 140 grams of food at a salt level of .6% has .84 grams or 840 milligrams of salt. Cost is about $22 including postage and handling. **Manufacturer:** 135. **Sources**: 347, 361.

Low-sodium dishes can be as flavorful as those with salt. Herbs, lemon juice, vinegar, and onion increase taste appeal without salt. Another solution is "sour salt," which is not a salt at all but a crystalline compound of powered citric acid extracted from the juice of citrus fruits. Because humans can distinguish only four main tastes—sweet, sour, salty, and bitter—this gives a sour taste that seems to be salty. Warn against using garlic salt or onion salt to which sodium has been added; instead use fresh or powdered garlic and onion.

Teach clients to read labels, avoiding sodium found in other forms. These include monosodium glutamate, baking powder, baking soda (sodium bicarbonate or bicarbonate of soda), brine, sodium benzoate (in condiments), sodium hydroxide (processing for fruits and vegetables, hominy, and ripe olives), and sodium propionate (in pasteurized cheeses and some breads and cakes). Plain frozen vegetables are better than salted canned ones, although some canned foods also come without salt. Use fresh tomatoes or no-salt-added canned tomatoes for seasoning stews and meat loaves. Rinse tuna fish and drain other foods to significantly reduce salt.

No one should use a salt substitute without first consulting his or her physician. One of the principal ingredients of salt substitutes is potassium. Taken in excess, potassium (a natural chemical in the body that controls muscle function) can cause nausea, diarrhea, muscle weakness, even cardiac arrest. Potassium bicarbonate may be substituted for baking soda in a low-sodium diet. It is usually available at drugstores and is sodium free. Note: Patients who have kidney dysfunction or are taking medications that disturb the body's potassium balance (beta-blockers for angina or ibuprofen) should avoid potassium.

Suggestions for lowering salt or sodium are given in *Mealtime Manual* and in this guide as well with two seasoning mixes on a reproducible sheet in Appendix G. Also see Resources.

DIABETES

Teaching a patient to control diabetes requires a multidisciplinary approach. The goal is to live a full life by adjusting lifestyle, diet, and exercise. The physician and nurse work together to find the best medication levels. The occupational and physical therapists, home economist, dietitian, and/or nutritionist teach about meal planning, weight control, exercise, and food habits.

Restricting sugar intake calls for developing new recipes that suit the patient's taste preferences. Each person's diet must be individualized to meet his or her needs and must be monitored until the client can independently handle the planning. Educating your patient about how insulin and insulin receptors work together to lower blood glucose levels and teaching methods of measuring blood and urine sugar levels at home are part of the program. Safety precautions should be taken because of possible lack of sensation, and instruction should be given in proper foot care for Type II diabetics.

Recent advancements that allow the patient to take more control of diabetes include new medications, the development of human insulin, the revolution of blood glucose monitoring, and new treatment for diabetic retinopathy. The attitude has also changed: people are having more confident, fuller lives even though diabetic.

For years, the rule for diabetics was no table sugar, no honey, no molasses. It was felt that eating any of these sugar-based sweeteners would make blood sugar surge. New research indicates that small amounts of sugar eaten with other foods does not send blood-sugar levels soaring. The American Diabetes Association relaxed its stand on use of sweeteners in recipes for diabetics. The new rule allows one teaspoon of any sugar-based sweetener per serving. Note: Some individuals are more sensitive to sugar than others, so any person with diabetes must check with the physician before accepting this finding.

The American Diabetes Association distributes teaching aids and materials. Magazines and cookbooks for the self-motivated patient are also available. See Resources on diabetes at the end of this chapter.

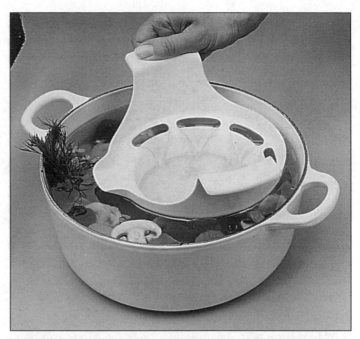

Figure 29-3. The Skim-It fat separator can be used with two hands. (Photo courtesy of East Hampton Industries, Inc., East Hampton, NY.)

If your patient has progressed to the point of visual loss, called diabetic retinopathy, adaptations in handling equipment, including glucometers and insulin injection, may be necessary. See Chapter 18 in this book and Chapter 9 in *Mealtime Manual*.

DIGESTIVE PROBLEMS

Loss of appetite, nausea, and irritable bowel often affect patients. Some problems are due to lessened physical activity and lack of fiber in food; others are due to depression, medication, stress, or age. Any serious reactions should be reported directly to the physician. A consultation with a dietitian or nutritionist leads to better meal planning.

Angina, a symptom of serious heart disease, may be experienced by a patient following a meal. Five million Americans experience chest pains and seek medical treatment. If your patient complains of chest pain after a meal, during or after vigorous activity, while lying in bed, when under emotional stress, or in response to cold temperatures, make sure that an appointment is made with the physician to discuss the matter. The pain may come at the same time every day. A doctor will be able to treat the pain and teach ways to manage angina effectively.

MODIFYING RECIPES

Home recipes can be modified by reducing or eliminating the amount of salt and substituting small amounts of oil or margarine for butter or solid shortening. Egg substitutes or egg whites may be used in place of whole eggs. Look for new ideas, such as fruit whips or applesauce and egg whites used in place of oil and whole eggs in recipes and mixes. See Chapter 31. Use non-stick pans, which require no extra fat.

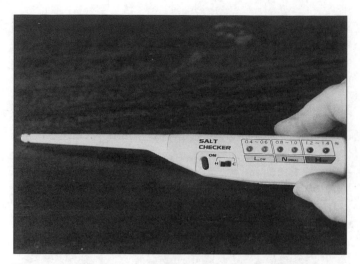

Figure 29-4. This unit helps a patient see what is being eaten while learning about salt content or when eating away from home. (Composite International, Inc., Worthington, OH. Photo by J.K.)

Convenience foods are often high in salt and fat. Reading labels is your client's best defense. To increase convenience of fresh foods made at home, instruct the client to make up double or triple amounts ahead of time, wrap in serving portions, and freeze for later.

RESOURCES

Addresses for publishers, periodicals, and organizations are given in Section Four.

One of your first sources for information may be your local supermarket. Many chains offer free hand-outs on nutritional issues, budget cooking, wise use of foods, low-sodium cooking, etc. These make excellent take-home teaching guides for patients.

A second source is the Government Printing Office. Write to the U.S. Consumer Information Center for a listing of nutrition and meal planning publications. Some government publications available through the Superintendent of Documents or U.S. Consumer Information Center, as well through your county home economist, Cooperative Extension Service, include the following:

Calories and Weight (108Y). (1990). USDA. 114 pages, $1.75. Caloric tables for hundreds of popular foods and beverages.

Cooking for People with Food Allergies (001-000-04512-1). (1988). Selecting and preparing foods that do not contain milk, eggs, corn, or wheat; tips on recognizing these ingredients in prepared foods; recipes to help avoid them. $1.50.

Nutrition and Your Health: Dietary Guidelines for Americans. U.S. Department of Agriculture/U.S. Department of Health and Human Services. HG-232 Bulletin. $.50 from the Superintendent of Documents. Or you may access the home page of the USDA Center for Nutrition Policy and Promotion at http://www.usda.gov/fcs/cnpp.html or the HHS home page at http://www.os.dhhs.gov.

Also from the U.S. Department of Agriculture, Human Nutrition Information Service: *Dietary Guidelines and Your Diet*, HG 232-1 through 7. Each pamphlet focuses on one of the Dietary Guidelines, giving practical tips on how to make changes in your diet. And *Dietary Guidelines and Your Diet*, HG 232-8 through 11. Pamphlets focus on specific ways to use all of the Dietary Guidelines together with choosing and preparing foods—Preparing Foods and Planning Menus; Making Bag Lunches, Snacks, and Desserts; Shopping for Food and Making Meals in Minutes; and Eating Better When Eating Out.

Food Guide Pyramid. U.S. Department of Agriculture/U.S. Department of Health and Human Services. HG-252 Bulletin. Free.

Fat Substitutes, (528Y). (1990). What they are, how different types are made, how they help cut fat, cholesterol, and calories. Free.

The American Heart Association distributes books and pamphlets on fat-controlled, low-cholesterol meal plans and cooking to reduce the risk of heart attack. These include *The American Heart Association Cookbook*, $25; *The American Heart Association Low-Salt Cookbook*, $20; *The American Heart Association Low-Fat, Low Cholesterol Cookbook*, $23; *The American Heart Association Kids' Cookbook*, $15; *The American Heart Association Quick and Easy Cookbook*, $25; *Hispanics and Heart Disease*, kit includes 15-minute video of two Hispanic families and the changes they made in their diets and lifestyles to promote heart health, $15; *Cholesterol and Your Heart*, $9.50 for 50 brochures; *Easy Food Tips for Heart-Healthy Eating*, $7 for 50 brochures; *Facts About the New Food Label*, $5.50 for 25 brochures. Call or write for full publications list.

The American Dietetic Association has a toll-free Consumer Nutrition Hotline: 800-366-1655. Nutritionists and dietitians handle questions.

Many food companies distribute books and pamphlets that recommend ways to reduce fat and cholesterol in the diet or to increase fiber. When using these, you may find that the focus is on one type of product and that other problems are overlooked, like low fat but high sugar or vice versa. Use your judgment and edit when using with your clients to follow the basic guidelines of low fat, low cholesterol, low sugar, and high fiber and calcium.

PUBLICATIONS

Aspen Reference Group (Roe, S. N. [Ed.], & Lawrence, K. E. [Director].) (1991). *Dietitian's Patient Education Manual.* Vols. 1 and 2. Frederick, MD: Aspen. Two loose-leaf binders, tabbed, $245. Excellent reference for not only dietitians but other allied health care professionals. Major topics include diabetes, obesity/weight control, coronary heart disease, renal and gastrointestinal diseases, hypertension, pulmonary disease, cancer, geriatrics, AIDS/HIV, rehabilitation and developmental disabilities. Gives background, nutritional requirements, patient teaching materials, related organizations, and references.

Baskin, R., & the Editors of Consumers Reports® Books. (1992). *How Many Calories? How Much Fat?: Guide to Calculating the Nutritional Content of the Foods You Eat.* Yonkers, NY: Consumers Reports® Books. $13.95. Facts on nearly 3000 foods, brand-name fresh and frozen, packaged, and fast foods. Charts show nutritional composition; help substitute foods lower in fat and sodium. Tips on reading food labels and general nutritional guidelines.

Better Homes & Gardens Eating Well with Your Food Guide

Pyramid Guide. (1996). Des Moines, IA: Meredith. $9.95. Easy-to-understand guide on using the Food Pyramid Guide, based on individual calorie needs. 73 recipes, quick recipe ideas, week of suggested menus.

Better Homes & Gardens Healthy Family Cookbook. (1995). Des Moines, IA: Meredith. $29.95. Recipes, tips, and techniques to reduce fat, cholesterol, sodium, and calories. Symbols identify recipes as low calorie, low sodium, and high fiber. How to make nutritional labels on packaged foods work to the cook's advantage, how to flavor foods with citrus juices, salsa, herbs, and more, how to substitute low-fat ingredients for high-fat, high-calorie ingredients.

Betty Crocker's Low Fat, Low Cholesterol Cookbook. (1991). New York: Prentice Hall, Simon & Schuster. $17.95. Recipes and guidelines for lowering cholesterol and fat.

Burlant, A. (1995). *Secrets of Lactose-Free Cooking.* Garden City Park, NY: Avery. $13.95. More than 150 recipes for lactose-free foods. Explains what lactose intolerance is, which foods are most likely to cause irritation, and which foods can be easily substituted.

Burt, L. & Mercer, N. (1989). *High Fit Low Fat.* Ann Arbor, MI: MedSport, University of Michigan Medical Center. $13.95 plus $2.40 shipping and handling. Cookbook emphasizes food low in fat, high in fiber, and stresses the importance of regular physical activity. Gives nutrition information and tips, new and original recipes. Includes diabetic exchanges to help with meal planning and a guide for cardiac rehabilitation patient. **Source:** 547.

Diet, Nutrition & Cancer Prevention: The Good News. National Cancer Institute. Dietary Guidelines for cancer prevention along with charts of high-fiber and low-fat foods. To order, call 800-4-CANCER.

Eating Smart Fat Guide. Washington, DC: Center for Science in the Public Interest. $3.95. Teaches how to reduce fat percentage in foods to the 25% to 30% range. **Source:** 112.

Gardner, L. (1993). *Health and the Hispanic Kitchen (La Salud y La Cocina Latina).* Potomac, MD: Precepts, Inc. Healthy cooking with Hispanic foods. Large-print, illustrated, step-by-step basic recipes for soups, main dishes, vegetables, and desserts. $12. Available through Para la Salud. **Source:** 400.

Gershoff, S., et al. (1990). *The Tufts University Guide to Total Nutrition.* Scranton, PA: Harper & Row. $22.50. Scientific findings on nutrition, role of fiber and cholesterol, advice on staples and equipment for a healthy kitchen, quizzes on nutrition.

Gines, D. J. (1990). *Nutrition Management in Rehabilitation.* Frederick, MD: Aspen. $46. Tells how to maximize client nutritional care in rehabilitation. Includes head injury, spinal cord injury, muscular dystrophy, cerebral palsy, geriatric disorders, multiple sclerosis, arthritis, stroke, dysphagia. Gives community resources, related organizations, information services.

Goldbeck, D. (1992). *The Good Breakfast: Making Breakfast Special.* Woodstock, NY: Ceres. $9.95.

Goulder, L., & Lutwak, L. (1988). *The Strong Bones Diet: The High Calcium Way to Prevent Osteoporosis.* Gainesville, FL: Triad. $14.95. How to prevent osteoporosis, recipes, methods of cooking, finding calcium in the grocery store and fast food chains. For women of all ages.

Healthy Heart One-Dish Meals. (1995). Birmingham, AL: Oxmoor House. $29.95. Low-fat, low-sodium recipes including

diabetic exchanges for each recipe. In most recipes, less than 30% of the calories are obtained from fat. One-third of the recipes are super-quick. Other Oxmoor low-fat cookbooks include ones on weight control, stir-frying, meat, pasta, chicken, and dessert.

Herbert, V., & Subak-Sharpe, G. J. (Eds.). (1990). *The Mount Sinai School of Medicine Complete Book of Nutrition.* New York: St. Martin's. $35.

Hermann-Zaidins, M., & Touger-Decker, R. (1989). *Nutrition Support in Home Health.* Frederick, MD: Aspen. $39.50. Practical guide for dietitians including clinical management of oral, enteral, and parenteral nutrition.

Jacobson, M., & Fritschner, S. (1991). *The Fast-Food Guide* (2nd ed.). New York: Center for Science in the Public Interest, Workman. $7.95. Ingredient listings and nutrition charts with the best and worst offerings. Helps educate client for eating out as well as at home.

Jamaieson, P., & Dorschner, C. (Eds.). (1993). *Recipe Rescue Cookbook.* Charlotte, VT: Camden House. $18.95. Healthy new approaches to traditional foods.

Katahn, T., & Martin. (1991). *The Low-Fat Good Food Cookbook.* New York: Norton. $8.95

Krummel D. A., & Kris-Etherton, P. M. (1996). *Nutrition in Women's Health.* Frederick, MD: Aspen. $49. Normal preventive and research findings. Topics include eating disorders, the elderly, obesity, osteoporosis, diabetes, and cancer.

Lactose-Free Foods: A Shopper's Guide. Wellesley, MA: Bullseye Information Services. Lists more than 1000 lactose-free national brand products. $6.95 plus $1.50 handling. **Source:** 102.

Mateljan, G. (1992). *Cooking Without Fat.* Irwindale, CA: Health Valley Foods. $15. Methods for reducing fat, shopping for low-fat foods, recipes. **Source:** 253.

Mantero-Atienza, E., et al. (1995). *Nutritional Considerations of Parkinson's Disease: The Route to Better Management of Parkinson's Disease.* Miami, FL: National Parkinson Foundation, Inc. Free through local chapter or write main office. Booklet covers modifications in protein, exchange system of meal planning, sample meal plan for patient on medication, and references.

Melvin, S., & Stone, M. (1990). *Snack to Your Heart's Content: The Low-Fat, Low-Cholesterol, Low-Calorie Quick and Easy Cookbook.* Gainesville, FL: Triad. $9.95. By authors of *Not Just Cheesecake*; uses non-fat yogurt cheese for ice cream, pizza, cream cheese, and more. Good way to help patient stay on diet. Also sells yogurt cheese maker.

Notelovitz, M., & Ware, M. (1985). *STAND TALL! The Informed Woman's Guide to Preventing Osteoporosis.* Gainesville, FL: Triad. $12.95. Medical explanation of osteoporosis in terms patient can understand. Guidelines for nutrition and exercise.

Ornish, D. (1996). *Everyday Cooking with Dean Ornish.* New York: HarperCollins. $25. Introduction to changing cooking patterns. Low- to no-fat recipes by season. Vegetarian, designed to reverse heart disease.

Page, H. C., Shroeder, J. S., & Dickson, T. C. (1996). *The Stanford Life Plan for a Healthy Heart.* San Francisco, CA: Chronicle Books. $29.95. Reference cookbook with low-fat recipes helps teach how to understand nutrition advice and implement a healthier lifestyle.

Piscatella, J. C. (1994). *Don't Eat Your Heart Out Cookbook* (rev. ed.). New York: Workman. $17.95. Information and motivation for clients to take care of their heart health whether as part of cardiac rehabilitation or preventive medicine. Recipes and tips.

Preventing Osteoporosis. Washington, DC: The American College of Obstetricians and Gynecologists. Free booklet describing problem, treatments, and giving table of calcium in foods.

Rogers, J. (Ed.). (1995). *Prevention's Quick and Healthy Low Fat Cooking.* Emmaus, PA: Rodale. $15.95.

Roth, E. M., & Streicher, S. L. (1990). *Good Cholesterol, Bad Cholesterol.* Rocklin, CA: Prima. $8.95. Cardiologist and cardiovascular nurse show patients how to painlessly adapt to a low-cholesterol lifestyle.

Schlesinger, S. (1994). *500 Fat-Free Recipes: A Complete Guide to Reducing the Fat in Your Diet.* New York: Villard, Random House. $23. 500 recipes from soup to dessert with one gram of fat or less.

Simko, M., Cowell, C., & Hreha, M. (1989). *Practical Nutrition: A Quick Reference for the Health Care Practitioner.* Frederick, MD: Aspen. $35.95. Interdisciplinary reference for health promotion and maintenance. Nutrition assessment by age and needs groups, environmental management. Dietary assessment tools, food preparation tips, nutrient and food source information.

Snetselaar, L. G. (1988). *Nutrition Counseling Skills: Assessment, Treatment and Evaluation* (2nd ed.). Frederick, MD: Aspen. $42. Nutrition counseling for prevention and treatment of coronary heart disease, hypertension, diabetes, weight control, cancer risk prevention, anorexia nervosa and bulimia, stress.

Sonberg, L. (1993). *The Complete Nutrition Counter.* New York: Berkley, Putnam Berkley. $5.99. A-to-Z listing of brand name foods and basic foods—calories, fat, sodium, fiber, cholesterol, Vitamin A, Vitamin C, protein, carbohydrates, calcium, and iron.

Stern, B. (1994). *Simply Heart Smart.* Toronto: Heart and Stroke Foundation of Canada and the Bonnie Stern Cooking Schools Ltd., Random House. Explains what healthy eating is, gives tips for adjusting diet for heart and diabetic clients. Gives more than 200 recipes in larger print, clearly presented, with both cup- and metric-based measurements. **Source:** 433.

Svetkey, L. P., et al. (1996). *Eating Well, Living Well with Osteoporosis: Dietary Approaches to Healthy Living from Duke University.* New York: Viking, Penguin.

University of California Wellness Letter editors and Sheldon, M. (1992). *The Wellness Encyclopedia of Food and Nutrition.* Berkeley, CA: Health Letter Associates. Distributed by Random House. $29.95. Excellent reference pertaining to all areas of nutrition, written for the consumer.

Wilson, J. W. (1988). *Eating Well When You Just Can't Eat the Way You Used To Cookbook.* New York: Workman. $12.95. Recipes and techniques for cutting back on fat, cholesterol, salt, sugar, and calories.

Witt, C., & Wirth, C. (1996). *Bodystat.* New York: Viking, Penguin. $22.95. Book is recommended for low-fat strategies and recipes that can become staples.

Woodruff, S. (1995). *Secrets of Fat-Free Baking.* New York: Avery, Garden City Park. $13.95. More than 130 simple-to-make, larger-print recipes, most having less than one gram of fat per serving.

Also see Resources in Chapter 30 and Chapter 24 in *Mealtime Manual.*

PERIODICALS

Appendix D gives rates and addresses.

American College of Nutrition Journal. Wiley.

American Dietetic Association Journal.

Cancer Smart. Quarterly newsletter.

Cooking Light. Combines health articles with low-fat, healthy recipes, teaches conversion of traditional recipes. See *Mealtime Manual,* Periodicals.

Newsletters on nutrition are listed in Appendix F. Also see Periodicals in *Mealtime Manual* and Resources in Chapter 4.

AUDIOVISUALS

Eating for Your Health: A Guide to Food for Healthy Diets. Washington, DC: American Association of Retired Persons. 13-minute, VHS video. Deli owner discusses how to lower sodium in the diet plus fat and cholesterol. Gives guidelines. Comes with Presenter's Guide and an excellent hand-out for each participant. This includes diagram of food labels, nutrition labels, unit pricing, daily charts for sodium, calories and cholesterol, recipes for low-sodium diet, low-calorie diet, and low-cholesterol diet. Free loan, request 90 days in advance from the Program Office of AARP.

How Does Your Nutrition Measure Up? (1987). Washington, DC: American Association of Retired Persons. 14 minutes, 22 seconds, VHS video. Comes with Presenter's Guide and brochures for participants. Free loan, request 90 days in advance from the Program Office of AARP. Large-print, excellent hand-out includes evaluation of one's nutritional health, suggestions for losing weight, gaining weight, maintaining good nutrition, shopping and cooking tips for one, adapting recipes for weight gain or loss, keeping a food diary, balancing a diet, food groups, eating well when eating out, using nutritional sense when shopping, and resources for further information.

Lower Your Cholesterol Now! with Leni Reed, and special comments by Scott M. Grundy, MD. $24.95 plus $3 shipping from Family Experiences Productions, Inc. **Source:** 199. Registered dietitian takes viewer through a 6-part video-guide to label reading, shopping, and cooking. Shows how to make wiser choices for lower calories, saturated fat, and cholesterol. Key points are reinforced with "quizzes." May be used for self-instruction or group programs.

Posters: these give a quick guide to clients working or waiting in your clinic—Sodium Scoreboard, Anti-Cancer Eating Guide, Sugar Scoreboard, Heartguard: CSPI Cholesterol Scoreboard, Rough It Up: Fiber Scoreboard, Fast Food Eating Guide, Nutrition Scoreboard. Cost is $4.95 each; $9.95 laminated from the Center for Science in the Public Interest. **Source:** 112.

Also see Audiovisuals in Chapter 30.

COMPUTER PROGRAMS

Dine Right: The Complete Diet Solution. Computer program for PCs (Dine Right) and Macs (Mac DINE Perfect) contains nutrition information on more than 5500 foods. May be used as clinic teaching tool. Client enters recipe, then asks for how much of what is in it, i.e., calories, protein, saturated and non-saturated fat, cholesterol, complex carbohydrates, dietary fiber, sugar, iron, calcium, vitamins A and C. Cost is about $99. For further information, write the Center for Science in the Public Interest. **Source:** 112.

Additional nutrition computer programs are available from other publishers, including Country Technology, Inc. Send for catalog. **Source:** 148.

DIABETES

The American Diabetes Association distributes materials for health care professionals and patients. These include Exchange Lists for Meal Planning and Exchange Lists for Weight Management. Write for current publications and costs.

The Buyer's Guide to Diabetes Products. Alexandria, VA: American Diabetes Association. $2.50. Catalog of electronic devices, supplies, and new technologies for management of diabetes.

The National Institute of Diabetes and Digestive and Kidney Diseases, National Institutes of Health distributes materials plus a monthly free newsletter: *Diabetes Dateline.* Write the National Diabetes Information Clearinghouse.

Better Homes & Gardens Diabetic Cookbook. Des Moines, IA: Meredith. $12.95. More than 140 recipes to fit diabetic's special needs as well as the family's.

Caditz, J. (1991). *Diabetes, Visual Impairment, and Group Support.* Santa Monica, CA: The Center for the Partially Sighted. $10.95 in regular and large-sized type.

Controlling Type II Diabetes Through Meal Planning and Exercise. Krames Communications. 75 color illustrations emphasize self-control of diabetes by adjusting lifestyles, diet, and exercise. **Source:** 308.

Diabetes Forecast. 12 issues per year, $24 per year includes magazine, membership in the ADA with services at the affiliate level—classes, support groups, workshops, family programs, summer camps, counseling. Magazine provides research updates, articles on how diabetes affects body, food and fitness, handling stress, and has special section for children with diabetes. See Periodicals, *Mealtime Manual.*

Diabetes Self-Management. $18 bi-monthly issues per year. Excellent magazine for diabetics. Advice on nutrition, new products, exercise, and all phases of life. See Periodicals, *Mealtime Manual.*

Diabetes Self-Management pocket reference guides: *Charting: The Systematic Approach to Achieving Control*, $3.95, and *Eating Out: Your Guide to More Enjoyable Dining*, $4.95. Add $1.50 handling and postage per copy. **Source:** 167B.

Dyer, N. (1979). *A Practical Education Program for the Diabetic Client Within the Rehabilitation Setting*, An AFB Practice Report, PRP970. New York: American Foundation for the Blind. $8.95. Information enables instructor with background in biology or health sciences to teach client with diabetes how to maintain good control of condition.

Franz, M., et al. (1991). *Learning to Live Well with Diabetes* (rev. and updated ed.). Minneapolis: DCI, Chronimed. International Diabetes Center. $24.95.

Kipnis, L., & Adler, S. *You Can't Catch Diabetes From a Friend.* Gainesville, FL: Triad. $9.95. Written for the young diabetic. Helps family and friends understand the disease and the child's need for independence.

Learning to Live with Diabetes, Patient Information Series, $3 from Medicine in the Public Interest. **Source:** 355.

Powers, M. A. (1996). *Handbook of Diabetes Medical Nutrition Therapy.* Frederick, MD: Aspen. Classic reference. Nutrition recommendations, practice guidelines, monitoring techniques, making food choices, setting and achieving management goals.

Schneider, C. (1991). *The Diabetes Brand Name Food Exchange Handbook* (2nd ed.). Philadelphia: Running Press. $14.95.

University of Alabama at Birmingham. *Complete Step-by-Step Diabetic Cookbook* (2nd printing). (1996). Birmingham, AL: Oxmoor House.

Walters, N. (1991). *Diabetes and Doing Your Best.* Baltimore: Olde Maryland Publishing Co. $9.20. Written by a 13-year-old boy who has diabetes, with two chapters by his physicians. Management tips, coping, dealing with problems, famous people who have had diabetes, how to help find a cure.

Also see *Mealtime Manual*, Chapter 24.

Audiovisuals

In Balance In Control: Personal Diabetes Management Series. Boehringer Mannheim Diagnostics. Six patient-oriented videotapes convey what patients need to know about diabetes and their role in its management. **Source:** 88.

30

Teaching About Shopping

AT-HOME PLANNING

Many facets of shopping must be assessed when working with your client. Going to the store is only one part. With the overwhelming array of foods in a market as well as difficulties caused by a disability ranging from weakness and incoordination to limited vision, low energy, and cognitive disturbances, planning ahead is essential.

Home is where good nutrition management and wise buying begin. Tasks involved in shopping include planning nutritious meals, compiling a list of what is needed for those meals, making up a consolidated list that includes non-food items, working within a budget, making selections from grocery store ads, handling money, getting out of and back into one's residence independently, using a form of transport to get to the store, carrying groceries, and putting them away.

Handling a budget is a part of home management training often ignored. Limited resources affect many patients—the elderly on fixed incomes, the young growing family, the person on welfare, and the individual who finds that medical necessities eat up more funds than expected. The person just starting to live independently has no experience with the decision making that comes with working out a food budget, especially if having lived within an institution. The client who is alone for the first time finds it difficult making decisions for one and has to learn to ask the store for smaller portions or to divide at home for several meals. In each case, nutrition may be affected.

Concrete training sessions teach best. The client should first see what is already at home. Sitting down with local grocery store flyers concretely teaches the person how to plan. A stockpile of bulk foods and foods available through welfare programs, like cheese, dry milk, and peanut butter, may be translated into immediate meal plans and recipes. See Resources for some books that may help. The "super shopper" checklist, in Appendix G, will help your client determine in which areas help is needed when learning to shop.

Making the grocery list itself is a major teaching goal. The person with weak or incoordinated grasp or severe arthritis may find it hard to write down items. The elderly shopper may forget. A master list lets the shopper check-off items needed as they come to mind. The check-off shopping list in Appendix G may be reproduced and given to your patients as a planning aid. It has been edited to encourage reduction of fat and cholesterol and may be enlarged on a copy machine for easier reading. Unedited lists are available through mail-order firms.

A writing device, such as the Writing Bird, helps when fingers are weak or affected by arthritis (Figure 30-1). Cost is about $15 from self-help firms. **Source:** 383. See *Mealtime Manual*, Chapter 20.

The patient with aphasia or developmental delay may not be able to read, so he or she may need a picture method of listing items. See Chapter 21.

To reduce walking and increase efficiency while shopping, the list should be designed to follow the floor plan of the major grocery store. More than 75% of shoppers use one grocery store, and more than 50% shop once a week. Organizing a list may be done so the person can follow it within the store. Sorting coupons by food groups before going to the store helps extend the budget and reduces frustration.

Some family service magazines, like *Family Circle*, provide a "Checkout Checklist" when giving new recipes. This allows the individual to see which items might be missing from the pantry shelf.

AT THE STORE

Efficiency is helped with a cart caddy or a consolidated unit for carrying lists, coupons, and a pen to check-off items (Figure 30-2). Caddies are available from variety stores and mail-order firms for about $5 and up.

A rolling walker with a large basket may provide extra stability for the client with difficulty ambulating. Many models have a seat so that the shopper can rest when tired or while waiting in line. See Chapter 13 and Chapter 26.

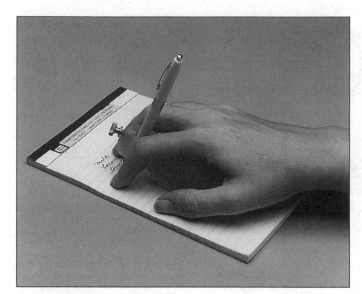

Figure 30-1. This Writing Bird helps when fingers are weak or affected by arthritis. (Photo courtesy of North Coast Medical, Inc., San Jose, CA.)

With the decreased length of stay and the lack of time or staff to make home visits, rehabilitation centers must provide extended training for handling one's community but often within the confines of an institution.

Easy Street Environments® is a concept that helps patients face the physical challenges of everyday life during their rehabilitation (Figure 30-3A,B). The typical community may be physically recreated and custom-designed within the institution in an area as small as 900 square feet. Modular parts include common barriers, surfaces, and props. Clients practice shopping, car transfer, boarding a bus, marketing, going to a restaurant, bank, etc. Staff personnel work with each patient teaching techniques, role playing as cashiers or tellers, and making suggestions for adaptations when needed. For further information, write **source** 267.

Within the grocery store, a cart may be used as an ambulatory aid after training by the therapist. If a client is a wheelchair user, your input can encourage the store to provide wheelchair grocery carts. See Chapter 25 in *Mealtime Manual*. A reacher gives access to items placed beyond one's reach. An alternative is to ask a passing shopper to give a hand. Part of the ADA regulations states that if one knows the store layout, the shopper can give a list to the store manager so that everything may be collected at one time by store personnel.

A reacher is especially helpful when upper extremity range is limited or when using a wheelchair (Figure 30-4). It should not be used for lifting heavy or breakable items from higher shelves.

The "Activ" reacher has a strong grip handle that is easier to use by people who have limited grasp (Figure 30-5). The inner surface of the jaws are covered with striated rubber to increase friction while holding. Hooks on the outside of the jaws allow the user to push and pull items. An adjustable lower arm support reduces strain on the wrist. It also comes in a folding model that fits in a pocketbook. **Manufacturer:** 191. Cost is about $35 and up from self-help and rehabilitation equipment suppliers. **Sources:** 191, 383.

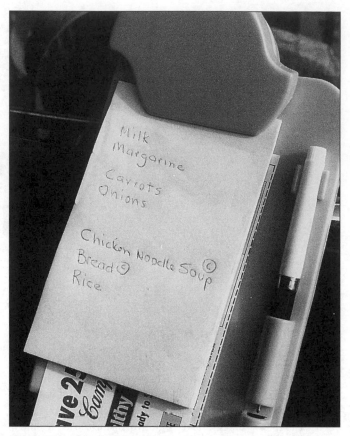

Figure 30-2. This organizer clips to the grocery cart. (Photo by J.K.)

A senior companion makes it possible for older or frail shoppers to get out and do their own shopping (Figure 30-6).

An over-the-shoulder hook reduces stress on the hands for carrying a bag or light groceries (Figure 30-7). Cost is about $13 from self-help firms. **Sources:** 383, 461.

When upper extremity strength is poor, one answer for getting around the grocery store is an electric scooter (Figure 30-8). For use at home as well as away, it conserves energy. Several large chains, especially in retirement areas, provide an electric scooter as a courtesy for shoppers who are limited in mobility and energy. The client should be carefully evaluated in relation to the scooter, the type of seat and support it offers, and the location and ability to handle the controls. **Source:** 47. Also see scooters in Chapter 16 and Chapter 19, as well as in *Mealtime Manual*.

On return home, a cart or other unit on wheels can help the shopper with a disability move the groceries from the car to inside the residence. Garden carts, "Pop-karts," and collapsible carry-alls that are used to transfer goods from the car to a private boat can be adopted for use at home. If there are steps or if handling the bags is too difficult, suggest that the shopper plan ahead for a family member or neighbor to do the transferring.

The use of a service dog as an assist in daily activities is gaining increased attention. Not only may the canine companion fetch and pick up items, but he or she can pull the wheelchair, hand money to the cashier, help carry light parcels including mail, groceries, and books to and from stores and other locations, get items from the refrigerator at home, and obey up to 70 or 80 additional commands (Figure 30-9). Since many of these are generic com-

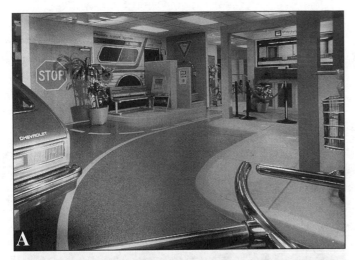

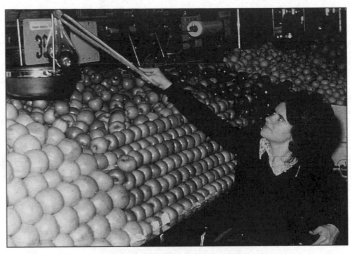

Figure 30-4. A reacher is especially helpful when upper extremity range is limited or when using a wheelchair. (Photo courtesy of the O.T. Dept., Rancho Los Amigos Medical Center.)

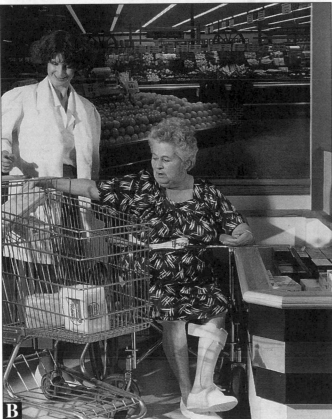

Figure 30-3A,B. Easy Street Environments® is a concept that helps patients face the physical challenges of everyday life during their rehabilitation. (Photos courtesy of Health Services Marketing, Ltd., Tempe, AZ.)

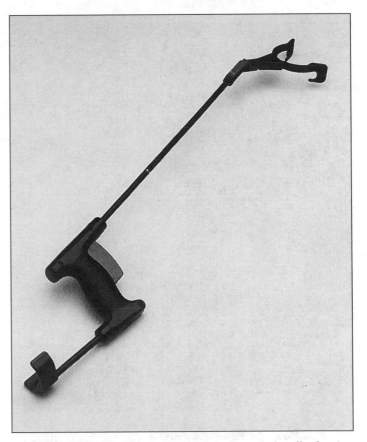

Figure 30-5. This "Activ" reacher has a strong grip handle that is easier to use by people who have limited grasp. (Photo courtesy of Etac USA, Inc., Waukesha, WI.)

mands, like fetch or pull, the possibilities are endless. One woman is able to drive a van but does not have the power because of post-polio syndrome to get into her wheelchair from the driver's seat. By hanging onto her canine companion, he pulls her over into the wheelchair. For further information on obtaining a dog, contact Canine Companions for Independence, Handi-Dogs, Inc., and Support Dogs, Inc., or one of the other groups listed under Animal Assistance. Addresses are in Appendix C. See also Chapter 20 for information on hearing dogs.

DRIVING EVALUATION AND AIDS

Getting back behind the wheel is a top priority for many patients. Practicality and safety must be carefully evaluated in each case by the physician and health care professionals. A post-stroke patient with perceptual losses requires an assessment of his

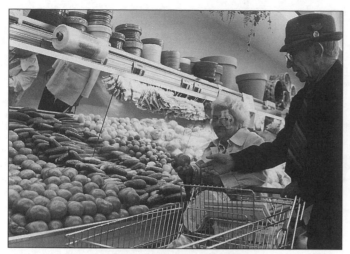

Figure 30-6. This man takes his companion who has poor vision to the store, helps her shop, does the driving, and carries in the grocery bags. (Senior Companion Program, photo courtesy of ACTION®, Washington, DC.)

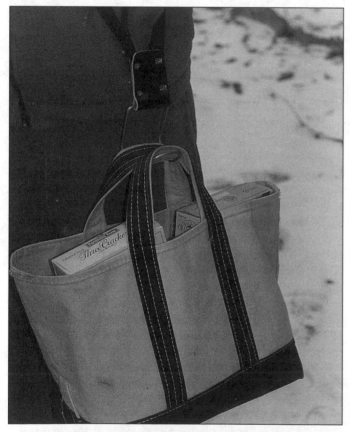

Figure 30-7. This over-the-shoulder hook reduces stress on the hands for carrying a bag or light groceries. (Photo by J.K.)

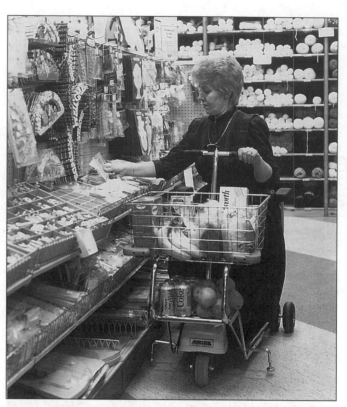

Figure 30-8. An electric scooter conserves energy for the person with multiple sclerosis or other disability. (Photo courtesy of Amigo® Mobility International, Inc.)

or her abilities as they relate to perception, reaction time, peripheral fields, and physical capabilities. People with Parkinson's, diabetes, and epilepsy need careful evaluation, because they may black out, lose consciousness, or control over bodily movements. All states require drivers with epilepsy to be barred from driving for periods ranging from three months to two years following their last seizure. Most states also require a diabetic to carry a letter from the physician saying the person is not prone to blackouts. Many hospitals and rehabilitation centers have Driver Assessment Programs. Check locally or through the Handicapped Driver's Mobility Guide from AAA, listed under Resources.

Clients who have sustained a stroke or have progressive or traumatic neurological disorders should be tested and, if necessary, receive training before taking to the road. The trainer must identify deficiencies that could hamper performance on the road, evaluate the need for adaptive equipment, and when there are limitations determine what therapy or training would help the client improve operation of a motor vehicle. In a Driver Assessment Program, the client will be tested for vision, perception, reaction time, and physical ability to handle an automobile. There are a number of driver training simulation products.

A driver assessment system may include a control console with the system computer, a computerized driver simulator station, projector, and printer (Figure 30-10). It comes with an Assessment Program, Evaluator's Manual, and operational training that teaches the health care professional how to use the system. Programs cover driver readiness, basic skills, perceptual skills, traffic interaction, high-speed travel, emergency situations, collision avoidance, and skill evaluation. For information, contact **source** 504.

The person with weak upper extremities or arthritis requires a physical evaluation of ability to handle the car and possible adaptations to make it easier. Standard options, such as power brakes and steering, decrease the strength needed and reduce fatigue. Modifications, such as a swivel seat, wide-view mirror, blind spot

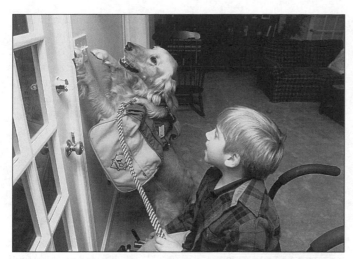

Figure 30-9. At the grocery store, a trained canine companion can carry light parcels, even hand money to cashier. (Photo courtesy of Canine Companions for Independence, Inc., Santa Rosa, CA.)

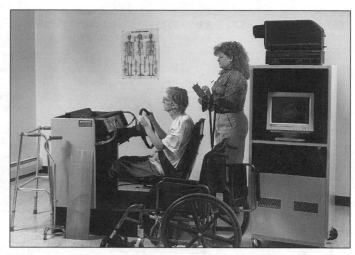

Figure 30-10. This driver assessment system includes a control console with the system computer, a computerized driver simulator station, projector, and printer. (Photo courtesy of Doron Precision Systems, Inc., Binghamton, NY.)

mirrors that attach onto regular side mirrors, added side mirrors when neck motion is limited, built-up key turners, and adapted safety belts, may be done locally. The person with limited hearing who is wearing a hearing aid may also gain more control over driving skills with the addition of right and left hand mirrors. Mirrors are available from auto part stores and mail-order firms, including 96, 235, 239, 278. Make sure that the mirror quality is good and that the reflection is not distorted.

Proper posture in the car conserves energy and reduces pain to the back or strain on weakened muscles (Figure 30-11). The Auto Riser wedge-shaped seat cushion keeps the person from sinking into the car seat. It raises the driver up to 3 inches for unobstructed, safer vision over the steering wheel. This is a solution for a common problem with older women who have lost height due to osteoporosis. The slanted foam cushion has a removable cover. You can make one by sculpting a piece of foam, or you can buy a cushion for about $7 and up from mail-order firms. **Manufacturer:** 290. **Sources:** 171, 241, 361, 495, 508, 561B.

For automobile controls and extensive adaptations, companies across the country are trained to help. Programs to assist drivers with physical handicaps get behind the wheel are sponsored by Chrysler Motors, General Motors, and the Ford Motor Company. Chrysler's Physically Challenged Resource Center offers information and advice on adaptive equipment manufacturers and installers. They also offer up to a $500 reimbursement for the installation of adaptive equipment on a new Chrysler product. General Motors Mobility Assistance Center is involved in similar studies and has a mobility video available. **Sources:** 121, 208B, 222. A list of driving programs and driving control manufacturers is given in *The Disabled Driver's Mobility Guide*. See Resources.

Adapted automobile controls allow people with severe physical disabilities to drive (Figure 30-12A,B). A rotary, hand-operated driving control combines a twist-type throttle with a thrust-style braking system to give the driver independent, simultaneous, one-hand control of both the throttle and brake. Cost is about $300 and up. A portable left foot accelerator installs in minutes; some models may be transferred from vehicle to vehicle. It allows the person

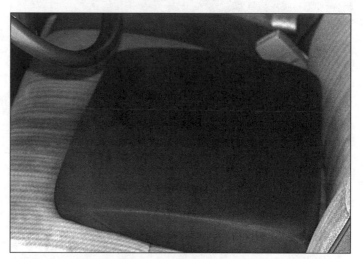

Figure 30-11. This Auto Riser wedge-shaped seat cushion keeps the person from sinking into the car seat. (Photo by J.K.)

with loss of function in the right leg and foot to drive safely. Cost is about $120.

Manufacturers of adaptive automobile controls include Automobility (64), Drive-Master (173), dSi (174), Gresham Driving Aids (232), Keith Howell (266B), Kroepke Kontrols (309), Mobility Products & Designs, Inc. (365), and Wells-Engberg, Inc. (568). Brochures are available from each company.

THE OLDER DRIVER

More than 12% of drivers on the road today are older than 65. Functional rather than chronological age is the best predictor of driving performance. Based on the fewer miles they tend to travel, seniors do have a higher serious accident rate than most other driver groups. The National Research Council found that drivers 75 and older are involved in more fatal crashes than any group except teenagers. Reaction times, peripheral vision, ability to track a mov-

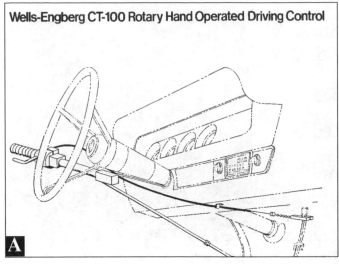

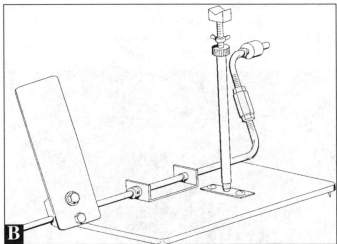

Figure 30-12A,B. Adapted automobile controls allow people with severe physical disabilities to drive. The portable left foot accelerator installs in minutes and transfers from vehicle to vehicle. (Illustrations courtesy of Wells-Engberg, Inc., Rockville, IL.)

ing object, perceptual speed, grip strength, neck flexibility, hearing loss, and short-term memory do not deteriorate at the same speed for all drivers. Adapting to conditions, such as roads, signs, and low cars designed with youth in mind becomes harder.

Teaching your older client flexibility exercises designed to improve older driver performance helps maintain the ability to turn the head and rotate the trunk. This translates to greater control on the road. The exercises are available in a brochure called *A Flexibility Training Package For Improving Older Driver Performance* from the AAA Foundation for Traffic Safety and might be incorporated into therapy as part of a patient's rehabilitation program. See Resources.

Ninety-five percent of the sensory input needed for driving comes through the eyes. Older individuals need more light to see clearly and find it harder to adjust to glare from approaching headlights. Depth perception is also weaker. Medications can also affect driving, so checking with the physician or pharmacist is important. Overconfidence because of "experience" masks problems. Because of age-related declines in vision, hearing, and

reflexes, more Motor Vehicle Departments are requiring drivers over a certain age to be re-tested before renewing a license.

Recommending use of public transportation or help from a volunteer driver is strengthened by using a self-rating performance form. Developed by Columbia University, the test asks questions that help a person evaluate whether driving should be curtailed or discontinued. Responses or reactions include "Intersections bother me because there is so much to watch out for from all directions" and "My thoughts wander when I am driving" or "My children and other family members are concerned about my driving ability." It also offers safety tips geared toward the older driver. Cost is about $2 from the AAA Foundation for Traffic Safety. Address is in Appendix C. You can also recommend that your older patient brush up by re-reading the free driver manual from the Motor Vehicle Department, or contact the local AAA office, senior center, adult education courses, or AARP chapter for re-education courses in your area.

Recommendations to older clients who are driving are given in reproducible form in Appendix G: Rules to Increase Your Safety When Driving.

CAR EMERGENCIES

Any client with physical limitations should be prepared for an automobile emergency. This includes a sign declaring that help is needed, a flashlight, and flares. Signs are available commercially through mail-order firms. **Distributor:** 71. **Sources:** 239, 457. A cellular phone is a wise safety investment if the person lives in a rural area or is severely limited in mobility. Police say they can respond faster to an emergency call made directly from a car.

TRANSITION TO ASSISTED OR PUBLIC TRANSPORTATION

Suggestions regarding the inability of an individual to safely handle an automobile may be made but cannot be legally enforced by a health care professional. In some states, doctors are required to report any physical condition that might impair driving ability to the Motor Vehicle Department. This is not always done, however, because of the doctor/patient relationship and vagueness of the laws.

Losing the freedom to drive, moreover, is a painful experience. Helping to make a transition may be done in several ways. Familiarize the person with municipal and private transportation services. Go on a practice bus run to and from the shopping areas or medical facilities as part of training. Suggest the patient arrange car pools with other seniors, having adult children or a volunteer do the driving. Have the group hire a private driver and share the costs. Talk with the local senior center about arranging driving for shopping on certain days.

Wheelchair-accessible buses have become more common following the passage of the ADA (Figure 30-13).

For the ambulating older shopper, especially in urban areas, crossing the street has its own hazards. Focusing on injury prevention within your community can markedly increase safety at little expense. Changes to be considered include more highly visible street markings for traffic lanes, traffic directions and crosswalks, lengthening the time of stoplight signals for crossing the street, increased police enforcement of the speed limit, and safety education presentations at senior centers. When a program like this was carried out in one area of New York City, the number of pedestrians killed dropped by 43%, even though the volume of traffic increased by 19%.

LIFTS

For the wheelchair user, getting a chair in and out of the car is often difficult for the patient and/or family member. Lighter weight wheelchairs reduce the strain, but for older individuals and those with chronic conditions a lifter may be indicated.

Lifts to put manual wheelchairs and powered scooters into a vehicle, an electric wheelchair into a van, or to carry a wheelchair or scooter on the outside of the vehicle are available in a range of designs and prices. Reviews of different types and ads are found in periodicals such as *Accent on Living*, *Mainstream*, *Paraplegia News*, *Spinal Network*, and *Team Rehab*. See Appendix D and Appendix F as well as Periodicals in *Mealtime Manual*.

Lifts, vans, and adapted controls are sometimes covered by Vocational Rehabilitation agencies, depending on the use to which the client will be putting the equipment. The Veterans' Administration will fund a van and lift for an individual who was disabled in a service-connected incident. Check with local DME representatives who have samples to try and may also have suggestions on funding.

Vehicles designed for carrying wheelchairs allow easier entrance and egress (Figure 30-14). A Volkswagen Eurovan CL-Mobility Access is equipped with a lift to bring the wheelchair into the van. For further information, see your local dealer or contact Volkswagen USA. **Source: 560B.**

A ramp or lift offers ways to get into and out of vans (Figure 30-15). The person who has marked weakness in the upper extremities or who has a caregiver with limited strength may prefer a lift. The fully automatic, electro-hydraulic, Lift-a-Way wheelchair lift shown allows independent mobility through total command of raising, lowering, folding, and unfolding. A semi-automatic model raises and lowers by a button control but requires an attendant to fold and unfold the platform.

A ramp may also be used with a manual or powered chair. Both units store completely within the vehicle when not in use. Options include automatic door operators, wheelchair tie-down system, powered chair tie-down, remote control systems, lowered floors, and raised roofs or doors. A six-way power seat base permits the person with a disability to transfer more easily from the wheelchair to the driver or passenger seat. **Manufacturer: 91.**

Also see lifts in Chapter 2. Some lift **manufacturers** include 10, 91, 100, 155, 237, 342, 444, 527, 534. Wheelchair lifts for pick-up trucks are available from Life Essentials, 320, and from General Motors, 222, for several models of their small and larger pick-ups, both of which offer a wheelchair storage compartment inside the wheelchair accessible cab. General Motors also reimburses a customer with a disability up to $1000 toward the purchases of devices that make driving easier.

A companion swivel seat allows the person with limited mobil-

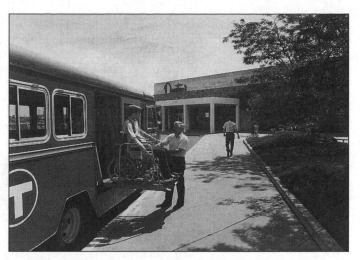

Figure 30-13. This bus is part of the public transit system in Minneapolis. (Photo courtesy of Sam Jacobs.)

ity or arthritis to get into and exit from the passenger's seat of a Dodge Caravan or Plymouth Voyager minivan with greater ease (Figure 30-16). The seat extends 20 inches and tilts forward six inches to make boarding safe and easy. Once seated, the occupant pushes a switch and is raised into the vehicle, then manually turns himself or herself to the left. **Source: 91.** Chrysler offers a cash rebate toward the purchase of adaptive equipment.

RESOURCES

Addresses for publishers, periodicals, and organizations are given in Section Four.

SHOPPING GUIDES

Bellerson, K. J. (1995). *The Shopping Guide to Fat in Your Food: A Carry-Along Guide to the Fat, Calories, and Fat Percentages in Brand Name Food*. Garden City Park, NY: Avery. $2.50.

Mercer, N., & Orringer, C. (1991). *Grocery Shopping Guide* (3rd ed.). Ann Arbor, MI: University of Michigan Press. Medsport, University of Michigan Medical Center Preventive Cardiology Program. $18.95. Gives basic background, then lists foods by brand and variety breaking them down into tables of Acceptable, Not Acceptable in different categories. **Source: 547.**

Shopping for Food and Making Meals in Minutes Using The Dietary Guidelines. U.S. Department of Agriculture, Human Nutrition Information Service, Home and Garden Bulletin No. 232-10. $2.50 from the Superintendent of Documents.

Also see Chapter 1, Chapter 3, and Chapter 29.

AUTOMOBILES AND DRIVING

Able Driving is Safe Driving. Bethesda, MD: American Occupational Therapy Association, Inc. Brochure.

American Association for Retired Persons. (1991). *55 Alive— Mature Driving* (3rd ed.). Washington, DC. American Association for Retired Persons. Courses are offered in communities on a rotating basis. Check with your local chapter.

The American Journal of Occupational Therapy has frequent articles on assessment of drivers with physical and cognitive dis-

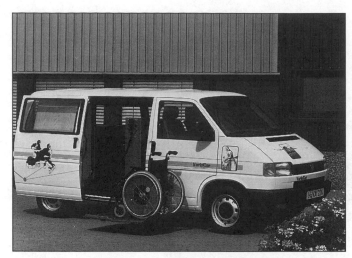

Figure 30-14. This Volkswagen Eurovan CL-Mobility Access is equipped with a lift to bring the wheelchair into the van. (Photo courtesy of Volkswagen USA, Auburn Hills, MI.)

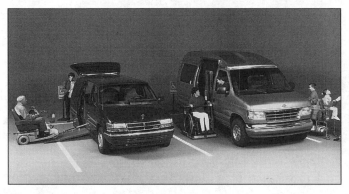

Figure 30-15. A ramp or lift offer ways to get into and out of vans. (Photo courtesy of The Braun Corporation Inc.™, Winimac, IN.)

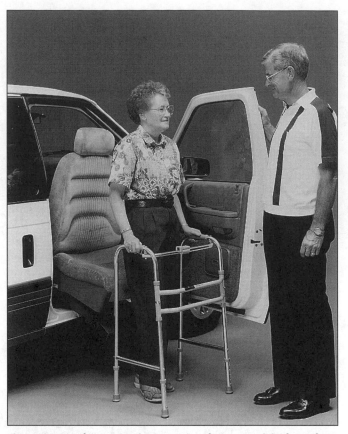

Figure 30-16. The companion seat uses the van's original seat but replaces it with a power base. (Photo courtesy of The Braun Corporation™, Winimac, IN.)

abilities. American Occupational Therapy Association, Inc., Bethesda, Md. Check annual indexes.

The Braun Corporation's newsletter, called *The Road to Mobility*, updates information in the area of transportation for people with disabilities. Free, **Source:** 91.

Brenton, M. *The Older Person's Guide to Safe Driving*, Public Affairs Pamphlet No. 641. $1 from AAA Foundation for Traffic Safety. Excellent pamphlet covers all aspects of driving for the older person. Might be given to patient as "required reading" and used in follow-up discussions as a teaching tool.

Driver Rehabilitation Resource Guide. Bethesda, MD: American Occupational Therapy Association, Inc. $10 AOTA members, $20 non-members. Books, articles, journals, software, and organizations related to driver assessment and training for drivers with disabilities. Includes partial listings for equipment and training, suppliers, commercial and van conversion, and hospital-based evaluation and training programs.

Evaluating Driving Potential of Persons with Physical Disabilities, $2.75; *Teacher's Preparation Course in Driver Education for the Physically Disabled*, $3.25; *Teaching Driver Education to the Physically Disabled,* $3.75; and *Hand Controls and Assistive Devices for the Physically Disabled Driver*, $2.75.

Albertson, NY: National Center for Disability Service. All are available from Director of Driver Education.

A Flexibility Fitness Training Program for Improving Older Driver Performance. Washington, DC: AAA Foundation for Traffic Safety. Single copy free with a stamped, self-addressed, business-sized envelope. Recommended exercises to maintain flexibility and increase safety when driving.

Galski, T., Bruno, R. L., & Ehle, H. T. "Driving After Cerebral Damage: A Model With Implications for Evaluation," *American Journal of Occupational Therapy*, 46:1 Vol. 46, No. 1, 324-332. Focus on evaluation of people with cerebral vascular disorders and head injuries.

Garee, B. (Ed.). (1982). *Going Places in Your Own Vehicle.* Bloomington, IL: Accent. $6.50. Discusses assessment of driving ability, transfers, driving, carrying a wheelchair, use of a van. Sources for equipment, lifts, automobile controls. **Source:** 8.

Hamada, K. (Ed.). (1995). *The Disabled Driver's Mobility Guide.* Heathrow, FL: American Automobile Association. $5. Controls and equipment, approved hand control and wheelchair lift manufacturers. Discusses learning to drive, lists agencies that teach driving by state and province.

Pierce, S. Legal considerations for a driver rehabilitation program. (1993, March). *Physical Disabilities: Special Interest Section Newsletter*, Vol. 16, No. 1. Bethesda, MD: American Occupational Therapy Association.

Plank, B. (1992). *Disabled Doesn't Mean Immobile: Adaptive*

Aids for Transportation. Matching Disability, Vehicle and Equipment. Bloomington, IL: Accent. $10 plus $1.25 handling from **source** 8.

Tips on Car Care and Safety for Deaf Drivers. Washington, DC: U.S. Department of Transportation, National Highway Administration. Free.

ORGANIZATIONS

Adaptive Mobility Services. **Source:** 25B.
American Automobile Association.
American Driver and Traffic Safety Education Association.
Association of Driver Educators for the Disabled.
National Mobility Equipment Dealers Association.
RESNA.
Society of Automotive Engineers.

AUDIOVISUALS

Chrysler Automobility Program. Free video explains assistive program for people with disabilities. Call 800-255-9877.

General Motors Mobility Program. Video focuses on GM's program to assist physically challenged individuals. Shows a local driver assessment center, installers of adaptive driving devices, and vehicle modifications as well as sources that may help fund the adaptation. Available through General Motors® Mobility Program. **Source:** 222.

Supermarket Savvy. $24.95 plus $3 shipping from Family Experiences Productions, Inc. **Source:** 199. Registered dietitian conducts a 52-minute video through the supermarket. Aisle by aisle, she points out methods and provides clues to a group with varying dietary interests. Topics cover choosing cheese and meats with lowest fat, figuring calories from fat, glossary of terms on package labels, sodium, cholesterol, and role of nutrition in cancer prevention. Backs up statements with quotes from reputable sources and separates fact from fiction.

31

Teaching Recipes

Every individual has taste preferences based on personal likes and dislikes and ethnic and cultural background. Using dishes a client is familiar with increases motivation. Over a period of time, the homemaking rehabilitation professional can find some basic recipes that meet both the needs for physical skills training and nutritional learning.

A recipe collector book helps create a custom cookbook of training recipes (Figure 31-1). It allows division by tasks or cultural preferences and inclusion of large-print recipes for people with visual or cognitive losses. The binder opens to form an easel to display the recipe while cooking. Cost is about $14.95 and up for binder and vinyl pages. **Source:** 539.

The recipe chart shown in Figure 31-2 is given as a reference for combining a variety of kitchen tasks and techniques. The recipes are designed to incorporate basic kitchen techniques and use common fresh and convenience foods.

You may find a sample chart to set up in Appendix G. Try setting one up for your clients, perhaps using a different one for each and letting them fill in individual meals or recipes that they would like to prepare during therapy sessions.

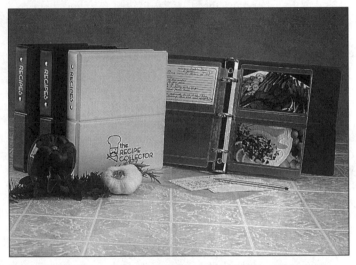

Figure 31-1. This recipe collector book lets one create a custom cookbook with nutritionally selected and large-print recipes. (Photo courtesy of Twentieth Century Plastics®, Brea, CA.)

SWEDISH TURKEY MEATBALLS

The low-fat ground turkey used in this recipe tastes like veal. Encourage your client to select all white meat ground turkey for lowest fat content. Skills involve mixing meat and using a portable electric skillet or the range top. Moderate hand dexterity and safety precautions are required to brown the meatballs. They could be browned in the oven if preferred or formed into a meat loaf, which requires a cooking time of about 45 minutes at 350°.

1 pound ground turkey

1 egg or equivalent egg substitute

¼ cup ketchup

¾ cup bread crumbs, dry or fresh

1 tablespoon fresh dill, or ½ teaspoon dried dillweed

Dash of nutmeg

1 small onion, finely diced, or 2 tablespoons dried onion

2 tablespoons canola or vegetable oil

1 10¾-ounce can or 1 12-ounce jar mushroom gravy

Dice onion by hand or in food processor.

Mix all ingredients except gravy in large bowl.

Form turkey mixture into walnut-sized meatballs and set on large plate until all are formed.

Measure 1 tablespoon of oil into skillet, and let heat over medium until hot.

Add meatballs, several at a time, not crowding them, and keep turning them in rotation until they are browned. As they become browned, remove with slotted spoon to bowl or plate.

If necessary, add a second tablespoon of oil and continue until all the meatballs are browned.

Return them to the pan; lower heat to medium low, and pour gravy over the meatballs, stirring lightly to cover them all.

Recipe/Techniques Chart	
Opening can	Using electric mixer
Opening box	Using food processor or blender
Opening jar	
Measuring liquids	Transferring batter
Measuring dry ingredients	Using stove top
Using measuring spoons	Setting oven
Preparing vegetables/fruits	Putting pan in oven
Breaking egg	Removing from oven
Beating egg	Using broiler
Cutting up meat	Using electric skillet
Mixing batter by hand	Using microwave

Figure 31-2. This recipe chart is given as a reference for combining a variety of kitchen tasks and techniques. See sample in Appendix G.

Heat until gravy begins to simmer.

Serve over rice, potatoes, or noodles, with a vegetable or salad.

Makes four servings that can be divided by your client for several meals.

If not eating immediately, refrigerate or freeze in covered container.

STIR-FRIED CHICKEN AND VEGETABLES

This recipe allows use of stove top or portable appliances and uses a variety of cutting tasks. A knife and board or kitchen shears may be used for the chicken. Freezing the chicken for 20 minutes will make it easier to cut. Vegetables may be varied, using broccoli, zucchini, or frozen, cut-up vegetables instead of a green pepper.

2 halves of a boneless chicken breast, cut in thin strips
1 small onion thinly sliced or cut in slivers
1 green pepper, thinly sliced
1 clove garlic, chopped, or ½ teaspoon garlic powder
1 teaspoon ground ginger
1 cup mushrooms or broccoli flowerets
1 cup snow peas or mushrooms
2 tablespoons canola or vegetable oil
¼ cup low-sodium soy sauce

Gather all ingredients, plus skillet, and turning utensil.

Prepare the chicken and vegetables and place on separate plates to one side.

Pour oil into skillet and heat on medium high until hot enough to brown meat. Add chicken, garlic, and ginger, and cook quickly until chicken is done.

Add onion; continue to cook for 2 minutes.

Add remaining vegetables and soy sauce and continue to stir and cook for two to three minutes longer or until vegetables are desired consistency.

SPICED APPLE AND ORANGE SAUCE

Preparing the ingredients for this sauce helps increase dexterity and coordination, develops tactile discrimination and teaches use of the stove top.

2 large cooking apples
1 large orange
¼ cup water
¼ cup sugar
⅛ teaspoon ground cinnamon

Peel, core, and slice apples. Place in a small saucepan.

Peel orange, cut into sections. Add with water to saucepan.

Cover and cook over medium heat until tender, about 10 minutes.

Remove from heat; and stir in sugar and cinnamon.

Cool slightly; serve plain or over frozen yogurt.

LIGHT CINNAMON SOUR CREAM COFFEE CAKE

This popular recipe has been modified to reduce fat and cholesterol content by using egg substitute, light sour cream, and margarine. The cooking tasks involved provide a test of the client's ability to handle measuring, mixing, transferring batter, and using an oven. This coffee cake keeps well and makes about 12 servings.

1 cup regular margarine, softened
1¼ cups sugar
Egg substitute to equal two eggs
1 cup low-fat sour cream
2 cups regular flour
1½ teaspoons baking powder
½ teaspoon baking soda
1 teaspoon vanilla
¾ to 1 cup finely chopped walnuts or sliced almonds, combined with
1½ teaspoons ground cinnamon and
¾ cup sugar

Grease and flour a 10-inch tube cake pan.

Measure all ingredients. Mix nuts with the cinnamon and sugar in a small bowl. Set aside.

Mix flour with baking powder and baking soda. Set to one side.

In large bowl of electric mixer, combine softened margarine, sugar, and egg substitute. Beat until light and fluffy.

Add vanilla and blend in half of the flour mixture with half of the sour cream. Mix well.

Add remaining flour and cream; mix on medium speed just until completely blended.

Spoon half of batter into prepared tube pan, and sprinkle half of the nuts mixture evenly over the dough. Spoon remaining dough into pan and smooth lightly.

Sprinkle remaining nuts mixture on top.

Place pan in cold oven, then set for 350°.

Bake for 50 minutes, or until done when tested with a toothpick.

Remove from oven and set on rack to cool completely.

Other meal preparation recipes might include teaching your client to make cookies or cake with applesauce or fruit puree instead of oil. Banana bran or a similar loaf requires measuring, mixing, and handling batter and an oven.

Section Four

HELP FOR THE HEALTH CARE
PROFESSIONAL AND THE
CAREGIVER

Funding and Resources for Home Management Training, Equipment, and Home Modifications

Finding adequate funding to meet training and equipment needs of clients is one of the most time-consuming and frustrating (next to paperwork) aspects of a health care professional's job. You know what is needed, but how to finance it remains a mystery to untangle or solve. This chapter will hopefully start you thinking along some very traditional as well as overlooked and unusual lines.

Sources for help fall into four main categories: government or public, non-profit, private or foundation, and volunteer. At times these overlap.

GOVERNMENT/PUBLIC LOCAL, COUNTY, AND STATE PROGRAMS

One of the most basic aids to any health care worker is the *County Guide to Programs and Services for the Aging and People with Disabilities*. The title varies, but all the government programs are listed with contact telephone numbers. To obtain one, call your local or area Agency on Aging or County Executive's Office.

Programs listed may include the following:
- Advocacy.
- Alcohol and Drugs.
- Clothing and Household Goods.
- Consumer Information and Protection.
- Counseling.
- Crisis Intervention.
- Day Care (for children and adults).
- Death and Dying (including hospice).
- Discount Programs.
- Education.
- Employment.
- Energy Assistance.
- Family Services.

- Financial Assistance/Financial Counseling (benefits, emergency help, tax assistance).
- Foods, Groceries, and Nutrition (counseling, emergency, food stamps, meal programs, grocery shopping assistance).
- Handicapped (including vision and hearing).
- Health (agencies, organizations, support groups, clinics, dental services, financial assistance, health education and information, medical equipment, and loans of same).
- Pharmacy/Medication (programs for those unable to afford).
- Home Care (assessment, planning, companions/helpers, friendly visitors, therapy services).
- Physical Security and Emergency Response Systems.
- Housing (complaints, financial assistance, shared living, supervised living arrangement/group homes, subsidized apartments, private apartments).
- Legal Aid and Services.
- Library Services.
- Nursing Homes.
- Recreation/Leisure.
- Senior Centers.
- Transportation (information, escorted, vans, discounts).
- Veterans.
- Volunteer Opportunities.

These are some federal and state agencies with offices that offer resources:
- Commission on the Aging.
- Crippled Children Programs.
- Department of Income Maintenance.
- Family and Children's Aid.
- Food Stamp Program.
- Home Care Programs.
- Internal Revenue Service.
- Medicare.

- Medicaid (managed by the state).
- Public library: Talking Books, reading machines, and aids, funded from Washington but administered locally.
- Senior Community Services Employment Program: places low-income individuals in social and community-service agencies in their neighborhoods, a good chance to set up a chore or household repair service position.
- Social Security Administration.
- Soldiers, Sailors and Marines Fund.
- State Association for the Blind.
- State Department of Social Services.
- State Employment Services.
- State Office for the Aging, State Senior Citizen Program.
- State Tax Relief for Senior Citizens.
- State Unemployment Compensation.
- Supplemental Security Income.
- Tax Assessor.
- Veterans Administration: regional office may authorize rehabilitation programs of short duration as well as equipment.
- Veterans Advisory Center: check if getting full compensation, ask about assistance for equipment.
- Vocational Rehabilitation Agency (Rehabilitation Services Administration).
- Workman's Compensation Board.

Although a nationwide program, the Division of Vocational Rehabilitation, which has various names, is run and budgeted by the state. The purpose is to make the individual employable. They will set up a plan for the client that eventually leads to attaining that goal. This includes education, books, medical supplies, surgery, and medical equipment. If transportation is keeping the person from going to a job or school, the cost of the modifications for an adapted vehicle or lift may be covered. An office with modifications to meet physical needs will be funded for the person who obtains a homebound job.

Homemaking is recognized as an occupation. As such, the Division of Vocational Rehabilitation also finances modifications within a residence to make it possible for the individual to be independent and responsible in caring for a family. In this case, the kitchen is the office. Obtaining funds for this takes time and documentation. The individual usually cannot have a degenerative disease that will limit abilities within a short period of time. Younger candidates are accepted more easily. For further information, contact your state vocational rehabilitation program, which is listed in the telephone book. Be prepared to do a carefully documented evaluation for the vocational rehabilitation office before the patient sees the counselor. Acceptance by the state also depends on the amount of money in the budget at the time of your client's application.

NATIONAL GOVERNMENT PROGRAMS

Medicare covers nursing and therapy in the hospital and home and hospice including some respite provisions. Coverage of durable medical equipment is limited to rental or purchase of wheelchairs, ambulation aids, hospital beds, and commodes. They do not cover items for use in the bathroom like raised toilet seats or safety bars. Lifting chairs may be covered when prescribed by the physician.

The Veterans Administration assists with payment of training, durable medical equipment, and home modifications for veterans. They cover vans and lifts for veterans with service-connected disabilities who use wheelchairs. The client must be evaluated for the equipment at the Veterans Administration hospital.

For senior citizens, the Federal Housing Administration (FHA)-insured reverse mortgages are designed to convert home equity into a monthly income or a line of credit from which they may withdraw cash. Applicants must be at least 62 and own their homes free and clear or have minimal debt to pay. Additional information on current status may be obtained through your nearest Housing and Urban Development (HUD) field office.

Other entitlements are available but are not listed here because they change fairly quickly. A social worker can wend a path through the various programs. If you do not have a social worker, talk with local town officials about social workers to which your client might be entitled or referred.

NON-PROFIT AND PRIVATE ORGANIZATIONS OR FOUNDATIONS

Private health insurance carriers vary in what equipment costs they cover. In many cases, the policy parallels that of Medicare. In cases of traumatic accidents, they may cover more items but this usually takes a lot of perseverance on the part of both the client and you.

Non-profit organizations that focus on a single disability or group of disabilities vary in the items they cover. They also differ in what their national headquarters offers versus local chapters. The Muscular Dystrophy Association funds a wide selection of specified equipment and transportation for people with a variety of dystrophies, including amyotrophic lateral sclerosis. They run free regional clinics with their own physicians. Most local chapters have support groups and patient-to-patient programs; some have a loan closet for equipment including wheelchairs. Request their booklets on assistance and programs.

The Arthritis Foundation offers self-help support and exercise classes as well as educational materials. These services are distributed through local chapters. In your area, the chapter may also provide equipment from a loan closet or have special endowments that cover purchase of a limited amount of new equipment when there is no third-party payment available. In some areas, they provide partial financial assistance through home health care agencies for homebound patients who have a primary diagnosis of arthritis. Services are limited to those provided by the agency and for patients who are not eligible to meet the financial costs determined by the agency or the chapter. The regional chapters of the Association of Rheumatology Health Professionals of the Arthritis Foundation have annual seminars and programs.

The American Cancer Society® provides publications on diet and nutrition, guides to handling chemotherapy, loan equipment, and has a call-back service for information. They also provide volunteers through local agencies to help with respite programs, with support to women who have undergone mastectomies, and with support to those who have cancer and their families. See Chapter 23.

The Multiple Sclerosis Society distributes publications on home exercises, treatment updates, and equipment. They have a fund for aids and often have local loan closets. Support groups in local communities provide assistance, exercise classes, and socialization.

The American Heart Association distributes publications on stroke, diet, lifestyle, and rehabilitation from a stroke through local chapters. Support groups are found across the country. Some are sponsored by local chapters, others by visiting nurses associations and hospitals.

The American Foundation for the Blind, the National Council for the Blind, local Lighthouse Associations, the National Association to Prevent Blindness, and other vision groups all offer educational materials for self-help and training. They will also guide you to sources for mobility training and recommended aids.

The Paralyzed Veterans' Association has developed wheelchair house plans for their members and have the experience, knowledge, and tenacity to find funding.

Groups such as United Cerebral Palsy, the Parkinson's Disease Society, Alzheimer's Society, Easter Seals, March of Dimes, American Lung Association, Cystic Fibrosis, and Hospice also provide support groups, educational courses, and materials. Locally, they may have loan closets or endowments. When a specific need is expressed, a social worker or counselor within the agency will try to find a benefactor to fund a certain project. Addresses for all groups are given in Appendix C. Also see specific chapters, such as Chapter 18, for disability-specific organizations.

Church-based organizations also help with funding. The Christian Fund for the Disabled matches the amount given by a local church. Started by Joni Eareckson Tada, who sustained a high-level spinal cord injury, the group develops fund raising and inspirational materials. See Joni and Friends, Spinal Cord Injuries and Paralysis, Section II, Appendix C.

For terminally ill patients, several organizations offer support and help. These include the Make-A-Wish Foundation, the Starlight Foundation, and local organizations. See Chapter 23 and Chapter 5.

The AARP has a wide variety of innovative programs to assist individuals. Check with the chapter in your area.

Approaching a local service club is another answer. If the person has been a member of any of the groups, support is usually forthcoming. Membership is not imperative; need is. Groups include the Lions, Kiwanis, Moose, Rotary, Jaycees, Junior League, the American Association of University Women, Knights of Columbus, Shriners, sororities, and fraternities.

VOLUNTEER

Many of the non-profit organizations listed above are sustained by the dedicated work of volunteers. Reach for Recovery from the American Cancer Society®, the Candlelighters for families of terminally ill children, and self-help groups under local chapters of The Arthritis Foundation all use volunteers.

LOOKING WHEN THERE IS NO MONEY

When there is need for a specific item for a patient, like a microwave oven or parts to build a device, but no money, there are

several possibilities. Notices on local bulletin boards sometimes bring a reply. Request donations from boards of local nursing associations and other groups. Search through garage sales, tag sales, and similar events. Talk to store owners about the availability of floor models when the season is over or the item no longer needed. Along the way, graciously accept donations that come in. That toaster oven, microwave, or food processor will find a home with exactly the right patient one day, even if you have to adapt the switch to make it work.

HOME MODIFICATIONS

Finding adequate funding for home modifications takes perseverance and ingenuity. Harnessing the skills of the family and friends is a first step. The State Vocational Rehabilitation Department may be a potential helper. Community Block Development Funds are another source. Distributed to states to assist in helping with home modifications, they are released through grants, low-cost loans, or home equity arrangements. There are income restrictions.

Next is to move on to other community organizations. In some communities, a business group of contractors will take on a special project. In others, church groups offer assistance, either physical or financial. Sometimes, a Boy Scout working for an Eagle badge may be tapped.

There are also national groups that work on projects for the needy. One of these is Habitat for Humanity International, which does not discriminate between housing for the non-handicapped and barrier-free housing. Christmas in April USA is a nationwide, annual, one-day event. Thousands of volunteers, working in groups, help low-income families, the elderly, and people with disabilities rehabilitate or renovate their homes. In 1992, a force of 60,000 volunteers gave 2400 homes across the nation various types of face lifts. For information about lending a hand or starting a program, write Christmas in April USA. Address is in Appendix C.

TAX RULES ON HOME MODIFICATIONS

Modification of a personal residence to accommodate the individual with a handicap may qualify for a medical deduction on the family income tax return. The Internal Revenue Service has ruled that the following costs are eligible in full when made for the primary purpose of accommodating a personal residence to the needs of the handicapped taxpayer, the taxpayer's spouse, or the dependents who live there:

- Ramps for entering or exiting.
- Widening doorways at entrances and exits to a home.
- Modifying areas so there is room for a wheelchair to turn and open door at front entrance and other exit doorways.
- Re-grading ground for safer access to residence.
- Porchlifts and other lifts, not including elevators.
- Wider hallways and interior doorways.
- Modified door hardware.
- Lowering of cabinets or other modifications to kitchen equipment.
- Relocated electrical outlets.
- Modified fire alarms, smoke alarms, or other warning systems.

- Installation of railings, support bars, or other modifications to bathrooms.
- Handrails and grab bars.
- Modifying stairs.

Other expenses made to adapt a personal residence for a person with a disability may be fully deductible as long as they do not increase the market value of the residence. An elevator does increase the value of a house, so it is not eligible. For detailed information and a full listing, see Revenue Ruling 87-106, Section 55,075, or call the Internal Revenue Service.

ORDERING EQUIPMENT

A quick phone call to the physician for a prescription for a cane, a commode, or other aid, and we feel that our job is done. This is not sufficient if the health care professional wants to ensure that the equipment covered by insurance will be reimbursed. The physician has a long form to fill out for wheelchairs, commodes, ambulation aids, and non-specified items covered by Medicare. As a therapist, you make the job easier when requesting a prescription by being aware of the questions that are asked and relaying the information to the physician. Durable medical equipment suppliers take responsibility for following up with this form, but your input raises the success rate. See Appendix G for a reproducible example of the Medicare form for non-specified items.

BRAINSTORMING FOR IDEAS

When no funds seem available, sit down with a group of colleagues for a concentrated think tank. Here's a list from a group of therapists involved in a course on self-help equipment. Many of the ideas may not bear fruit in your situation, but it's worth a try!

- ACTION provides senior companions and helpers to the elderly and homebound.
- Association of Community Health Service Agencies: Put the problem in their collective lap and see what avenues are recommended.
- Associations for children with disabilities: It is not always adults who need assistance or modifications in the home, but growing children who are becoming independent.
- Children's and teenagers' associations like the Boy Scouts, Campfire Girls, 4-H, Girl Scouts, Future Business Leaders of America, Future Farmers of America, Future Homemakers of America, Vocational Industrial Clubs of America, Junior Achievement, or Junior Chamber of Commerce. They will make items, shop for seniors and the homebound, clean, read, etc. Some may make it part of a Handicapped Awareness Badge or a pre-vocational program.
- Church programs, such as Catholic Charities, the Council of Catholic Women, Lutheran Social Services, and Jewish Vocational Services are sources for possible equipment funding and manual assistance as well as emergency food supplies and volunteers.
- Clubs: Newcomers, Postcomers, Block or Neighborhood Associations. One Junior League ran a fashion show to benefit a self-help aids loan closet.

- County extension agents.
- College and high school vocational programs: They will make items or do simple home adaptations and repairs. College design and engineering classes may take on more complicated projects. Architecture students could do the designing of house modifications for a specific individual. State college home economics students might set up nutrition and energy conservation programs.
- Colleges and schools who prepare health care professionals perhaps will work a special need into their curriculum as a teaching project. This usually has to be set up ahead of time and have a definite date for completion. Try departments and schools of occupational therapy, certified occupational therapy assistants, physical therapy and nursing, departments or schools of family and consumer sciences or human ecology. State associations of occupational therapists, physical therapists, and other allied health professionals may also take on a special project.
- Community recreation programs: Activities can be coordinated toward a project goal.
- Consumer movement: The organization of consumer groups in every walk of life means that some association out there has the same focus as your patient.
- Contractors' Association: See Home Modifications, earlier in this chapter.
- Corporations: Try local representatives of home appliances and building materials; offer them offer them publicity in local newspapers and professional journals once the project is done. Try international companies like 3M, AT&T, IBM, Toyota.
- Elder citizens employment programs.
- Equipment suppliers: Source for unneeded equipment, source to plan seminars on new equipment, such as Reimbursement of Post-Hospitalization Non-Medical Equipment.
- Firemen's Benevolent Association.
- Foster grandparents: Works both ways, the elderly client helps the child and/or the child helps the older individual with household chores, gardening, reading, shopping, etc.
- FISH—Friends in Sympathetic Help: Respite services, shopping, and medical appointment aid.
- Grange.
- Green Thumb.
- Health Day: Perfect time to educate the public about not only your programs but projects and needs.
- Homebound patients with time and guidance can make items for others.
- Homemakers with time.
- Housing Authority: Mentioned under several agencies above, but worth a direct approach when help is required.
- Individuals.
- Insurance companies: Beyond the individual patients, on a generic basis will sometimes support a new program.
- Merchants: Local shop owners set aside a day to give a percentage to sponsor a van for a client, aids for the elderly.
- Newspaper column: List needs as part of a local column that also gives advice on health and related matters.
- Nursing homes can run reassurance programs and help with construction of small aids like bibs and aprons or walker and wheelchair bags.

- Opportunity Programs for the Aging.
- Patients can help one another with emotional as well as physical support, each lending a different kind of talent.
- Professional organizations: Health- and non-health-related will develop projects.
- Programs for the developmentally delayed.
- Red Cross: Reassurance program and transportation.
- Rehabilitation centers.
- Retirees groups such as the AT&T Pioneers, RSVP.
- Salvation Army and Good Will Industries will make needed items.
- Senior citizens who have talents needed, such as companionship, transportation assistance, woodworking, and home repair skills.
- Seniors Clubs.
- Sheltered workshops will make aids.
- Sunshine Clubs International.
- Unions will take on a project or may have funds to support client's needs.
- United Way may have discretionary funds that can be applied.
- YMCA and YWCA.

BEYOND FUNDING FOR THE INDIVIDUAL PATIENT

Often, we think of new approaches or needed services for more than a single patient. A group of Parkinson's patients need an active support group. Those with arthritis need a self-help program to encourage them to do more. The post-stroke patients require a transition program, because they feel stuck in a morass of worry about how they are progressing and when the next stroke will occur. The elderly in the community have home repairs and small jobs they can no longer do, and they have no family to help. Enthusiasm may be present, but the lack of funds is a barrier. This does not need to be true for the committed health care professional who seeks channels to implement an idea.

For innovative approaches to treatment and programs, research grants are available from professional organizations. The American Occupational Therapy Foundation, for example, accepts proposals from AOTA members. These include "innovation grants" for $5000 or less and "impact studies" for $15,000. Deadlines are October 15 and January 15, respectively. Student grants for $1000 are available, due by November 10. For further information, write the organization. Address is in Appendix C.

RESOURCES

Addresses are given in Appendix G unless otherwise noted.

PUBLICATIONS

Assistive Technology Funding Workbook. (1991). Washington, DC: RESNA. $25 plus $3.50 handling. Part I: A Roadmap to Funding Sources explores what is possible with state and federal funding, including hints to potential solutions. Part II: An Outline of Federal Laws and Rules describes three principal sources of support for assistive technology development, including delivery of assistive technology devices.

Cahn, E. & Rowe, J. (1992). *Time Dollars.* Emmaus, PA: Rodale Press. $19.95. Workable plan for people to turn their time into wealth and establish volunteerism in cities and towns. May give new thoughts and approaches to get patients helped and projects funded. **Source:** 447.

Directory of State Vocational Rehabilitation Agencies. Washington, DC: Department of Health and Human Services. Free.

Exceptional Parents. When it comes to finding equipment, perhaps no one is as determined and creative as a parent with a child who has a disability. Frequent suggestions on how to obtain equipment and methods that have been used are given. See Appendix D.

Guide to Health Insurance for People with Medicare. (1991). Washington, DC: National Association of Insurance Commissioners, and Health Care Financing Administration of the U.S. Department of Health and Human Services, HCFA-02110. Superintendent of Documents. Free from the U.S. Consumer Information Center. Basic information, types of health insurance, tips on buying private health insurance, what Medicare does and does not pay for. Addresses and telephone numbers of each state agency on aging and state insurance departments.

Handicapped Funding Directory. Margate, FL: Research Grant Guides. Updated annually. Approximately $35. **Source:** 440.

Medicare Handbook. Superintendent of Documents. $2.25. Information for beneficiaries on medicare benefits, description of benefits, health insurance to supplement.

Poliaszek, S. *Managing Your Health Care Finances.* Washington, DC: United Seniors Cooperative. $10. How to get the most out of Medicare and Medigap insurance.

Team Rehab Report. Free magazine gives information on newest technology, recommendations on customized equipment funding. See Appendix D.

The Social Security Book: What Every Woman Absolutely Needs to Know. (1990). Washington, DC: American Association of Retired Persons. Free. Explains types of benefits and how to receive them. Many women do not understand what is available to them under varying circumstances, such as when a spouse becomes disabled.

Understanding Social Security. (1991). Washington, DC: Social Security Administration, Superintendent of Documents. Free from the U.S. Consumer Information Center. Overview of the system, explains disability and survivor's benefits, Medicare coverage, and Supplemental Security income.

AUDIOVISUALS

Funding Assistive Technology. Washington, DC: RESNA. Third-Party Payor Program, Department 4006. Program consists of seven 30-minute videos designed to help explain client's needs to funding sources. Topics include communication, assessment, seating, back aids, manual mobility, powered mobility, augmentative communication. Cost is $30 each or $150 for all seven. For further information, call 703-524-6686.

B

Assessment and Evaluation Forms

Every agency has its own needs and focus when working with clients. Within an institution, equipment for objective evaluation and testing may be readily available, and a program may be in place for weekly, even daily, rounds or conferences on patient progress. For the home health care professional, however, supplies are often more limited, settings for evaluation varied, and the chance for team meetings often constrained by distance and time.

The forms included here are courtesy of the Home Management Training Program, Occupational Therapy Department, Howard A. Rusk Institute of Rehabilitation Medicine, New York University Medical Center and the Visiting Nurse Association of Ridgefield Inc., Ridgefield, CT. We hope that they will give a baseline on which to plan your own home management rehabilitation program.

RESOURCES

Asher, I. E. (1996). *Occupational Therapy Assessment Tools: An Annotated Index* (2nd ed.). Bethesda, MD: American Occupational Therapy Association. Order No. 1020. $30 AOTA members, $40 non-members. 200 profiles on all practice areas, and reviews more than 100 new assessments. Includes Activities of Daily Living and Home Management, Cognitive, Environmental and more.

Clarke, E. N., & Peters, M. *Scorable Self-Care Evaluation*. San Antonio, TX: Therapy Skill Builders. $29.95. For adolescent and adult assessment, covers personal care, housekeeping, financial management, work and leisure skills. **Source:** 522.

Howard A. Rusk Institute of Rehabilitation Medicine
New York University Medical Center
Occupational Therapy Department
400 East 34th Street, New York, NY 10016

<u>DAILY LIFE SKILLS</u>

<u>Self Rating Check List</u>

Name: _____ Rm. #:_____

Address: _____

Please rate yourself at the skill level you are most comfortable. Please state the personal goal(s) you would like to most achieve. Your self rating along with your personal goals will help us to plan your program.

DAILY LIFE SKILLS

KEY: (1) Easy   (2) Difficult   (3) Unable   (4) Not Tried

	Date Initial						Date D/C				
	1	2	3	4	NA		1	2	3	4	NA
HYGIENE/GROOMING											
Wash hands and face _____	___	___	___	___	___		___	___	___	___	___
Brush teeth _____	___	___	___	___	___		___	___	___	___	___
Brush or comb hair_____	___	___	___	___	___		___	___	___	___	___
Care of nails _____	___	___	___	___	___		___	___	___	___	___
Shave or put on makeup_____	___	___	___	___	___		___	___	___	___	___
Use toilet paper _____	___	___	___	___	___		___	___	___	___	___
Arrange clothes at toilet _____	___	___	___	___	___		___	___	___	___	___
Bathe self _____	___	___	___	___	___		___	___	___	___	___
Apply deodorant_____	___	___	___	___	___		___	___	___	___	___
Shampoo hair _____	___	___	___	___	___		___	___	___	___	___
Manage catheter _____	___	___	___	___	___		___	___	___	___	___
DRESS/UNDRESS											
Put on/remove cardigan _____	___	___	___	___	___		___	___	___	___	___
Put on/remove slip over garment _	___	___	___	___	___		___	___	___	___	___
Put on/remove coat_____	___	___	___	___	___		___	___	___	___	___
Put on/remove bra _____	___	___	___	___	___		___	___	___	___	___
Put on/remove underpants _____	___	___	___	___	___		___	___	___	___	___
Put on/remove trousers _____	___	___	___	___	___		___	___	___	___	___
Put on/socks _____	___	___	___	___	___		___	___	___	___	___
Put on/remove shoes_____	___	___	___	___	___		___	___	___	___	___
Tie shoe laces _____	___	___	___	___	___		___	___	___	___	___
Button/snaps/zippers _____	___	___	___	___	___		___	___	___	___	___
MOBILITY-BED/W/C/STANDING											
Turn over in bed _____	___	___	___	___	___		___	___	___	___	___
Sit up in bed _____	___	___	___	___	___		___	___	___	___	___
Transfer from bed to W/C _____	___	___	___	___	___		___	___	___	___	___
Transfer from W/C to toilet _____	___	___	___	___	___		___	___	___	___	___
Transfer from W/C to tub/shower _	___	___	___	___	___		___	___	___	___	___
Get in and out of chairs _____	___	___	___	___	___		___	___	___	___	___
Get in and out of car _____	___	___	___	___	___		___	___	___	___	___
Wheelchair up/down ramps _____	___	___	___	___	___		___	___	___	___	___
Get down/up from floor _____	___	___	___	___	___		___	___	___	___	___
Pick up objects from floor _____	___	___	___	___	___		___	___	___	___	___
Open and go through doors _____	___	___	___	___	___		___	___	___	___	___
Cross street with traffic light _____	___	___	___	___	___		___	___	___	___	___
Get W/C in/out of car _____	___	___	___	___	___		___	___	___	___	___
Walk carrying objects _____	___	___	___	___	___		___	___	___	___	___
Do bus steps _____	___	___	___	___	___		___	___	___	___	___

KEY: (1) Easy   (2) Difficult   (3) Unable   (4) Not Tried

	Date Initial					Date D/C				
	1	2	3	4	NA	1	2	3	4	NA
MARKETING:										
Push shopping cart _____	___	___	___	___	___	___	___	___	___	___
Reach high/low shelf _____	___	___	___	___	___	___	___	___	___	___
Negotiate check out counter_____	___	___	___	___	___	___	___	___	___	___
Pay cashier _____	___	___	___	___	___	___	___	___	___	___
Carry groceries_____	___	___	___	___	___	___	___	___	___	___
MEAL PREPARATION:										
Pour hot liquids _____	___	___	___	___	___	___	___	___	___	___
Open package goods _____	___	___	___	___	___	___	___	___	___	___
Carry pot: sink to range _____	___	___	___	___	___	___	___	___	___	___
Remove item from fridge_____	___	___	___	___	___	___	___	___	___	___
Get items from cupboard _____	___	___	___	___	___	___	___	___	___	___
Prepare a snack _____	___	___	___	___	___	___	___	___	___	___
Prepare a light hot meal _____	___	___	___	___	___	___	___	___	___	___
Prepare a full hot meal_____	___	___	___	___	___	___	___	___	___	___
MEAL SERVICE:										
Set table _____	___	___	___	___	___	___	___	___	___	___
Carry hot food to table _____	___	___	___	___	___	___	___	___	___	___
Clear table _____	___	___	___	___	___	___	___	___	___	___
Wash and put away dishes _____	___	___	___	___	___	___	___	___	___	___
CLEANING ACTIVITIES:										
Wipe up spills (counter/floor) ____	___	___	___	___	___	___	___	___	___	___
Change bed linen _____	___	___	___	___	___	___	___	___	___	___
Use dust mop/broom _____	___	___	___	___	___	___	___	___	___	___
Use dust pan_____	___	___	___	___	___	___	___	___	___	___
Dust high/low surfaces_____	___	___	___	___	___	___	___	___	___	___
Use wet mop_____	___	___	___	___	___	___	___	___	___	___
Carry cleaning materials _____	___	___	___	___	___	___	___	___	___	___
Clean range_____	___	___	___	___	___	___	___	___	___	___
Clean refrigerator _____	___	___	___	___	___	___	___	___	___	___
Vacuum_____	___	___	___	___	___	___	___	___	___	___
Clean bathroom _____	___	___	___	___	___	___	___	___	___	___
LAUNDRY:										
Hand wash _____	___	___	___	___	___	___	___	___	___	___
Household wash _____	___	___	___	___	___	___	___	___	___	___
Fold clothes _____	___	___	___	___	___	___	___	___	___	___
Iron _____	___	___	___	___	___	___	___	___	___	___
Hang clothes in closet _____	___	___	___	___	___	___	___	___	___	___
LEISURE ACTIVITIES:										
Care of pets _____	___	___	___	___	___	___	___	___	___	___

DAILY LIFE SKILLS

In the space below, write goals that you want to accomplish during the group session: _____

_____
_____
_____
_____
_____
_____
_____
_____
_____

Level of functioning at completion of 10 week session: _____

_____
_____
_____
_____
_____
_____
_____
_____
_____
_____

Comments: _____

_____
_____
_____
_____
_____
_____
_____
_____
_____
_____
_____
_____
_____
_____
_____

**Howard A. Rusk Institute
of Rehabilitation Medicine
New York University Medical Center**

OCCUPATIONAL THERAPY DEPARTMENT
HOMEMAKING PRE-TRAINING EVALUATION

Name: _____

Chart #: _____ Date: _____

Diagnosis: _____ Disability: _____

Age: _____ Sex: _____

Doctor: _____ OT: _____

1. Has patient been primary homemaker? _____

_____

_____

Future plans: _____

_____

_____

_____

2. Homemaking activity analysis:
   a. Safety _____

_____

_____

   b. Perception _____

_____

_____

   c. Technical aids _____

_____

_____

3. Present function level of independence in homemaking tasks:
   a. Tested in standard kitchen _____   Adapted kitchen _____
   b. Independent homemaker _____
   c. Supervision required _____
   d. Unsafe _____

4. Learning potential: _____

_____

_____

5. Recommendations: _____

_____

_____

_____

_____

_____

_____

HOWARD A. RUSK INSTITUTE OF REHABILITATION MEDICINE
NEW YORK UNIVERSITY MEDICAL CENTER
OCCUPATIONAL THERAPY SERVICE

REEVALUATION/PROGRESS

Date: _____ Date of ADM: _____

Attendance: _____Indiv: _____ Group: _____

Short term goals: _____

_____Met: _____ Unmet: _____

Reason not met: _____

Self Care Day: yes _____ no _____; with _____ without _____ Caregiver; Safe: yes _____ no _____

Patient/Family Education: yes _____ no _____ Training In: _____

Patient/Family participate in setting goals: yes _____ no _____

FUNCTIONAL STATUS

STATUS:	IND	MOD. I	SUP.	MIN. A	MOD. A	MAX. A	Total A
	7	6	5	4	3	2	1

I. PERFORMANCE AREAS	TREATMENT OUTCOMES			COMMENTS
	Current status	Impv	Unchg	
Eating/Drinking	7 6 5 4 3 2 1			
Swallowing Status	7 6 5 4 3 2 1			
Dressing UE	7 6 5 4 3 2 1			
LE	7 6 5 4 3 2 1			
Grooming/Hygiene	7 6 5 4 3 2 1			
Oral Hygiene	7 6 5 4 3 2 1			
Home Management: Meals Budget Shop	7 6 5 4 3 2 1			
Functional Communication (call bell, phone, typewriter, writes)	G F P			
Functional Mobility Walker/ Wheelchair	G F P			
Community Mobility	G F P			
Prevocational/Educational Activities	G F P			

Safety judgment for performance areas: _____ Good _____ Fair _____ Poor _____

Orthosis provided: _____; Patient educated in wear and care: yes _____ no _____

Assistive devices provided: _____; Patient educated: yes _____ no _____

Electronic Assistive Tech. assessed: yes _____ no _____ not indicated _____

Powered mobility assessed: yes _____ no _____ not indicated _____ Order submitted: yes/no

Home modifications recommended: yes/no Home visit: yes _____ no _____ not indicated _____

Community Excursion: yes _____ no _____; Outcome: _____

II. PERFORMANCE COMPONENTS THAT
IMPACT FUNCTION

Patient: _____

Dominance: L   R

FUNCTIONAL SITTING BALANCE	Current Status	I	U	Current Status	I	U	COMMENTS
Static	G F P			G F P			
Dynamic	G F P			G F P			
	Left			Right			
FUNCTIONAL REACH	Non-Functional			Non-Functional			
• Arm overhead	G F P			G F P			
• Hand to mouth	G F P			G F P			
• Hand behind back	G F P			G F P			
• Forward reach-pronated	G F P			G F P			
• Forward reach-supinated	G F P			G F P			
PREHENSION (grasp/release)	G F P			G F P			
• Palmar grip (cube 1")	G F P			G F P			
• Cylindrical (full soda can)	G F P			G F P			
• Lateral (key)	G F P			G F P			
• Pinch to Pinch	G F P			G F P			
CO-ORDINATION							
Gross	min mod severe			min mod severe			
Fine	impairment			impairment			
MUSCLE TONE	WFL Hypotonic Hypertonic			WFL Hypotonic Hypertonic			
SYNERGY PATTERNS (Brunnstrom)	STAGE 1 2 3 4 5 6			STAGE 1 2 3 4 5 6			
CONTRACTURE	min mod severe			min mod severe			
SUBLUXATION	min mod severe			min mod severe			
EDEMA	mid mod severe			mid mod severe			
SENSORY AWARENESS: (differentiate sensory stimuli)	min mod severe impairment						
SENSORY PROCESSING: tactile, proprioception, auditory (interpret sensory stimuli)	mid mod severe impairment						
VISUAL PROCESSING: Ocular alignment control	min mod severe impairment						
PERCEPTUAL PROCESSING: topographical, R/L Disc, body scheme, stereognosis	min mod severe impairment						
COGNITION: (Orientation, attention, sequencing, memory problem solves)	7 6 5 4 3 2 1 (FIM)						
ENDURANCE	G F P						

III. FUNCTIONAL SUMMARY:
   (Use for theInterdisciplinary Report)

Patient: _____

Goals (Met/Unmet): _____
_____
_____
_____

Outcome of Treatment (translate clinical goals to functional outcome): _____
_____
_____
_____
_____
_____
_____
_____

Goals for Next Review Will Be: _____
_____
_____

Patient/Family Have Participated in: _____
_____
_____

Anticipated Functional Outcome for Discharge: _____
_____
_____

**Howard A. Rusk Institute of
Rehabilitation Medicine
New York University Medical Center**

Name: _____

Therapist: _____

Date: _____

OCCUPATIONAL THERAPY SERVICE
HOMEMAKING UNIT
HOME FOLLOW-UP GUIDELINES

WORK SIMPLIFICATION

<u>Getting a Close Look at Your Work Patterns</u> (Being Motion Conscious):

<u>Re-Arranging Your Storage Space</u>:

<u>Evaluating Your Work Space</u>:

<u>Electrical Appliances You Used During Your Training</u>:

<u>Assistive Devices You Used During Your Training in the Homemaking Unit</u>:

<u>Miscellaneous Notes</u>:

HOME INFORMATION
Barrier Free Design Service
Occupational Therapy Department

Dear family member:

In order to help the team focus treatment and plan equipment, we need to know specifics about the physical environment of the patient's home. Please fill out ALL of this form as completely as possible.

PLEASE RETURN TO: _____

Patient's name: _____Room #: _____

1. ACCESS TO THE OUTSIDE OF THE RESIDENCE:

This is: _____ an apartment in an apartment building
_____ an apartment in a two-family house
_____ a private house

The residence is: a rental _____ owned _____.

A. Front entrance has how many steps to enter_____?
There are railings on: one side _____ both sides _____ no railings _____.

B. Are there other entrances to the building? Please note:
Side entrance _____: how many steps _____? Railings_____?
Back entrance _____: how many steps _____? Railings_____?

2. ACCESS WITHIN THE RESIDENCE:

A. STAIRS INSIDE THE HOUSE (Check all that apply):
_____ One short flight from the entrance door to the living level.
_____ One straight flight from the first floor to the second floor.
_____ A flight from first to second floor, that turns, and is broken by a landing, either at the
bottom _____ middle _____ or top _____.
_____ Other configuration. Please describe: _____

_____

B. DOORWAYS: Measuring the "clearance" through doorways is important, as sometimes as little as 1 or 2 inches make the difference between wheelchair access and no access. Please look at the directions to the right, below, and give us the following doorway measurements:

What is the CLEARANCE through:
_____ entrance door(s)
_____ bedroom door
_____ bathroom door

To enter a doorway, sometimes one must make a right- or left-hand turn from a hallway. Is this the case with either the bedroom doorway _____ or the bathroom doorway _____? If yes, how wide is the hallway _____?

DOORS AND HALLWAYS: HOW TO MEASURE THE CLEARANCE AT A DOORWAY:
(if possible, use a metal measuring tape)

BATHROOM:

SEVERAL TYPICAL BATHROOM FLOOR PLANS ARE SHOWN BELOW. CIRCLE THE
LETTER OF THE ONE WHICH IS SIMILAR TO THE LAYOUT OF THE BATHROOM
THE PATIENT WILL USE.

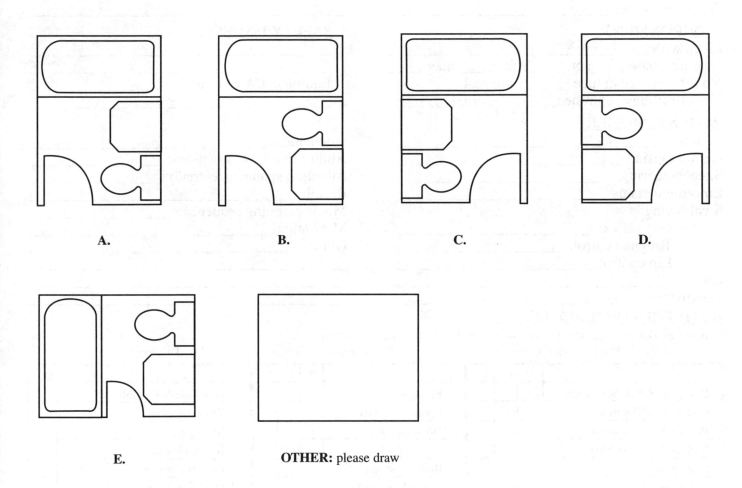

A.   B.   C.   D.

E.   **OTHER:** please draw

1. Does the sink have a cabinet below it, or is it open underneath? _____.

2. Are there doors or a shower curtain on the tub? _____.

3. Is there a shower stall in addition to, or instead of the tub?_____.
    Please measure the walls inside the shower stall, to let us know how big it is:_____ by _____.
    Does the shower stall have a door or a curtain? _____.
    If it has a door, how wide is the opening? _____ inches.

VISITING NURSE ASSOCIATION OF RIDGEFIELD, INC.
OCCUPATIONAL THERAPY EVALUATION AND PLAN OF TREATMENT

Initial _____ Recert. _____ Discharge _____ SOC Date _____ Cert. Period _____

Patient Name: _____ Patient Number: _____

Diagnosis 1: _____ Patient Phone: _____

Other Diagnoses: _____

ENVIRONMENT:
Lives with: _____

Live in: house ____ apt. ____ rm. ____ other ____

No. of steps: entrance _____ internal _____

No. of railings: entrance _____ internal _____

SAFETY ISSUES:
_____

_____

Equipment/Aids in use: _____

_____

PATIENT PROFILE
Vision: _____

Hemianopsia: _____

Speech/hearing: _____

Emotional status: _____

Swallowing:

    Gag reflex: _____

    Tongue control: _____

    Lip control: _____

Diet: _____

Continence: _____

Orientation: _____

Ability to follow directions: _____

Attention span/concentration: _____

Recall: _____

Motor-planning sequence: _____

Motivation: _____

Other: _____

_____

_____

ACTIVITIES OF DAILY LIVING
Indicate assistance code and equipment aids used, if any, for each activity.

P = Prior to admission   C = Current   D = Discharge

	P	C	D		P	C	D		P	C	D
Gen Status-BB, WC, amb				Feeding-solids				Hmaking-WC, amb			
Bed mob. roll s to s				Feeding-liquids				Trnsp of foods			
Bed mob. come to sit				Dressing - UE				Meal prep			
Bed mob. bridge hips				Dressing - LE				Kitch. cleanup			
Sitting bal. short				Buttons, snaps, etc.				Cooking, stvtop			
Sitting bal. long				Grooming/oral hyg				Cooking, oven			
Transfers to wc				Bathing				Laundry			
Transfers to bed				Handwriting				Shopping			
Tfers to toilet/comm				Dial phone				Safety			
Tfers to tub/shower				Handle money							
Wheelchair mobility				Personal hygiene							

1. Independent
2. Guarding by
3. Minimal assistance by
4. Moderate assistance by

5. Dependent on
6. N/A

F. Family/S.O.
V. Nurse of other pro.
A. Aide
E. Adaptive equipment

PERCEPTION

Spatial Relationships	
Auditory	
Body Image Scheme	
Unilateral Neglect	
Figure Ground	
Apraxia (motor pl. dysfunc.)	
Remarks	

UPPER EXTREMITY CLINICAL PICTURE

Dominant Hand: L R

Grade: N = Normal   G = Good   F = Fair

P = Poor   T = Trace   O = Zero

Joint Tested	Arom L	Arom R	Prom L	Prom R	Mmt L	Mmt R		L	R
Shoulder: flexion							Opposition		
extension							Coordination - Gross		
abduction							Coordination - Fine		
adduction							Muscle Tone		
int. rotation							Synergy Patterns		
ext. rotation							Contractures		
Elbow: flexion							Subluxation		
extension							Edema		
Forearm: sup							Orthotic or Asst. Dev		
pronation							Gross Grasp/Release		
Wrist: flexion							Lateral Prehension		
extension							**UPPER EXTREMITY SENSATION**		
ulnar deviation							Intact, impaired, abs, & loc.		
radial deviation							Deep Pressure		
Fingers: flexion							Proprioc./Pos. sense		
extension							Stereognosis		
abduction							Light Touch		
adduction							Pain		
Thumb: flexion							Temperature		
extension									
abduction									
adduction									

Equipment Needs:_____

_____

Remarks: _____

_____

_____

Goals: _____

_____

_____

OCCUPATIONAL THERAPY PLAN OF CARE:

_____

_____

_____

The OT Plan of Treatment is recommended pending physician approval:

_____   _____

Occupational Therapist   Date

The OT Plan of Treatment is recommended and or approved by:

_____   _____

Physician   Date

PLEASE SIGN AND RETURN THIS COPY

Helpful Organizations and Agencies

Many organizations and agencies offer information and additional support. Before contacting a national office, check with local resources. Frequently, groups have chapters that offer programs and services to nearby residents. These include education, volunteer help, transportation, referral to other agencies, and funding. Hospitals, medical clinics, and social service agencies can provide referrals and listings. Check your local telephone book for hotline numbers.

I. FEDERAL, STATE, AND LOCAL RESOURCES

Check the government pages in your telephone book for offices near you.

ACTION
1100 Vermont Ave. NW
Washington, DC 20525
202-606-5135
Through its Senior Companion Program in partnership with visiting nurse associations, local volunteers assist in home care, shopping, and socialization for the homebound or those limited by disabilities.

ADMINISTRATION ON AGING—see Section IV.

AGENCY FOR HEALTH CARE POLICY AND RESEARCH PUBLICATIONS CLEARINGHOUSE
P.O. Box 8547
Silver Spring, MD 20907
800-358-9295
410-594-1364
http://www.ahcpr.gov/

ALZHEIMER'S DISEASE EDUCATION AND REFERRAL CENTER—see Section IV.

ARCHITECTURAL AND TRANSPORTATION BARRIERS COMPLIANCE BOARD
1331 F St. NW, Ste. 1000
Washington, DC 20004
800-872-2253
202-514-0301
Distributes information on barrier-free planning and laws.

CENTER FOR CHRONIC DISEASE PREVENTION AND HEALTH PROMOTION
Building 1 South
Room SSB249
1600 Clifton Rd., N.E.
Atlanta, GA 30333
404-639-3492
Plans, directs, and coordinates programs for prevention of premature mortality and disability due to chronic illnesses.

CENTERS FOR DISEASE CONTROL AND PREVENTION
Public Inquiries
1600 Clifton Rd. NE
Atlanta, GA 30333
800-311-3435
404-639-3311
Distributes publications and makes referrals to agencies for specific condition or problem.

CLEARINGHOUSE FOR THE HANDICAPPED
Office of Special Education and Rehabilitative Services
U.S. Department of Education
330 C St. SW
Room 3132, Switzer Building
Washington, DC 20202
202-708-5366
Provides information and referral to federal and private services for people with disabilities.

U.S. CONSUMER INFORMATION CENTER
P.O. Box 100
Pueblo, CO 81009
719-948-9724
TDD: 800-492-8104 (MD)
Fax: 719-948-9724
E-mail: catalog.pueblo@gsa.gov
http://www.pueblo.gsa.gov
Distributes government publications on topics such as finance, nutrition, homemaking, disabilities, and health. Free catalog.

DEPARTMENT OF AGRICULTURE, HOME ECONOMICS EXTENSION
Check for area office in government pages of telephone book.

FANNIE MAE
3900 Wisconsin Ave. NW
Washington, DC 20016-2892
202-752-4330
http://www.fanniemae.com
Has developed HomePartners, a mortgage loan program for low- and moderate-income borrowers with disabilities or with at-home dependents who are disabled.

FEDERAL COUNCIL ON AGING—see Section IV.

FEDERAL TRADE COMMISSION
Office of Public Affairs
Room 421
Sixth St. and Pennsylvania Ave. NW
Washington, DC 20580
202-326-2180

FOOD AND DRUG ADMINISTRATION
Department of Health and Human Services
Office of Consumer Affairs
1390 Piccard Dr.
Silver Spring, MD 20850-4332
301-443-3170

FOOD AND NUTRITION INFORMATION CENTER
National Agricultural Library Building
Room 304
Beltsville, MD 20705
301-504-5719

MEDICAID

Federal and state program provides health care services to people with low incomes. Services vary by state. Contact state or local welfare, social service, or public health agency. Consult government pages of your telephone book.

MEDICARE

U.S. Department of Health and Human Services
Health Care Financing Administration (HCFA)
7500 Security Blvd.
Baltimore, MD 21244-1850
800-638-6833 (Medicare Hotline)

Health insurance program is for people 65 years or older and some individuals younger than 65 who have a disability making them eligible for Social Security Disability Insurance. Medicare helps pay for medically necessary physician services, outpatient hospital services, and therapy plus other medical services and supplies. Medicare Part B covers the cost of some types of durable medical equipment. Contact a state or local welfare, social service, or public health agency for information. Consult government pages of your telephone book.

MILITARY BENEFITS

Veterans hospitals around the country have pilot programs to deliver home health services. The Veterans Administration (VA) provides prosthetic and other equipment to eligible disabled veterans through local VA Medical Centers. The health plan for military dependents, CHAMPUS, also provides coverage for many home services.

NATIONAL ARTHRITIS, MUSCULOSKELETAL AND SKIN DISEASES INFORMATION CLEARINGHOUSE (NIAMS)—see Section II, Arthritis and Rheumatic Diseases.

NATIONAL CLEARINGHOUSE OF REHABILITATION TRAINING MATERIALS

5202 North Richmond Hill Dr.
Oklahoma State University
Stillwater, OK 74078-4080
800-223-5219
405-624-7650
Fax: 405-624-0695
TDD: 405-624-3156
http://www.nehrtm.okstate.edu

NATIONAL DIABETES INFORMATION CLEARINGHOUSE—see Section II under Diabetes.

NATIONAL DIGESTIVE DISEASES INFORMATION CLEARINGHOUSE

U.S. Public Health Service
2 Information Way
Bethesda, MD 20892-3570
E-mail: nddic@aerie.com
http://www.niddk.nih.gov

Service of the National Institute of Diabetes and Digestive and Kidney Diseases. Provides information to consumers and professionals, responds to inquiries, distributes publications.

NATIONAL HEALTH INFORMATION CENTER

Office of Disease Prevention and Promotion
U.S. Department of Human Services
P.O. Box 1133
Washington, DC 20013-1133
800-336-4797

Distributes materials on health-related organizations and makes referrals for professionals and consumers to specific agencies.

NATIONAL INFORMATION CENTER FOR CHILDREN AND YOUTH WITH DISABILITIES

P.O. Box 1492
Washington, DC 20013-1492
800-999-5599
703-893-6061 (DC)
V/TDD: 703-893-8614

National information clearinghouse is authorized by Congress to provide assistance to parents, educators, caregivers, advocates, and others working to improve the lives of children and youth with disabling conditions. Services include personal responses to specific questions, referral to other organizations, and technical assistance for parents and professional groups. Materials are available, upon request, in large-print, Braille, or tape.

NATIONAL INSTITUTE OF MENTAL HEALTH—see Section II under Mental Health.

NATIONAL INSTITUTES OF ARTHRITIS, MUSCULO-SKELETAL AND SKIN DISEASES—see Section II under Arthritis and Rheumatic Diseases.

NATION INSTITUTES OF NEUROLOGICAL DISORDERS AND STROKE—see Section II under Heart Disease and Stroke.

NATIONAL INSTITUTE ON AGING—see Section IV.

NATIONAL INSTITUTE ON DEAFNESS AND OTHER COMMUNICATION DISORDERS—see Section II under Deafness and Hearing Loss.

NATIONAL INSTITUTE OF HANDICAPPED RESEARCH

Office of Special Education and Rehabilitation Services
Washington, DC 20201

Focuses on research for people with disabilities; makes referrals to the appropriate agency.

NATIONAL LIBRARY OF MEDICINE
8600 Rockville Pike
Bethesda, MD 20894
800-638-8480
Prepares bibliographies on topics of interest to consumers, such as disease prevention, rehabilitation of the elderly, medication and the elderly, and sleep disorders and the elderly. Materials are available through the Superintendent of Documents, US Government Printing Office, listed further on.

NATIONAL LIBRARY SERVICES FOR THE BLIND AND PHYSICALLY DISABLED
The Library of Congress
1291 Taylor St., NW
Washington, DC 20542
202-707-5100
TDD: 202-707-0744
Fax: 202-707-0712
E-mail: NLS@loc.gov
http://www.loc.gov/nis or http://lcweb.loc.gov/nis
Available to people with loss of vision or with motion impairment; this organization can provide cassette players, talking books, braille books, and visual aids. Obtain application form for Library of Congress program and check services through local library.

NATIONAL   REHABILITATION   INFORMATION CENTER—see Section III.

PHYSICALLY IMPAIRED ASSOCIATION OF MICHIGAN
PAM Assistance Centre
Living and Learning Resource Centre
Media Centre
1023 S. U.S. 27
St. Johns, MI 48879
800-274-7426
V/TDD: 517-224-0333
Distributes information on independent living, including home adaptations and homemaking. Send for publication list.

REHABILITATION SERVICES ADMINISTRATION(RSA)
Department of Education
Switzer Building, Room 3024
330 C St. SW
Washington, DC 20202
202-732-1265
Program is administered through state offices. For qualified individuals, RSA provides training and other services, including assistive devices and home or office adaptations to allow accessibility and independence, thus relieving a caregiver to return to work. Homemaking is considered a remunerative occupation; thus training, kitchen changes, and some equipment may be covered. Eligibility depends on the state and results of evaluation by an RSA counselor or other professional, such as an occupational therapist. Contact state vocational rehabilitation office, listed under state government pages of your telephone book.

SOCIAL SECURITY ADMINISTRATION (SSA)
U.S. Department of Health and Human Services
Washington, DC 20201
Organization is responsible for Medicare and Medicaid, two major federal programs offering assistance to the aging and those with disabilities. For information, contact local office listed in government pages of your telephone book. See entries under Medicaid and Medicare in this section.

SUPERINTENDENT OF DOCUMENTS
United States Government Printing Office
Washington, DC 20402-9322
Distributes materials printed by government agencies. Request bibliographies for topics you wish to pursue.

U.S. CONSUMER INFORMATION CENTER
P.O. Box 100
Pueblo, CO 81009
Request catalog of publications.

U.S. CONSUMER PRODUCT SAFETY COMMISSION
Office of Information and Public Affairs
5401 Westbard Ave.
Bethesda, MD 20207
800-638-2772 (Consumer Product Safety Hotline)
TDD: 800-638-8270 (National)
Tests equipment and distributes materials on safety, such as electricity and selecting equipment for children. Free publications list.

U.S. DEPARTMENT OF HOUSING AND URBAN DEVELOPMENT
Office of the Secretary
451 Seventh St. SW
Washington, DC 20410-0001
800-795-7915
TDD: 800-927-9275
Provides information on adapting housing, finding accessible and affordable housing, and laws pertaining to people with disabilities and the aging. Address inquiry to Office of Elderly and Assisted Housing.

U.S. DEPARTMENT OF TRANSPORTATION
National Highway System
400 Seventh St. NW
Washington, DC 20591
800-424-9393
202-366-4000
TDD: 800-424-9153

II. GOVERNMENT AND VOLUNTARY AGENCIES WORKING WITH PEOPLE WITH SPECIFIC DISABILITIES

AIDS

AIDS ARC SWITCHBOARD
San Francisco AIDS Foundation
Box 426182
San Francisco, CA 94142-6182
415-864-5805
Answers questions and makes referrals to local agencies.

NATIONAL AIDS HOTLINE
Centers for Disease Control
Atlanta, GA 30333
800-342-AIDS
800-344-SIDA (Spanish)
TTY: 800-AIDS
Answers questions and provides local referrals. Operates 24 hours a day, 7 days a week.

PEOPLE WITH AIDS COALITION OF NEW YORK (PWAC) HOTLINE
800-828-3208
Women who are parents of children with AIDS are on helpline Mon., Wed., and Fri. from 2 p.m. to 6 p.m. to help others who have a child with HIV or AIDS or are trying to cope with a child's death.

AMPUTEES

AMERICAN AMPUTEE FOUNDATION
P.O. Box 250218
Hillcrest Station
Little Rock, AR 72225
501-666-2523
Fax: 501-666-8367
Provides information on training and prostheses. Publishes extensive resource guide helpful to people with any kind of disability.

AMERICAN ORTHOTIC AND PROSTHETIC ASSOCIATION—see Section IV.

AMPUTEE COALITION OF AMERICA
1932 Alcoa Highway, Ste. 365
Knoxville, TN 39720
423-524-8772
Fax: 423-525-7917
Advocate for amputees provides access through nationwide database dedicated to amputees for support groups, prosthetic and educational information, publishes quarterly magazine, *In Motion*, has lending library of videos, presents consumer-oriented annual meeting. Membership encompasses individuals, allied disability organizations, health professionals, and others.

NATIONAL AMPUTATION FOUNDATION
73 Church St.
Malvern, NY 11565
516-887-3600
Fax: 516-887-3667

ANIMAL ASSISTANCE GROUPS

ASSISTANCE DOGS OF AMERICA, INC.
8806 State Rte. 64
Swanton, OH 43558
419-825-3622

ASSISTANCE DOGS INTERNATIONAL
10175 Wheeler Rd.
Central Point, OR 97502
503-826-9229

CANINE COMPANIONS FOR INDEPENDENCE
P.O. Box 446
Santa Rosa, CA 95402-0446
800-767-2275
707-528-08030
Fax: 707-528-0146

DELTA SOCIETY
P.O. Box 1080
321 Burnett Ave. South 3rd Fl.
Renton, WA 98057-9906
800-869-6898
206-226-7357

DOGS FOR THE DEAF
Listed under Deafness and Hearing Loss.

GUIDE DOG FOUNDATION FOR THE BLIND
Training Center
371 Jericho Turnpike
Smithtown, NY 11787

HANDI-DOGS, INC.
P.O. Box 12563
Tucson, AZ 85732

INDEPENDENCE DOGS INC.
146 State Line Rd.
Chadds Ford, PA 19317
610-358-2723
Fax: 610-358-5314

INTERNATIONAL HEARING DOGS, INC.
Listed under Deafness and Hearing Loss.

PURINA PETS FOR PEOPLE PROGRAM
Ralston Purina Company
Checkerboard Sq. OCA
St. Louis, MO 63164
800-PURINA

SIMIAN HELPING HANDS FOR THE HANDICAPPED
1505 Commonwealth Ave.
Boston, MA 02135
617-787-4419
Program trains monkeys to assist people with severe disabilities.

SUPPORT DOGS, INC.
301 Sovereign Ct., Ste. 113
St. Louis, MO 63011
314-394-6163

ARTHRITIS AND RHEUMATIC DISEASES

AMERICAN LUPUS SOCIETY
2617 E Columbus Ave.
Spokane, WA 99207
800-331-1802 (information line for publications)
310-542-8891 (direct inquiries)
Assists patients with systemic lupus erythematosus and their families in coping with the disease. Works to obtain funds for lupus research. Call for local chapter. Publishes newsletter, *The Quarterly*, as well as other publications on lupus.

AMERICAN COLLEGE OF RHEUMATOLOGY—see Section VI.

THE ARTHRITIS FOUNDATION
1330 West Peachtree St.
Atlanta, GA 30309
800-283-7800
404-872-7100
Fax: 404-872-0457
National voluntary organization provides self-help and support groups; publishes newsletters and a magazine, *Arthritis Today*; distributes information; and advocates for those with arthritis in governmental affairs. Programs vary from chapter to chapter but may include physician referral, clinics, exercise programs, social services, transportation, loan closets, direct financial assistance, and educational and emotional support groups. Affiliated with the American Juvenile Arthritis Association (AJOA) and the Association of Rheumatology Health Professionals, a multidisciplinary organization of therapists, physicians, nurses, social workers, and other professional health care workers committed to improving care and treatment of people with arthritis. Local and regional chapters focus on care as well as training and education of health care professionals. Call for information on local chapter.

THE ARTHRITIS SOCIETY
250 Bloor St. East Ste. 901
Toronto, ON M4W 3P2
Canada
800-361-1112 (ON)
416-967-1414
Fax: 416-967-7171

LUPUS FOUNDATION OF AMERICA, INC.
1717 Massachusetts Ave. NW, Ste. 203
Washington, DC 20036
800-558-0121
Serves as central communication liason among lupus groups throughout United States, Canada, and Puerto Rico. Assists patients, provides referrals, and distributes publications, including *Lupus News*, on living with lupus.

MULTIPURPOSE ARTHRITIS CENTERS
Clinical and research centers are funded for basic and clinical research; professional, patient, and public education; and community-oriented activities. Request listing from the Arthritis Foundation, listed earlier.

NATIONAL ARTHRITIS, MUSCULOSKELETAL AND SKIN DISEASES INFORMATION CLEARINGHOUSE (NIAMS)
1 AMS Circle
Bethesda, MD 20892-3675
301-495-4484
Fax: 301-587-4352
Federal agency provides publications, bibliographies, and reference sheets. Makes referrals to proper agencies. Assists health care professionals in locating patient education materials.

NATIONAL INSTITUTES OF ARTHRITIS, MUSCULOSKELETAL AND SKIN DISEASES
National Institutes of Health
Building 31, Room 9A04
Bethesda, MD 20892
301-496-3583
Federal agency provides information on research and referrals to federally funded and other arthritis agencies.

SCLERODERMA FEDERATION
Peabody Office Bldg.
1 Newbury St.
Peabody, MA 01960
800-422-1113
508-535-6600
Fax: 508-535-6696
Composed of several scleroderma organizations; group supports medical research and provides education services to patients and caregivers. Distributes publications on living with scleroderma and treatment.

SCLERODERMA INTERNATIONAL FOUNDATION
704 Gardner Center Rd.
New Castle, PA 16101
412-652-3109
Disseminates information on scleroderma to patients, physicians, and others. Publishes newsletter, *The Connector*.

SPONDYLITIS ASSOCIATION OF AMERICA
P.O. Box 5872
Sherman Oaks, CA 91413
800-777-8189
Focuses on care of people with ankylosing spondylitis and support of research. Publications include newspaper, *AS News*, as well as other books and pamphlets.

CANCER

AMERICAN BRAIN TUMOR ASSOCIATION
2720 River Rd., Ste. 146
Des Plaines, IL 60018-4117
800-886-2282
847-827-9910
Fax: 847-827-9918
E-mail: abta@aol.com

AMERICAN CANCER SOCIETY®, INC.
1599 Clifton Rd. NE
Atlanta, GA 30329-4251
800-ACS-2345
404-320-3333
Fax: 404-329-5787
Makes referral to local chapter for specific programs and activities. Disseminates materials on cancer prevention, research, treatments, and the handling of the effects of chemotherapy and radiation. New York-based Reach to Recovery program pairs women who have had breast cancer with new patients to offer support and advice. See also Reach to Recovery.

CANADIAN CANCER SOCIETY
10 Alcorn Ave., Ste. 200
Toronto, ON M4V 3B1
Canada
416-961-7223
Fax: 416-961-4189

CANCER INFORMATION CENTER
National Cancer Institute
31 Center Drive MSC 2580
Building 31, Room 10A07
Bethesda, MD 20892-2580
800-4-CANCER
301-496-5583
Federal agency provides information on cancer treatment; makes local referrals; distributes materials on research, types of treatment for various kinds of cancer, living with cancer, and handling the side effects of chemotherapy.

LOOK GOOD...FEEL BETTER
800-395-LOOK
Or through local American Cancer Society office.

MAKE TODAY COUNT
1235 East Cherokee St.
Springfield, MO 65804-2203
800-432-2273
417-885-3324
Support program for people with cancer and their families. Will refer to local chapter, often affiliated with a hospital.

NATIONAL COALITION FOR CANCER SURVIVORSHIP
888-9037-6227
Information about treatment, insurance issues, and emotional support. No charge for call or materials.

NATIONAL LEUKEMIA ASSOCIATION
585 Stewart Ave., Ste. 536
Garden City, NY 11530
516-222-1944
Organization offers support to people with leukemia and their families and provides information on treatment and support groups.

NATIONAL LYMPHEDEMA NETWORK
2211 Post St., Ste. 404
San Francisco, CA 94115
800-541-3259
Fax: 415-921-4284

REACH TO RECOVERY
c/o American Cancer Society®
777 Third Ave.
New York, NY 10017
Provides peer support for women who have had mastectomies. For more information, contact local cancer society chapter.

SUSAN G. KOMEN BREAST CANCER FOUNDATION
800-462-9273

Y-ME
National Breast Cancer Organization
212 West Van Buren
Chicago, IL 60607
800-221-2141
800-986-9505 (Spanish)
Fax: 312-294-8597
Offers counseling, support, and publications. Has men's support group for spouses of women who have breast cancer.

CHRONIC FATIGUE SYNDROME

ASSOCIATION OF PROFESSIONAL SLEEP SOCIETIES
604 Second St. SW
Rochester, MN 55902
Accredits sleep clinics in US; provides consumer information on sleep disorders.

CHRONIC FATIGUE IMMUNE DYSFUNCTION SYNDROME SOCIETY
P.O. Box 320108
Portland, OR 97223
503-684-5261
CHRONIC FATIGUE IMMUNE DYSFUNCTION ASSOCIATION OF AMERICA
P.O. Box 220398
Charlotte, NC 28222-0398
800-442-3437
Fax: 704-365-9755
E-mail: cfids@vnet.net

NATIONAL CHRONIC FATIGUE SYNDROME AND FIBROMYALGIA ASSOCIATION
P.O. Box 18426
Kansas City, MO 64133
816-313-2000
Fax: 816-313-2001
Provides information on current status of research into chronic fatigue syndrome, methods of coping, and referrals to local support groups.

NATIONAL SLEEP FOUNDATION
1367 Connecticut Ave. NW, Ste. 200
Washington, DC 20036
202-785-2300
Fax: 202-785-2880
Non-profit organization dedicated to improving the quality of life for individuals who suffer from sleep disorders, supports sleep research, education and training, provides public information programs, and distributes information on healthy sleeping.

Also see ASTHMA AND ALLERGY FOUNDATION OF AMERICA under Chronic Obstructive Pulmonary Disease; DIZZINESS AND BALANCE DISORDERS ASSOCIATION OF AMERICA under Vestibular Disorders; as well as agencies listed under Mental Health and Pain. A further resource is the AMERICAN ACADEMY FOR ENVIRONMENTAL MEDICINE, and the AMERICAN SLEEP DISORDERS ASSOCIATION, listed in Section VI.

CHRONIC OBSTRUCTIVE PULMONARY DISEASE (COPD), ASTHMA, AND ALLERGIES

AMERICAN ACADEMY OF ALLERGY AND IMMUNOLOGY
611 East Wells St.
Milwaukee, WI 53202
800-822-ASMA
414-272-6071
Fax: 414-272-6070
http://www.aaai.org
Distributes pollen information and names of local allergists.

AMERICAN ALLERGY ASSOCIATION
Box 640
Menlo Park, CA 94026
415-855-8036
Provides information and referrals for people with food or chemical allergies.
AMERICAN LUNG ASSOCIATION
1740 Broadway
New York, NY 10019-4374
800-LUNG-USA (586-4872)
212-315-8700
Fax: 212-265-5642
Provides information on living with COPD and refers to local support groups.

AMERICAN THORACIC SOCIETY—see Section VI.

ASTHMA AND ALLERGY FOUNDATION OF AMERICA
1125 15th St. NW, Ste. 502
Washington, DC 20005
800-727-8462
202-466-7643
Fax: 202-466-8940
Distributes information on research into allergies and asthma, and living with these conditions; refers to medical centers and local support groups.

ASTHMA SOCIETY OF CANADA
130 Bridgeland Ave., Ste. 425
Toronto, ON M6A 1Z4
Canada
800-787-3880 (Canada)
416-787-4050
Fax: 416-787-5807
E-mail: asthma@myna.com

CYSTIC FIBROSIS FOUNDATION
6931 Arlington Rd.
Bethesda, MD 20814
800-344-4823
301-951-4422
Fax: 301-951-6378

HEALTH HOUSE®
American Lung Association
Minneapolis Affiliate
1829 Portland Ave.
Minneapolis, MN 55404
612-871-7332, ext. 204

NATIONAL HEART, LUNG, AND BLOOD INSTITUTE—
see Section I.

NATIONAL INSTITUTE OF ALLERGY AND INFECTIOUS
DISEASE (NIAID)
Building 31, Room 7A-50
Bethesda, MD 20892
301-496-5717
Distributes information and publications.

NATIONAL JEWISH CENTER FOR IMMUNOLOGY AND
RESPIRATORY DISEASES

DEAFNESS AND HEARING LOSS

The following groups promote research into causes and treatment of deafness and loss of hearing; distribute publications on living with hearing loss, methods of communication, and assistive devices; and will make referrals to local programs and support groups.

ALEXANDER GRAHAM BELL ASSOCIATION FOR THE
DEAF
3417 Volta Pl. NW
Washington, DC 20007-2778
V/TDD: 202-337-5220

AMERICAN ASSOCIATION OF THE DEAF-BLIND
814 Thayer Ave., Ste. 302
Silver Spring, MD 20910
TTY: 301-588-6545
Fax: 301-588-8705

AMERICAN DEAFNESS AND REHABILITATION ASSO-
CIATION (AADB)
P.O. Box 251554
Little Rock, AR 72225
501-868-8850

AMERICAN SPEECH-LANGUAGE-HEARING ASSOCIA-
TION—see Section VI.

DOGS FOR THE DEAF, INC.
10175 Wheeler Rd.
Central Point, OR 97502
V/TDD: 503-826-9220
Fax: 503-826-6696

HEAR YOU ARE, INC.
125 Main Street
Netcong, NJ 07857
V: 201-347-7662
TDD: 201-691-0663
Fax: 201-691-0611

HEARING AID HOTLINE
800-521-5247

HELEN KELLER NATIONAL CENTER FOR DEAF-BLIND
YOUTHS AND ADULTS
111 Middle Neck Rd.
Sands Point, NY 11050
Voice or TDD: 516-944-8900

INTERNATIONAL HEARING DOGS, INC.
5901 E. 89th Ave.
Henderson, CO 80640
V/TDD: 303-287-3277
Fax: 303-287-7886

NATIONAL ASSOCIATION FOR THE DEAF
814 Thayer Ave.
Silver Spring, MD 20910-4500
V: 301-587-1788
TTY: 301-587-1788
Fax: 478-2610

NATIONAL HEARING AID ASSOCIATION
20361 Middlebelt St.
Livonia, MI 48152
313-478-2610
Assists purchasing of proper hearing aids through distribution of consumer information.

NATIONAL INSTITUTE ON DEAFNESS AND OTHER
COMMUNICATION DISORDERS
Information Office
9000 Rockville Pike
Bethesda, MD 20892
301-496-5751
Distributes information and makes referrals to local agencies.

SHHH: SELF HELP FOR HARD OF HEARING PEOPLE,
INC.
7910 Woodmont Ave., Ste. 1200
Bethesda, MD 20814
301-657-2248
TTY: 301-657-2249
Fax: 301-913-9413
E-mail: national@shhh.org
http://www.shhh.org

DIABETES

AMERICAN DIABETES ASSOCIATION
1660 Duke St.
Alexandria, VA 22314
800-DIABETES (342-2383)
703-549-1500
Fax: 703-683-2890
http://www.diabetes.org
Promotes understanding of diabetes through distribution of materials, encouragement of support groups, and publishing of monthly magazine.

NATIONAL DIABETES INFORMATION CLEARING-HOUSE
1 Information Way
Bethesda, MD 20892-3560
301-468-2162
E-mail: ndic@aerie.com
http://www.niddk.nih.gov
Distributes materials, carries on research in diabetes, makes referrals to local agencies.

HEAD INJURY

BRAIN INJURY ASSOCIATION, INC.
1776 Massachusetts Ave. NW, Ste. 100
Washington, DC 20036-1901
800-444-6443
202-296-6443 (9 a.m. to 5 p.m. Eastern time)
Fax: 202-296-8850
National advocacy and support organization for people with head injuries and their families.

COMA RECOVERY ASSOCIATION
570 Elmont Rd., Ste. 104
Elmont, NY 11003
516-355-0951 (10 a.m. to 5 p.m. Eastern Standard Time)
Fax: 516-355-0961
Provides information on coma, including treatment techniques.

FAMILY CAREGIVER ALLIANCE FOR FAMILIES OF BRAIN IMPAIRED ADULTS
425 Bush St., Ste. 500
San Francisco, CA 94108
800-445-8106 (CA only)
415-434-3388
Fax: 415-434-3508 (9 a.m. to 5 p.m. Pacific time)
Focus is on issues for caregivers of brain-injured adults.

HEAD INJURY HOTLINE
c/o Constance Miller
P.O. Box 84151
Seattle, WA 98124
206-329-1371
206-621-8558
Fax: 206-623-4251
http://www.headinjury.com
(Formerly Phoenix Project.)

THE NATIONAL INSTITUTE OF NEUROLOGICAL DISORDERS AND STROKES—see under Heart Disease and Stroke.

NEW YORK STATE HEAD INJURY ASSOCIATION
855 Central Ave.
Albany, NY 12206
800-228-8201
518-459-7911

HEART DISEASE AND STROKE

AMERICAN ACADEMY OF APHASIA—see Section VI.

AMERICAN HEART ASSOCIATION
National Center
7272 Greenville Ave.
Dallas, TX 75231-4596
800-AHA-USA1 (242-8721)
214-373-6300
Fax: 214-706-1341
E-mail: chuckh@amhrt.org
http://www.amhrt.org
Distributes educational materials in print and audiovisual form. Catalog available through local chapters. Develops Stroke Clubs. Call for referral to local chapter, or check local phone book.

CORONARY CLUB
9500 Euclid Ave.
Cleveland, OH 44106
216-444-3690
Fax: 216-444-9385
For consumers and professionals. *Heartline*, monthly newsletter.

NATIONAL APHASIA ASSOCIATION
Murray Hill Station
P.O. Box 1887
New York, NY 10156-0611
800-922-4622
Fax: 212-727-9126

NATIONAL INSTITUTES OF NEUROLOGICAL DISOR-
DERS AND STROKE
Information Office
Building 31, Room 8A06
9000 Rockville Pike
Bethesda, MD 20892
301-496-5751
Federal agency offers publications and referrals.

NATIONAL STROKE ASSOCIATION
96 Inverness Dr. East, Ste.1
Englewood, CO 80112-5122
800-STROKES
303-649-9299
Fax: 303-649-1329
Distributes materials for stroke survivors and their families.
Free catalog.

STROKE CONNECTION
800-553-6321
Distributes materials for stroke survivors and their families;
makes referrals to local support groups; distributes newsletter.
Free catalog.

HOSPICE AND TERMINAL ILLNESS

CANDLELIGHTERS CHILDHOOD CANCER
FOUNDATION
7910 Woodmonst Ave., Ste. 460
Bethesda, MD 20814
301-657-8401
800-366-2223
Fax: 301-718-2686

CHILDREN'S HOSPICE INTERNATIONAL
1850 M St. NW, Ste. 900
Washington, DC 20036
800-242-4453
703-684-0330
Fax: 703-684-0226

COMPASSIONATE FRIENDS
P.O. Box 1064
Palmer, AK 99645-1064
907-746-6123

HOSPICE ASSOCIATION OF AMERICA
519 C St. NE
Washington, DC 20036
202-546-4759
Fax: 202-547-3540
Publish bimonthly *Hospice* Forum.

MAKE-A-WISH FOUNDATION OF AMERICA
100 West Clarendon Ave., Ste. 2200
Phoenix, AZ 85013-3518
800-722-WISH
602-279-9474

NATIONAL HOSPICE ORGANIZATION
1901 North Moore St.
Arlington, VA 22209
800-658-8898
703-243-5900
Fax: 703-525-5762

STARLIGHT FOUNDATION
12233 West Olympic Blvd.
Los Angeles, CA 90064
800-274-7827
310-207-5558
Fax: 310-207-2554
http://www.starbright.com

INCONTINENCE

AMERICAN MEDICAL DIRECTORS ASSOCIATION
10480 Little Patuxent Parkway, Ste. 760
Columbia, MD 21044
800-876-AMDA
410-740-9743
Fax: 410-740-4572

BLADDER HEALTH COUNCIL
c/o American Foundation for Urologic Disease
300 West Pratt St., Ste. 401
410-727-2908
Fax: 410-528-0550

NATIONAL ASSOCIATION FOR CONTINENCE
P.O. Box 8310
Spartanburg, SC 29305-8310
800-BLADDER (252-3337)
864-579-7900
Fax: 864-579-7902

SIMON FOUNDATION FOR CONTINENCE
P.O. Box 835
Willmette, IL 60091
800-237-4666
847-864-3913
Fax: 847-864-9758

MENTAL HEALTH

AMERICAN ASSOCIATION FOR GERIATRIC PSYCHIA-
TRY (AAGP)
7910 Woodmont Ave., 7th Floor
Bethesda, MD 20814
301-654-7850
Fax: 301-654-4137
E-mail: aagpaol@aol.com
Will send free directory of AAGP members around the country.

AMERICAN MENTAL HEALTH COUNSELORS ASSOCI-
ATION
801 North Fairfax, Ste. 304
Alexandria, VA 22314
800-326-2642
Fax: 703-751-1696
Call for referral to local agencies.

AMERICAN PSYCHIATRIC ASSOCIATION
APA Division of Public Affairs
1400 K St. NW
Washington, DC 20005
202-682-6000
Distributes pamphlets on mental disorders, drug abuse, and
how to select a psychiatrist.

AMERICAN PSYCHOLOGICAL ASSOCIATION
750 First St. NE
Washington, DC 20002-4242
202-336-5500
Publishes pamphlets on mental health problems and provides
list of psychological associations in area. Send SASE.

NATIONAL ASSOCIATION OF SOCIAL WORKERS—see
Section VI.

NATIONAL FOUNDATION FOR DEPRESSIVE ILLNESS
P.O. Box 2257
New York, NY 10116
800-248-4344
212-268-4260 (in NY)
Fax: 212-268-4434
http://www.depression.org
Distributes materials on depression and methods of treatment,
and list of centers specializing in treating depression.

NATIONAL MENTAL HEALTH ASSOCIATION
1021 Prince St.
Alexandria, VA 22314-2971
800-969-NMHA (6642)
703-684-7722
Fax: 703-684-5968
http://www.nmha@aol.org
Distributes materials on mental health and sources of help.

PUBLIC HEALTH SERVICE
Alcohol, Drug Abuse, and Mental Health Administration
Rockville, MD 20857
Distributes free pamphlet, *A Consumer's Guide to Mental
Health Services.*

NEUROMUSCULAR DISORDERS

AMERICAN PARKINSON'S DISEASE FOUNDATION, INC.
1250 Hylan Blvd.
Staten Island, NY 10305
800-223-2732
Non-profit organization is dedicated to research of Parkinson's
disease and help to those with Parkinson's disease and their
caregivers. Free materials on speech and swallowing, exercise,
and activities of daily living.

AMERICAN ACADEMY FOR CEREBRAL PALSY AND
DEVELOPMENTAL MEDICINE
1910 Byrd Ave., Ste. 100
P.O. Box 11086
Richmond, VA 23230-1086
804-282-0036

AMYOTROPHIC LATERAL SCLEROSIS (ALS) ASSOC-
IATION
21021 Ventura Blvd., Ste. 321
Woodland Hills, CA 91364
800-782-4747 (Patients)
818-340-7500
E-mail: eajc27b@prodigy.com
http://www.alsa.org
Provides referrals and literature on feeding, self-help equipment, handling of daily activities, and support groups.
Promotes research into causes and treatment of ALS. Call or
write for local chapter and materials.

GAZETTE INTERNATIONAL NETWORKING INSTITUTE
(GINI)
Listed under Post-Polio Syndrome.

HUNTINGTON'S DISEASE SOCIETY OF AMERICA
140 West 22nd St., Sixth Floor
New York, NY 10011-2420
800-345-4372
Promotes research into Huntington's disease and distributes
information on living with the disease and support groups.

MUSCULAR DYSTROPHY ASSOCIATION (MDA)
3300 East Sunrise Dr.
Tucson, AZ 85718-3208
800-572-1717
520-529-5300
Fax: 520-529-5300
Provides assistance to people with muscular dystrophy through
various programs, including loan closets for equipment, funding of
specific equipment, transportation, and outpatient clinics. Call or
check your telephone book for local chapter and support programs.

NATIONAL MULTIPLE SCLEROSIS SOCIETY
733 Third Ave., Sixth Floor
New York, NY 10017
800-624-8236 (information line for publications)
800-227-3166 (for specific inquiries or referral to local chapter)
212-986-3240 (NY)
Distributes information on living with multiple sclerosis, the role of nutrition and exercise, assistive devices, and support groups. Promotes increased focus on research into its causes.

NATIONAL PARKINSON FOUNDATION
1501 NW Ninth Ave. (Bob Hope Rd.)
Miami, FL 33136-9990
800-327-4545
305-547-6666
Distributes information on living with Parkinson's disease, including methods for coping by spouses and caregivers. Encourages research into the causes and treatment; makes referrals to local support groups.

THE NEUROLOGY ASSOCIATION, INC.
P.O. Box 2055
Lenox Hill Station
New York, NY 10021
800-247-6978
http://www.neuropathy.org/neuropathy
Self help organization with newsletter for persons with peripheral neuropathies and limitations credited by them.

PARKINSON'S DISEASE FOUNDATION
William Black Medical Research Building
Columbia University Medical Center
640-650 W. 168th St.
New York, NY 10032-9982
800-457-6676
212-923-4700
Foundation reports on research in Parkinson's disease, publishes a quarterly newsletter with suggestions for people with Parkinson's and their caregivers. Articles cover activities of daily living such as eating and traveling; includes reviews of pertinent books and programs.

SJOGREN'S SYNDROME FOUNDATION, INC.
29 Gateway Dr.
Great Neck, NY 11021
516-767-2866
Distributes information that includes treatment recommendations and location of support groups for people with Sjogren's Syndrome.

SPINA BIFIDA ASSOCIATION OF AMERICA (SBAA)
4590 MacArthur Blvd. NW, Ste. 250
Washington, DC 20007-4226
800-621-3141
202-944-3285
Fax: 202-944-3295
Promotes research into causes and treatment of spina bifida. Provides materials on handling children with spina bifida and activities of daily living; gives referrals for information and support groups through local organizations.

UNITED CEREBRAL PALSY ASSOCIATION
1660 L St. NW
Washington, DC 20036-5602
800-872-5827
V/TTY: 202-776-0406
Fax: 202-776-0414
E-mail: ucpainc@aol.com
Provides publications, courses, referrals, and direct services through over 150 affiliates for people with cerebral palsy and those with other disabling conditions.

UNITED PARKINSON FOUNDATION
833 West Washington Blvd.
Chicago, IL 60607
312-733-1893
Fax: 312-733-1896
Distributes information on research into Parkinson's disease, methods of treatment, and living with the disease.

PAIN

Local hospitals and clinics frequently have outpatient programs and support groups for pain management. Contact local physicians or hospitals for additional information.

AMERICAN CHRONIC PAIN ASSOCIATION
P.O. Box 850
Rocklin, CA 95677
916-632-0922
Distributes information on pain treatment programs and makes referrals to more than 800 chapter support groups.

AMERICAN COUNCIL ON HEADACHE MEDICATION
800-255-ACHE
609-845-0322 (in case of emergency)
Non-profit educational resource for headache sufferers and their families.

AMERICAN PAIN SOCIETY
4700 West Lake Ave.
Glenview, IL 60025
708-375-4715
Fax: 708-975-4777
Makes referrals to pain centers.

FIBROMYALGIA NETWORK
P.O. Box 31750
Tucson, AZ 85751-1750
800-853-2929
Fax: 520-290-5550
Publishes newsletter; refers individuals to local support groups.

NATIONAL CHRONIC PAIN OUTREACH ASSOCIATION INC.
7979 Old Georgetown Rd., Ste. 100
Bethesda, MD 20814-2429
301-652-4948
Non-profit organization operates information clearinghouse and offers publications, tapes, and videotapes. Free catalog is available. Publishes quarterly magazine, *Lifeline*, for chronic pain sufferers and health care professionals. Computerized Support Group Registry gives local referrals. Support Group Starter Kit helps those interested in beginning a group.

NATIONAL HEADACHE FOUNDATION
5252 North Western Ave.
Chicago, IL 60625
312-878-7715

POST-POLIO SYNDROME

GAZETTE INTERNATIONAL NETWORKING INSTITUTE (GINI)
International Polio Network
4207 Lindell Blvd., #110
St. Louis, MO 63108-2915
314-534-0475
Fax: 314-534-5070
E-mail: gini_intl@msn.com
Publishes newsletter and materials for individuals with severe disabilities and for people with post-polio syndrome. Request publications list.

POST-POLIO PROGRAM
National Rehabilitation Hospital
102 Irving St. NW
Washington, DC 20010

THE POLIO SOCIETY
4200 Wisconsin Ave. NW
Box 106273
Washington, DC 20016
301-897-8180
(Send SASE with $1 postage.)

POST-POLIO STUDY
National Institutes of Health
Building 10, Rm. 4 N. 248
Bethesda, MD 20892

SPINAL CORD INJURIES AND PARALYSIS

All of the organizations listed below distribute information on research into the treatment of and living with spinal cord injuries and paralysis.

AMERICAN PARALYSIS ASSOCIATION
500 Morris Ave.
Springfield, NJ 07081
800-225-0292
201-379-2690
Fax: 201-912-9433
http://www.apa.uci.edu/paralysis

AMERICAN PARAPLEGIC SOCIETY
7520 Astoria Blvd.
Jackson Heights, NY 11370-1178
718-803-3782

AMERICAN SPINAL INJURY ASSOCIATION
2020 Peachtree Rd. NW
Atlanta, GA 30309
404-355-9772
Fax: 404-355-1826

CANADIAN PARAPLEGIA ASSOCIATION
520 Sutherland Dr.
Toronto, ON M4G 3V9
416-422-5640

EASTERN PARALYZED VETERANS ASSOCIATION
75-20 Astoria Blvd.
Jackson Heights, NY 11370-1178
800-803-0414
Group serves as advocate for improvement in treatment of people with paralysis, and publishes materials, including wheelchair home plans and accessibility guides.

INTERNATIONAL MEDICAL SOCIETY OF PARAPLEGIA
National Spinal Injuries Centre
Stoke Mandeville Hospital
Aylesbury
Buckinghamshire, England

JONI AND FRIENDS
P.O. Box 3333
Agoura Hills, CA 91301
818-707-5664
Newsletter is for the person with severe disabilities. Organization is source of financial aid through the Christian Fund for the Disabled.

NATIONAL SPINAL CORD INJURY ASSOCIATION
8300 Colesville Rd., Ste. 551
Silver Spring, MD 20910
800-962-9629 (National Spinal Cord Injury Hotline)
301-588-6959
E-mail: nscia@aol.com
http://www.spinalcord.org
Non-profit organization promotes research into spinal cord injury treatment, provides information to clients and families on rehabilitation programs, living with spinal cord injury, and other related subjects.

PARALYSIS RESEARCH ORGANIZATION
147 King St., #601
Littleton, MA 01460
800-424-CURE
Focuses on finding a cure for spinal cord injuries, publishes newsletter.

PARALYZED VETERANS OF AMERICA (PVA)
2111 East Highland Ave.
Phoenix, AZ 85016-4702
and
801 18th St. NW
Washington, DC 20006
800-795-4327
202-872-1300
Fax: 202-785-4452
Advocates for research into treatment of spinal cord injuries and programs for those who have sustained injuries. Publishes two magazines. See Periodicals, *Mealtime Manual*.

SPINAL CORD SOCIETY CANADA/SPINAL CORD RESEARCH
120 Newkirk Rd., Unit 1
Richmond Hill, ON L4C 9S7
905-508-4000
Organization promotes both research and better treatment of people with spinal cord injuries. Distributes information on programs and on coping with day-to-day living with spinal cord injuries.

SPINAL INJURIES ASSOCIATION
Newpoint House
76 St. James Ln.
London N10 3DF, England
British organization serving similar purpose as National Spinal Cord Injury Association.

STRESS

AMERICAN INSTITUTE OF STRESS
124 Park Ave.
Yonkers, NY 10703
914-963-1200
Distributes publications with stress-reducing suggestions; makes referrals to local agencies.

Also see agencies under Mental Health.

VESTIBULAR AND BALANCE DISORDERS

DIZZINESS AND BALANCE DISORDERS ASSOCIATION OF AMERICA
Good Samaritan Hospital
1015 NW 22nd Ave., Room 300
Portland, OR 97210
503-229-7348
Offers publications, including newsletter; makes suggestions for coping, including ideas for nutrition and treatment. Makes referrals to local support groups.

EAR FOUNDATION
1817 Patterson St.
Nashville, TN 37203-2110
V/TTY: 800-545-4327
615-329-7807
Fax: 615-329-7935
E-mail: theearfld@aol.com

NATIONAL ATAXIA FOUNDATION
750 Twelve Oaks Center
15500 Wayzata Blvd.
Wayzata, MN 55371
612-473-7666

VESTIBULAR DISORDERS ASSOCIATION
P.O. Box 4467
Portland, OR 97208-4467
800-837-8428
503-229-7705
Fax: 503-229-8064
E-mail: veda@teleport.com
Offers publications and makes referrals to local groups.

VESTIBULAR DISORDERS GROUP
Box 1197, FDR Station
New York, NY 10150
Distributes publications and makes referrals to support groups.

VISUAL LOSS AND BLINDNESS

Consult local physicians for information about low-vision clinics and mobility training programs in area.
The organizations listed promote research into causes and treatment of vision loss, education, and increased opportunities in both employment and general living.

AMERICAN ASSOCIATION OF THE DEAF-BLIND (AADB)—see under Deafness and Hearing Loss.

AMERICAN ASSOCIATION OF OPHTHALMOLOGY—see Section VI.

AMERICAN BROTHERHOOD FOR THE BLIND
1800 Johnson St.
Baltimore, MD 21230
410-659-9315

AMERICAN COUNCIL OF THE BLIND
1155 15th St. NW, Ste. 720
Washington, DC 20006
800-424-8666
202-467-5081

AMERICAN FOUNDATION FOR THE BLIND
11 Penn Plaza
New York, NY 10001
800-232-5463
212-502-7600
Fax: 212-502-7773
Non-profit organization develops and disseminates information, provides referral services on education and training programs. Publications are available in print or braille. Free catalogs.

AMERICAN OPHTHALMOLOGICAL SOCIETY
Duke University Eye Center
Box 3802
Durham, NC 27710
919-684-5365
Fax: 919-684-2230
Professional organization whose primary concern is eye research and care.

AMERICAN OPTOMETRIC ASSOCIATION
243 North Lindbergh Blvd.
St. Louis, MO 63141

AMERICAN PRINTING HOUSE FOR THE BLIND
1839 Frandfort Ave.
P.O. Box 6085
Louisville, KY 40206-0085
800-223-1839
502-895-2405
Fax: 502-899-2274

BETTER VISION INSTITUTE
P.O. Box 77097
Washington, DC 20013
800-424-VICA
703-243-1537

GLADYS E. LOEB FOUNDATION, INC.
2002 Forest Hill Dr.
Silver Spring, MD 20903
301-434-7748
Non-profit organization provides publications and aids, including stove guard rings for blind.

GUIDE DOGS FOR THE BLIND
P.O. Box 151200
San Rafael, CA
94915-1200
415-499-4000
Guide Dog News, apply.

GUIDING EYES FOR THE BLIND
611 Granite Springs Rd.
Yorktown Heights, NY 10598
800-942-0149
914-245-4024
Fax: 914-245-1609

HELEN KELLER NATIONAL CENTER FOR DEAF-BLIND YOUTHS AND ADULTS (HKNC)—see under Deafness and Hearing Loss.

LEADER DOGS FOR THE BLIND
1039 South Rochester Rd.
Rochester, MI 48307
810-651-9011
Fax: 810-651-5812

THE LIGHTHOUSE NATIONAL CENTER FOR VISION AND AGING
111 East 59th St.
New York, NY 10020
800-334-5497
212-821-9200
Distributes information on programs for those with loss of vision, and distributes information about cataract treatment.

NATIONAL ASSOCIATION FOR PARENTS OF THE VISUALLY IMPAIRED
P.O. Box 317
Watertown, MA 02272
800-562-6265
617-972-7441
Fax: 617-972-7444

NATIONAL ASSOCIATION FOR VISUALLY HANDICAPPED
22 West 21st St., Sixth Floor
New York, NY 10010
212-889-3141
Fax: 212-727-2931
Provides materials on treatment options, methods for maximizing vision, and prevention of blindness. Catalog is free.

NATIONAL BRAILLE ASSOCIATION, INC.
3 Townline Circle
Rochester, NY 14623-2513
716-472-9260
Fax: 716-427-0263
Converts books into Braille.

NATIONAL EYE CARE PROJECT
P.O. Box 429098
San Francisco, CA 94142-9098
800-222-EYES
Gives free eye examinations for the elderly.

NATIONAL EYE INSTITUTE
Box 20/20
Bethesda, MD 20892
Distributes booklet on cataracts and cataract treatment.

NATIONAL FEDERATION OF THE BLIND
1800 Johnson St.
Baltimore, MD 21230
800-638-7513
410-659-9314

NATIONAL LIBRARY SERVICES FOR THE BLIND AND PHYSICALLY HANDICAPPED—see Section I.

PILOT DOGS
625 West Town St.
Columbus, OH 43215
614-221-6367
Fax: 614-221-1577

PREVENT BLINDNESS AMERICA
500 East Remington Rd.
Schaumberg, IL 60173
800-331-2020
847-843-2020
Distributes information on low-vision training and aids.

RESEARCH TO PREVENT BLINDNESS
645 Madison Ave.
New York, NY 10022
800-621-0026
Fax: 212-688-6231

STATE SOCIETY FOR THE BLIND
Provides mobility training and assistive devices. Assists in learning to manage home, education, and employment. Check state government pages in your telephone book.

OTHER RELATED ORGANIZATIONS

AMERICAN ASSOCIATION OF HOMES AND SERVICES FOR THE AGING
901 East St. NW, Ste. 500
Washington, DC 20004-2037
202-783-2242
Fax: 202-783-2255
Distributes publications on what to consider when choosing a nursing home.

AMERICAN ASSOCIATION OF PEOPLE WITH DISABILITIES
4401 Connecticut Ave. NW, Ste. 223
Washington, DC 20008
"First national cross-disability membership organization" representing an estimated 49 million people with disabilities in the United States. Private, non-profit, advocating productivity, independence, integration of people with disabilities, enforcement of non-discrimination laws, promotion of service availability in areas of medical equipment and mobility aids, and educating public on related issues.

ASSOCIATION FOR CHILDREN WITH DOWN SYNDROME
2616 Martin Ave.
Bellmore, NY 11710
516-221-4700
Fax: 516-221-4311
http://www.acds.org

ASSOCIATION FOR PERSONS WITH SEVERE HANDICAPS
29 West Susquehanna Ave., Ste. 210
Baltimore, MD 21204-5201
Distributes information on coping with daily life, employment, and education, and makes referrals to support groups.

CENTER FOR UNIVERSAL DESIGN
School of Design
North Carolina State University
Box 8613
Raleigh, NC 27695-8613
V/TTY: 800-647-6777
V/TTY: 919-515-3082
Fax: 919-515-2032
E-mail: cahd@ncsu.edu
Promotes universal design of barrier-free buildings and outdoor areas. Disseminates information about home adaptation, technical design, and development of housing solutions for persons with disabilities.

COUNCIL FOR EXCEPTIONAL CHILDREN
P.O. Box 3000, Dept. EP
Denville, NJ 07834
800-247-8080
Fax: 201-489-1240
http://families.com
Provides support to parents and caregivers of children through publications and referral to support groups.

CROHN'S AND COLITIS FOUNDATION OF AMERICA
386 Park Avenue South
New York, NY 10016-7374
800-932-2423
212-685-3440
Fax: 212-685-3440
Distributes materials on living with ileitis and colitis.

DISABILITIES RESOURCES INC.
4 Glatter Ln.
Centereach, NY 11720
516-585-0290
Guide to toll-free information for people with disabilities.

DISABILITY RIGHTS EDUCATION AND DEFENSE
FUND
2212 6th St.
Berkeley, CA 94702
510-644-2555
and
GOVERNMENTAL AFFAIRS
Disability Rights Center
1633 Q St. NW
Washington, DC 20036
202-986-0375
National disability rights law and policy center is dedicated to
equal rights for people with disabilities. Provides education and
training programs on disability civil rights issues, legal support,
and advocacy. Distributes publications and makes referrals to
local sources.

DREAMMS FOR KIDS
Dept. 301
2763 Tasha Dr.
Clearwater, FL 34621-1223
813-781-7711
E-mail: DREAMMS@aol.com

EPILEPSY FOUNDATION OF AMERICA
4351 Garden City Dr.
Landover, MD 20785-2267
800-332-1000
301-577-0100
TTY: 800-332-2070
Fax: 301-577-4941
E-mail: postmaster@efa.org
Promotes research into causes and treatment of epilepsy.
Distributes materials for those with epilepsy, their families, and
caregivers. Free catalog.

FRIENDS' HEALTH CONNECTION
Long Distance Love
P.O. Box 114
New Brunswick, NJ 08903
908-418-1811
http://www.48friend.com
Telephone support/helpline that matches people with similar
interests and medical conditions.

HANDICAPPED ORGANIZED WOMEN, INC.
P.O. 35481
Charlotte, NC 28235
704-376-4735
Promotes needs of women with disabilities. Distributes publi-
cations and makes referrals to local support groups.

LEARNING DISABILITIES ASSOCIATION OF AMERICA
4156 Library Rd.
Pittsburgh, PA 15234
412-341-1515
Distributes materials on programs in rehabilitation and education. Provides referrals to local agencies.

MARCH OF DIMES BIRTH DEFECTS FOUNDATION
1275 Mamaroneck Ave.
White Plains, NY 10605
914-428-7100
Focuses on research into causes of birth defects. Provides referrals and support for people with disabilities.

NATIONAL ASSOCIATION FOR DOWNS SYNDROME
P.O. Box 4542
Oak Brook, IL 60521
630-325-9112
Distributes publications and makes referrals to local groups.

NATIONAL ASSOCIATION OF HOME BUILDERS
NAHB Research Center
Prince George's Blvd.
Upper Marlboro, MD 20772
301-249-4000

NATIONAL ASSOCIATION FOR HOME CARE
288 7th St. SE
Washington, DC 20003-4306
800-896-3650
301-942-6430
Fax: 301-942-2302
Promotes better home care and hospice programs. Provides
information on types of services available and makes referrals to
area agencies and publishes magazines, *Homecare* and *Caring*.

NATIONAL ASSOCIATION FOR PRIVATE RESIDENTIAL
RESOURCES
Box 163270
Sacramento, CA 95816
416-455-0723

NATIONAL CENTER FOR YOUTH WITH DISABILITIES
Institute for Health and Disability
University of Minnesota
Box 721
420 Delaware St. SE
Minneapolis, MN 55455
612-626-2825
V/TTY: 612-626-3939
Fax: 612-626-2134
E-mail: ncyd@gold.tc.umn.edu
http://www.peds.umn.edu

NATIONAL CITIZENS COALITION FOR NURSING HOME REFORM
1424 16th St. NW, Ste. 202
Washington, DC 20036
202-332-2275
Fax: 202-332-2949
Advocates for residents of nursing homes and board and care facilities.

NATIONAL COUNCIL ON DISABILITY
800 Independence Ave. SW
Washington, DC 20591
202-267-3846
Advocates more and improved programs for education, employment, accessible housing, and rehabilitation. Distributes publications.

NATIONAL COUNCIL ON INDEPENDENT LIVING
2111 Wilson Blvd., Ste. 405
Arlington, VA 22201
703-525-3406
Advocates increased possibilities for accessible housing, independent living programs, rehabilitation, education, and employment. Publishes materials on living on one's own with a disability and on accessible housing.

NATIONAL EASTER SEALS SOCIETY
230 West Monroe, Ste. 1800
Chicago, IL 60606
312-726-6200
TDD: 312-726-4258
Fax: 312-726-1494
E-mail: nessinfo@seals.com
http://www.seals.com
Provides resource list of local and state chapters. Distributes publications on various aspects of disabilities. Chapters may provide funds for assistance or work with state and local agencies to meet needs. Some have a loan closet for wheelchairs and other aids.

NATIONAL HOUSING AND REHABILITATION ASSOCIATION
1726 18th St. NW
Washington, DC 20009
202-328-9171
Fax: 202-265-4435
Promotes accessible housing and means of obtaining it. Publishes materials on how to adapt housing units for barrier-free access.

NATIONAL INSTITUTE FOR BURN MEDICINE
909 East Ann St.
Ann Arbor, MI 48104
313-769-9000

NATIONAL KIDNEY FOUNDATION
30 East 33rd St.
New York, NY 10016
800-622-9010
Fax: 212-689-9261
Distributes information on kidney disease and treatment; suggests funding options, and makes referrals to local agencies.

NATIONAL MATERNAL AND CHILD HEALTH CLEARINGHOUSE
2070 Chain Bridge Rd.
Vienna, VA 22182-2536
703-821-2098
Provides publications and referrals to other organizations.

NATIONAL ORGANIZATION ON DISABILITY
910 16th St. NW, Ste. 600
Washington, DC 20006
800-248-2253
202-293-5960
TTY: 202-293-5960
Fax: 202-293-7999
Advocates increased programs for people with disabilities; distributes materials on education, rehabilitation, and related needs.

NATIONAL OSTEOPOROSIS FOUNDATION
1150 17th St. NW, Ste. 500
Washington, DC 20036-4603
800-223-9994
800-464-6700
202-223-2226
Fax: 202-223-2237
Focuses on research into prevention and treatment of osteoporosis. Distributes newsletter and other materials for women and the elderly.

NATIONAL REHABILITATION ASSOCIATION
633 South Washington St.
Alexandria, VA 22314
703-836-0850
TDD: 703-836-0849
Professional organization promotes increased rehabilitation programs and funding.

NATIONAL RESEARCH AND TRAINING CENTER ON FAMILIES OF ADULTS WITH DISABILITIES
2198 Sixth St., Ste. 100
Berkeley, CA 94710
800-644-2666
Fax: 510-644-4445
Studies and develops materials for parents who have disabilities, publishes materials.

OSTEOPOROSIS SOCIETY OF CANADA
33 Laird Dr.
Toronto, ON M4G 3S9
Canada
800-463-6842
416-696-2663

PERSPECTIVES NETWORK
7205 Pullman Pl.
Mobile, AL 36695-4321
800-685-6302
205-639-5037
Fax: 205-639-5037

POINTS OF LIGHT FOUNDATION
800-879-5400
Will make referral to a volunteer center near you and mail information on obtaining or being a volunteer.

P.R.I.D.E. FOUNDATION, INC. (Promote Real Independence for the Disabled and Elderly)
391 Long Hill Rd., Box 1293
Groton, CT 06340
860-445-1448
E-mail: DressPride@aol.com
http://members.aol.com/sewtique/pride.htm
Distributes information to individuals with disabilities, including materials on home management and self-care. Makes assistive devices.

ROYAL ASSOCIATION FOR DISABILITY AND REHABIL-ITATION
12 City Forum
250 City Rd.
London ECIV 8AF
England
0171-250-3222
Fax: 0171-250-0212
Distributes publications and information on living with a disability, many written for British market but adaptable to needs of consumers with disabilities anywhere.

TELEPHONE PIONEERS OF AMERICA
930 15th St., Room 1249
Denver, CO 80202
303-571-9270
Fax: 303-572-0520
Organization for retired telephone workers provides a variety of services, including technical and financial assistance to people with disabilities.

THROUGH THE LOOKING GLASS
2198 Sixth St., Ste. 100
Berkeley, CA 94710-2204
800-644-2666
510-848-1112
Advocacy and education program is for parents with disabilities. Services mainly the Berkeley, Calif., area but advises people across the country. Three issues a year newspaper, *Parenting with a Disability* is free.

VISITING NURSE ASSOCIATION
Non-profit organization provides nursing care, therapy, patient education, social services, home health aides. Programs vary from agency to agency. Check the yellow pages.

III. COMPUTERIZED INFORMATION SERVICES FOR PEOPLE WITH DISABILITIES

ABLEDATA
8455 Colesville Rd., Ste. 935
Silver Springs, MD 20910
800-227-0216
TTY: 301-608-8912
Fax: 301-608-8958
http://www.naric.com/naric
Computerized search service assists in finding over 21,000 self-help aids and equipment. Provides bibliographical lists of books, articles, and visual materials. $10 charge for a customized list of products.

ACCENT ON INFORMATION
P.O. Box 700
Bloomington, IL 61702
309-378-2961
Search service provides lists of self-help aids and sources for people with disabilities. Send for AOI topics search request form and fee schedule. $12 per topic. Fee waived for individuals who cannot afford to pay.

ACCESS/ABILITIES
P.O. Box 458
Mill Valley, CA 94942
415-388-3250
Search service provides listing of self-help aids and sources for people with disabilities.

ASSISTIVE DEVICE DATABASE SYSTEM
American International Data Search, Inc.
2326 Fair Oaks Blvd., Ste. C
Sacramento, CA 94825
916-925-4554
Computerized information system is for people with disabilities.

CLEARINGHOUSE ON THE HANDICAPPED
Office of Special Education and Rehabilitative Services
Department of Education
Switzer Building
Room 3119
Washington, DC 20202
202-732-1245

NATIONAL SPINAL CORD INJURY HOTLINE
2200 Kernan Drive
Baltimore, MD 21207
800-526-3456 (National)
E-mail: SCIHotline@aol.com
http://users.aol.com/SCIHotline
Computerized information service is for people with spinal cord injuries and other disabilities.

IV. GOVERNMENTAL LOCAL, FEDERAL, AND STATE AGENCIES WORKING WITH THE AGING

AREA AGENCY ON AGING
Under the Older Americans Act, everyone 60 years of age or older is eligible for various homemaker and alternative services. This includes hot meals (Meals-on-Wheels is the most well-known). Look for Area Agencies on Aging or under Aging or Senior Citizens in the government pages of your telephone book. Other benefits for the elderly, which vary from locale to locale, include reduced real estate taxes; reduced drug costs; generic drug laws; housing assistance, including fuel allotments and rent exemptions from increases; half- or free-fare passes on buses and trains.

ADMINISTRATION ON AGING
Department of Health and Human Services
330 Independence Ave. SW
Washington, DC 20201
202-619-0724
E-mail: AoA_ESEC@Ban-Gate.AoA.DHS.Gov
http://www.AoA.DHS.Gov
Federal agency coordinates programs carried out by states and towns.

ALZHEIMER'S DISEASE EDUCATION AND REFERRAL CENTER
P.O. Box 8250
Silver Spring, MD 20907-8250
800-438-4380
301-495-3311
Fax: 301-495-3334
E-mail: adear@alzheimers.org
http://www.alzheimers.org/adear
Federal agency provides information and programs for patients with Alzheimer's Disease.

FEDERAL COUNCIL ON AGING
330 Independence Ave. SW
Room 4280 HHS-N
Washington, DC 20201
202-245-2451
Federal agency. Contact your state Agency on Aging for a list of area offices.

NATIONAL ASSOCIATION OF AREA AGENCIES ON AGING
1112 16th St. NW, Ste. 100
Washington, DC 20036
800-677-1116
202-296-8130
Promotes increased programming for the elderly and oversees development of services. Makes referrals to local resources.

NATIONAL INSTITUTE ON AGING
Public Information Office
Federal Building
Room 6C12
9000 Rockville Pk.
Bethesda, MD 20892
301-496-1752
and
Information Center
P.O. Box 8057
Gaithersburg, MD 20890-8057
Publishes series of fact sheets, *Age Pages*, on health concerns of the elderly, including safety, falls, nutrition.

V. VOLUNTARY AGENCIES WORKING WITH THE AGING AND WIDOWED

AARP WIDOWED PERSONS SERVICE
601 E Street NW
Washington, DC 20049
Provides peer support for widows and widowers; is part of the American Association for Retired Persons. Request publication *On Being Alone*.

ALZHEIMER'S ASSOCIATION
919 North Michigan Ave., Ste. 1000
Chicago, IL 60611-1676
800-272-3900
Fax: 312-335-1000
http://www.alz.org
Provides information, publications, and referrals to more than 200 chapters. Resource library on Alzheimer's disease and related disorders is stored in a computer database. Direct access is available from anywhere in the United States by using micro-computer with a modem and appropriate software.

AMERICAN ASSOCIATION OF RETIRED PERSONS (AARP)
444 North Capitol St. NW, Ste. 846
Washington, DC 20001-1812
800-424-3688
202-387-1968
Fax: 202-387-2193
Nationwide voluntary organization for people older than 55, working or retired. Distributes publications including materials on organizations, programs for local presentation, such as 55 Alive driving course, laws affecting the elderly, and caregiving. Publishes *Modern Maturity* monthly magazine, has discount pharmacy. Call for referral to local chapters, for catalog, or information on activities.

AMERICAN SOCIETY ON AGING
833 Market St., Ste. 512
San Francisco, CA 94103
415-974-9600
Voluntary organization focuses on needs of the elderly.

BEVERLY FOUNDATION
44 South Mentor Ave.
Pasadena, CA 91106
818-792-2292
Fax: 818 792 6117
Develops programs and opportunities for creative aging.

BROOKDALE CENTER ON AGING
425 East 25th St.
New York, NY 10010
212-481-4350
Provides information for professional caregivers. Write Attn: Publications.

CENTER FOR THE STUDY OF AGING
706 Madison Ave.
Albany, NY 12208
518-465-6927
Distributes books, videotapes, and audiocassettes from more than 200 publishers on topics dealing with the aging, including caregiving, social work, counseling, housing, home care, respite care, and nutrition. Send for catalog.

CHILDREN OF AGING PARENTS (CAPS)
1609 Woodbourne Rd., Ste. 302A
Levittown, PA 19057
800-227-7294
215-945-6900
Provides publications and referrals.

COALITION OF ADVOCATES FOR THE RIGHTS OF THE INFIRM ELDERLY (CARIE)
1315 Walnut St., Ste. 1000
Philadelphia, PA 19107
215-545-5728
Advocates to help older citizens stay in their homes.

FAMILY SERVICE AMERICA, INC.
11700 West Lake Park Dr.
Milwaukee, WI 53224
800-221-2681
414-359-1040
E-mail: comms@fsanet.org
Non-profit association consists of almost 300 member agencies that help families solve complex problems of elder care through counseling, support groups, and specialized services such as meetings with experts on elder care. For location of nearest agency and a copy of the caregiver brochure, send a SASE to this address, or check for a local listing in your telephone book.

FOSTER GRANDPARENT PROGRAM
400 Montauk Highway
West Islip, NY 11795
516-669-5355
Pairs adult with child who needs help or emotional support. Call for local chapter.

FRIENDS AND RELATIVES OF INSTITUTIONALIZED AGED, INC.
11 John St., Ste. 601
New York, NY 10038
Non-profit consumer advocacy organization is dedicated to improving system of care for institutionalized elderly. Counsels families seeking a nursing home and teaches how to monitor and change conditions in nursing homes. Publishes *Consumer's Guide to Nursing Home Care* as well as newsletter, *The Home Guard*.

THE GERONTOLOGICAL SOCIETY OF AMERICA—see Section VI.

GRAY PANTHERS
P.O. Box 21477
Washington, DC 20009-9477
800-280-5362
202-466-3132
Fax: 202-466-3133
Intergenerational movement lobbies for better opportunities for the elderly. Publishes newspaper.

JEFFERSON AREA BOARD FOR AGING
Charlottesville, VA 22901
Produce publications and audiovisuals for caregivers of the aging.

LEGAL COUNSEL FOR THE ELDERLY
American Bar Association
1909 K St. NW
Washington, DC 20036
202-833-6720
Makes referrals to local lawyers or organizations. Distributes publications.

NATIONAL ALLIANCE OF SENIOR CITIZENS
1700 18th St. NW, Ste. 401
Washington, DC 20009
202-986-0117
Fax: 202-986-2974
Advocates better opportunities for senior citizens in housing, funding, employment, leisure activities, and more.

NATIONAL ASSOCIATION OF AREA AGENCIES ON AGING
1112 16th St. NW, Ste. 100
Washington, DC 20036
202-296-8130

NATIONAL ASSOCIATION OF PROFESSIONAL GERIATRIC CARE MANAGERS
1604 North Country Club Rd.
Tucson, AZ 85716-3102
520-896-8008
Fax: 520-325-7925

NATIONAL COUNCIL ON THE AGING, INC.
409 Third St. SW, Second Floor
Washington, DC 20024
800-424-9046
202-479-1200
TDD: 202-479-6674
Fax: 202-479-0735
E-mail: info@ncoa.org
Oversees three organizations: the National Institute on Adult Day Care, the National Institute on Community-Based Long-Term Care, and the National Center on Senior Citizens, all reachable through the above number. Distributes publications and provides services to assist professionals who work with older adults, including information for caregivers and referrals to support groups. Family Care Givers of the Aging helps locate community resources for caregivers of frail, older relatives, and friends.

NATIONAL COUNCIL OF SENIOR CITIZENS
8403 Colesville Rd., Ste. 1200
Silver Springs, MD 20910-3314
301-578-8800
Advocates equal opportunities for senior citizens, participates in social and political activities related to the elderly, sponsors workshops, develops programs for state and local groups, provides speakers, and distributes materials.

NATIONAL FAMILY CAREGIVERS ASSOCIATION
9621 East Bexhill Dr.
Kensington, MD 20895-3104
800-896-3650
301-942-6430
Fax: 301-942-2303
http://www.nfcacares.org
Provides publications, information, education, and referrals to support groups.

NATIONAL INSTITUTE ON ADULT DAY CARE
National Council on the Aging
409 3rd St. SW, 3rd Pl.
Washington, DC 20024
202-479-6682
Fax: 202-479-0735
Distributes publications on adult day care and makes referrals to local agencies.

OLDER WOMEN'S LEAGUE
666 11th St. NW, Ste. 700
Washington, DC 20001
202-783-6686
Fax: 202-638-2356
Focuses on special needs of the older woman. Advocates equality and increased programs.

THE SANDWICH GENERATION
P.O. Box 132
Wickatuck, NJ 07765-0132
908-536-6215
Publishes magazine dealing with financial, legal, medical, and emotional issues related to caring for elderly relatives.

THEOS FOUNDATION
322 Blvd. of Allies, Ste. 105
Pittsburgh, PA 15222
412-471-7779
Organization is for the widowed and their families.

UNITED SENIORS HEALTH COOPERATIVE
1331 H St. NW, Ste. 500
Washington, DC 20005-4706
202-393-6222
Fax: 202-783-0588
E-mail: 103134.2627@compuserve.com
http://www.ushc-online.org
Non-profit organization offering guidance on health care planning, long-term care insurance, housing alternatives, financial assistance, and other resources. Catalog of publications.

WELL SPOUSE FOUNDATION
610 Lexington Ave., Ste. 814
New York, NY 10022-6005
800-838-0879 (24 hour answering service)
212-644-1241
Fax: 212-644-1338
National organization has more than 50 regional support groups, serving the needs of 7 to 9 million well spouses who care for partners with chronic illness or disability.

VI. PROFESSIONAL ORGANIZATIONS WORKING WITH PERSONS WITH DISABILITIES

AMERICAN ACADEMY OF APHASIA
University of California at Los Angeles
Dept. of Linguistics
Los Angeles, CA 90024
310-206-3206

AMERICAN ACADEMY FOR ENVIRONMENTAL MEDICINE
Box 16106
Denver, CO 80216
303-622-9755
Promotes research into effects of environmental pollution on health; distributes materials on this and on conditions related to effects.

AMERICAN ACADEMY OF ORTHOPEDIC SURGEONS
6300 North River Rd.
Rosemont, IL 60018-4226
800-346-1105
708-823-7186

AMERICAN ASSOCIATION ON MENTAL RETARDATION
444 North Capitol St. NW, Ste. 846
Washington, DC 20001-1512
800-424-3688
202-387-1968
Fax: 202-387-2193
Interdisciplinary association of professionals and individuals is concerned about mental retardation. Helps review and shape public policies, encourages research and communication, and promotes quality services for people with mental retardation and their families. List of publications is available.

AMERICAN ASSOCIATION OF OPHTHALMOLOGY
655 Beach St.
San Francisco, CA 94109
415-561-8533

AMERICAN COLLEGE OF RHEUMATOLGY
60 Executive Park South
Atlanta, GA 30329
404-633-3777
Fax: 404-633-2870
Focus on treatment of and research in the field of arthritis and rheumatology. The Association of Rheumatology Health Professionals is a section of this group.

AMERICAN CONGRESS OF REHABILITATION MEDICINE
4700 West Lake
Glenview, IL 60025
708-375-4777
Interdisciplinary organization. Publishes *Archives of Physical Medicine and Rehabilitation.*

AMERICAN HOME ECONOMICS ASSOCIATION
1555 King St.
Alexandria, VA 22314
703-706-4600
Professional organization is involved in home economics education. Publishes newsletter as well as magazine with research findings and programs.

AMERICAN MEDICAL ASSOCIATION
515 North State St.
Chicago, IL 60610
312-464-5000
National professional association for physicians makes referrals to area physicians.

AMERICAN OCCUPATIONAL THERAPY ASSOCIATION, INC.
4720 Montgomery Ln.
P.O. Box 31220
Bethesda, MD 20824-1220
800-SAY-AOTA (for AOTA members)
301-652-AOTA
TDD: 800-377-8555
Professional organization for occupational therapists makes referrals to regional associations. Publishes materials for professionals on occupational therapy including resource packets, videos and books; and for consumers on environmental adaptations, various disabilities, stress, and activities after hip surgery. Assists in locating sources for adaptive devices; provides continuing education courses by seminar, computer or self-paced correspondence.

AMERICAN OPHTHALMOLOGICAL SOCIETY—see Section II under Visual Loss and Blindness.

AMERICAN ORTHOTIC AND PROSTHETIC ASSOCIATION
1650 King St., Ste. 500
Alexandria, VA 22314
703-836-7116
Fax: 703-836-0838

AMERICAN PAIN SOCIETY—see Section II under Pain.

AMERICAN PHYSICAL THERAPY ASSOCIATION
1111 North Fairfax St.
Alexandria, VA 22314
703-684-2782
800-999-3212
Fax: 703-706-3396
Organization for physical therapists. Distributes publications; makes referrals to area therapists.

AMERICAN PODIATRIC MEDICAL ASSOCIATION
9312 Old Georgetown Rd.
Bethesda, MD 20814
301-571-9200
Distributes materials on care of feet and proper footwear.

AMERICAN PSYCHIATRIC ASSOCIATION—see Section II under Mental Health.

AMERICAN PSYCHOLOGICAL ASSOCIATION—see Section II under Mental Health.

AMERICAN SLEEP DISORDERS ASSOCIATION
1610 14th St. NW, Ste. 300
Rochester, MN 55901
Promotes research into sleep disorders and distributes materials on methods of coping. Makes referrals to area organizations.

AMERICAN SOCIETY OF NEUROREHABILITATION (ASNR)
5841 Cedar Lake Rd., #204
Minneapolis, MN 55416
612-545-6324
Fax: 545-6073
Organization for physicians and other health care professionals who deal with neurologically disabled persons. Focuses on improvement of patient care, research, teaching, and training in areas of neurorehabilitation.

AMERICAN SPEECH-LANGUAGE-HEARING ASSOCIATION
10801 Rockville Pike
Rockville, MD 20852
800-638-TALK
V/TDD: 301-897-5700
Professional organization for speech therapists distributes materials on communication and education. Makes referrals to local agencies.

AMERICAN THORACIC SOCIETY
1740 Broadway
New York, NY 10019-4374
212-315-8700

ASSOCIATION OF DRIVER EDUCATORS FOR THE DISABLED
P.O. Box 49
Edgerton, WI 53534
608-884-8833
Fax: 608-884-4851

ASSOCIATION OF REHABILITATION NURSES
5700 Old Orchard Rd.
Skokie, IL 60017-1057
708-966-3433
Fax: 708-966-9418

ASSOCIATION OF RHEUMATOLOGY HEALTH PROFESSIONALS
60 Executive Park South, Ste. 150
Atlanta, GA 30329

CANADIAN ASSOCIATION OF OCCUPATIONAL THERAPIST
110 Englinton Ave. West, 3rd Fl.
Toronto, ON M4R 1A3
416-487-0480

FOUNDATION FOR HOSPICE HOME CARE
519 C St. NE
Washington, DC 20002
202-547-7424
Distributes literature on hospice programs and makes referrals to area hospices.

THE GERONTOLOGICAL SOCIETY OF AMERICA
1275 K St. NW, Ste. 350
Washington, DC 20005-4006
202-842-1275
Fax: 202-842-1150
Focus is on research, practice, and education in aging. Divided into interest groups. Publishes several journals.

HUMAN FACTORS AND ERGONOMICS SOCIETY
P.O. Box 1369
Santa Monica, CA 90406-1369
310-394-1811
Fax: 310-394-2410

NATIONAL ASSOCIATION OF SOCIAL WORKERS
750 First St. NE
Washington, DC 20002
202-408-8600
Makes referrals to a licensed practitioner in local area.

NATIONAL MOBILITY EQUIPMENT DEALERS ASSOCIATION
914 East Skagway Ave.
Tampa. FL 33604
813-932-8566
Fax: 813-931-4683

RESNA (Rehabilitation Engineering Society of North America)
1700 North Moore St.
Arlington, VA 22209-1903
703-524-6686
TTY: 703-524-6639
Fax: 703-524-6630
Non-profit organization founded for the advancement of rehabilitation and assistive technologies.

SOCIETY OF AUTOMOTIVE ENGINEERS
400 Commonwealth Dr.
Warrendale, PA 15096-0001
412-776-4841
Fax: 412-776-5944

VISITING NURSE ASSOCIATION OF AMERICA
3801 East Florida Ave., Ste. 806
Denver, CO 80210
800-426-2547
Distributes literature on programs and makes referrals to local visiting nurse agencies.

VII. CONSUMER ORGANIZATIONS WORKING WITH PEOPLE WITH DISABILITIES AND THE AGING

ADAPTIVE ENVIRONMENTS CENTER
The National Center for Access Unlimited
374 Congress St., Ste. 301
Boston, MA 02210
V/TTY: 617-695-1225
Fax: 617-482-8099
E-mail: adaptive@interramp.com

AMERICAN AUTOMOBILE ASSOCIATION (AAA)
1000 AAA Dr.
Heathrow, FL 32746-5063
407-444-7961
Fax: 407-444-7955
Publishes book on driving and automobile controls for people with disabilities, which is updated annually and gives contacts for mobility equipment in all 50 states. Available at most AAA offices.

AMERICAN DRIVER AND TRAFFIC SAFETY EDUCATION ASSOCIATION
I.U.P. Highway Safety Corner
R&P Building
Indiana, PA 15702-1093
412-357-4051
FAX: 412-357-7595

AAA FOUNDATION FOR TRAFFIC SAFETY
1440 New York Ave. NW, Ste. 201
Washington, DC 20005
800-305-7233
202-638-5944
Fax: 202-638-5943
Distributes materials to increase traffic and automobile safety, including recommendations for older drivers.

AMERICAN RED CROSS
Seventeenth and D Streets
Washington, DC 20006
202-737-6300
Call local chapter for listing of services.

ASSOCIATION OF HOME APPLIANCE MANUFACTURERS
20 North Wacker Dr., Ste. 1231
Chicago, IL 60606
800-621-0477
312-984-5800
Fax: 312-984-9950
If a problem arises with an appliance, contact the authorized service agency or manufacturer of the appliance first. If it is not resolved, consumer may call for assistance.

CANADIAN COUNCIL ON SOCIAL CONCERN SELF-HELP UNIT
P.O. Box 3505
55 Parkdale Ave.
Ottawa, ON
Canada
613-728-1865
Self-help clearinghouse includes more than 200 organizations across Canada.

CHRISTMAS IN APRIL
4713 Wisconsin Ave. NW, Second Fl.
Washington, DC 20016
202-362-1611
Volunteer agency that repairs and modifies homes of the aging and those with disabilities nationwide, set up in advance and done on one day in April.

COMMUNITY ACTION NETWORK
600 Madison Ave.
New York, NY 10022
212-702-0944
Fax: 212-702-0932
Volunteer, non-profit, public service finding solutions to community social problems; publish booklets on a range of topics including elderly care, handicapped, AIDS. Send for full list.

CONSUMER FEDERATION OF AMERICA
1424 16th St. NW, Ste. 604
Washington, DC 20036

COUNCIL OF BETTER BUSINESS BUREAUS
4200 Wilson Blvd., Eighth Floor
Arlington, VA 22209
703-276-0133
Provides assistance with problems regarding purchases and poor or fraudulent business practices. Check for local office in your telephone book.

HABITAT FOR HUMANITY INTERNATIONAL
121 Habitat St.
Americus, GA 31709-3498
Helpline: 912-924-6935
Fax: 912-924-6541
Volunteers build and renovate homes for people with and without disabilities.

INSTITUTE FOR TECHNOLOGY DEVELOPMENT
Advanced Living Systems Div.
428 North Lamar Blvd.
Oxford, MS 38655
601-234-0158
Distributes materials on adapting homes and equipment design.

MEDIC ALERT FOUNDATION
2323 Colorado Ave.
Turlock, CA 95381-1009
800-344-3226
Provides identification tags for people with medical problems.

MEDICARE RIGHTS CENTER, INC.
1460 Broadway
New York, NY 10036

NATIONAL ASSOCIATION OF THE REMODELING INDUSTRY
4301 North Fairfax Dr., Ste. 310
Arlington, VA 22203-1627
703-276-7600
Fax: 703-243-3465

NATIONAL BURGLAR AND FIRE ALARM ASSOCIATION
7101 Wisconsin Ave., Ste. 1390
Bethesda, MD 20814
Distributes materials on types of and setting up of alarm systems. For information, send $2.

NATIONAL CONSUMERS LEAGUE
1701 K St. NW, #1200
Washington, DC 20006
800-876-7060
202-835-3323
Fax: 202-835-0747

NATIONAL FIRE PROTECTION ASSOCIATION
1 Batterymarch Park
Quincy, MA 02269
800-344-3555
Distributes publications on planning for fire safety.

NATIONAL KITCHEN AND BATH ASSOCIATION
687 Willow Grove St.
Hackettstown, NJ 07840
908-852-0033
Fax: 908-852-1695
Focus is on kitchen and bath design; publishes materials on accessible and barrier-free kitchens as well as equipment.

NATIONAL SAFETY COUNCIL
1121 Spring Lake Dr.
Itasca, IL 60143-3201
708-285-1121
Fax: 708-285-1315
Evaluates equipment, distributes publications on safety subjects.

PROMATURA
428 North Lamar
Oxford, MS 38655
601-234-0158
Fax: 601-234-0288
E-mail: mwyldc@promatura.com
Distributes materials on adapting homes and equipment design.

SELF HELP CLEARINGHOUSE
Northwest Covenant Medical Center
25 Pocono Rd.
Denville, NJ 07834
201-625-9565
Major self-help groups are often listed in the yellow pages of the telephone book under "social service organizations." This organization provides comprehensive lists of groups nationwide and can also offer guidance on setting up a group if one does not already exist in the area. For information, send a stamped, self-addressed envelope.

TELE CONSUMER HOTLINE
P.O. Box 27207
Washington, DC 20005
800-332-1124
V/TTY: 202-347-7208
http://www.teleconsumer.org/hotline
Non-profit, impartial telephone consumer service. Send stamped, self-addressed envelope for information on telephone products and services.

THE USAA FOUNDATION
9800 Fredericksburg Rd.
San Antonio, TX 78284-9894
Division of large insurance and financial corporation. Distributes materials on financial planning for the aging as well as selection of nursing homes and other consumer affairs.

UNITED WAY
Call local office for listing of organizations and referral.

VIII. ORGANIZATIONS CONCERNED WITH NUTRITION

AMERICAN DAIRY ASSOCIATION
O'Hare International Center
10255 West Higgins Rd., Ste. 900
Rosemont, IL 60018-5616
847-803-2000
Fax: 847-803-2077
Distributes materials for consumers' use of dairy products and responds to dietary questions.

AMERICAN DIETETIC ASSOCIATION
216 West Jackson Blvd., Ste. 800
Chicago, IL 60606-6995
312-899-0040
Responds to consumers' questions on nutrition and makes referrals to area organizations.

AMERICAN SEAFOOD INSTITUTE'S FISH AND
SEAFOOD HOTLINE
800-EAT-FISH
Seafood industry experts respond to inquiries about nutrition, purchase, storage, and preparation of fish and seafood. Monday to Friday, 9:00 a.m. to 5:00 p.m., Eastern Time.

CANNED FOOD INFORMATION COUNCIL
500 North Michigan Ave., Ste. 300
Chicago, IL 60611
312-836-7279

CENTER FOR SCIENCE IN THE PUBLIC INTEREST
1501 16th St. NW
Washington, DC 20036
Consumer advocacy group promotes better nutrition. Publishes books, posters, such as low-fat and anti-cancer guides, as well as a newsletter, *Nutrition Action Healthletter*. Listed under Periodicals.

FOOD MARKETING INSTITUTE
Publication Sales
800 Connecticut Ave. NW
Washington, DC 20006

NATIONAL ASSOCIATION OF ANOREXIA NERVOSA AND RELATED DISORDERS
Box 7
Highland Park, IL 60035
708-831-3438
Fax: 708-433-4632

NATIONAL ASSOCIATION OF MEAL PROGRAMS (NAMP)
1414 Prince St., Ste. 202
Alexandria, VA 22314
703-548-5558
Information on starting a meals program in local area.

NATIONAL CENTER FOR NUTRITION AND DIETETICS
Consumer Nutrition Hotline
800-366-1655
Registered dietitians provide referrals to area consulting dietitians, take questions, and send free materials. Monday to Friday, 10:00 a.m. to 5:00 p.m., Eastern Time. Recorded messages in English and Spanish available 24 hours.

NATIONAL FOOD SAFETY DATABASE
http://www.foodsafety.org

NUTRITION INFORMATION SERVICE
University of Alabama at Birmingham
800-231-DIET
Sponsored in part by the National Cancer Institute. Experts from the Department of Nutrition Sciences answer calls about nutrition, diet and food, Monday through Friday, 9:00 a.m. to 4:00 p.m., Central Time.

OVEREATERS ANONYMOUS
6075 Zenith Ct. NE
Rancho Rio, NM 87124-6424
505-891-2664
Fax: 505-891-4320
Provides peer support and programs for overweight individuals to combat compulsive overeating. Write for local support groups.

SECOND HARVEST
National Office
116 South Michigan Ave., Ste. 4
Chicago, IL 60603
800-532-FOOD
Refers caller to a local food bank for assistance, or gives location at which to offer your time and donations of food.

SOCIETY FOR NUTRITION EDUCATION
2001 Killebrew Dr., No. 340
Minneapolis, MN 55425-1820
612-854-0035

U.S. FOOD AND DRUG ADMINISTRATION'S CENTER FOR FOOD, SAFETY AND APPLIED NUTRITION HOTLINE
800-332-4010

USDA MEAT AND POULTRY HOTLINE
800-535-4555
202-720-3333 (in Washington, DC)
Staff responds to inquiries about labeling, nutrition, safety, storage, and preparation of meat and poultry. Monday to Friday, 10:00 a.m. to 4:00 p.m., Eastern Time.

IX. LOCAL ORGANIZATIONS THAT OFFER VOLUNTEERS, POSSIBLE FUNDING, AND/OR OTHER ASSISTANCE TO PEOPLE WITH DISABILITIES AND THE AGING

Many organizations provide a variety of services and programs at the local level. Benefits may include transportation, respite help, volunteer shoppers or companions, education, and funds for equipment or home modifications. Call local chapter for area information and services.

B'NAI BRITH

EASTER SEALS
See NATIONAL EASTER SEAL SOCIETY—Section II, Other Related Organizations.

ELKS
Benevolent Protective Order of Elks
P.O. Box 159
Winston, NC 27986
919-358-7661
Local chapters often provide funding to people with disabilities. Contact the national organization for an active chapter in your area.

FRATERNAL ORDER OF EAGLES

FRIENDS FOR IMMEDIATE AND SYMPATHETIC HELP (FISH)
Call local chapter for transportation, shopping, and other services.

JAYCEES

JUNIOR LEAGUE

KIWANIS

KNIGHTS OF COLUMBUS

LIONS

LOYAL ORDER OF MOOSE

OPTIMIST

ROTARY CLUB

UNITED WAY

WHEELS FOR KIDS
206-863-4659
Program that modifies electronic systems so children in wheelchairs can operate them. What began as a local project is spreading.

YMCA/YWCA

X. REHABILITATION FACILITIES AND HOSPITALS

This is a list of institutions who have contributed to this publication. An extensive list of rehabilitation facilities may be obtained through the Commission on the Accreditation of Rehabilitation Facilities, listed below.

CHILDREN'S HOSPITAL AT STANFORD
Rehabilitation Engineering Center
Palo Alto, CA 94300

COMMISSION ON THE ACCREDITATION OF REHABILITATION FACILITIES
4891 East Grant Rd.
Tucson, AZ 85712
520-325-1044
Fax: 520-318-1129
Creates standards for home- or community-based programs as well as rehabilitation facilities.

GOOD SAMARITAN MEDICAL CENTER
Publication Service
1130 East McDowell Rd., Ste. A-7
Phoenix, AZ 85006-2675.

THE HEBREW HOME FOR THE AGED AT RIVERDALE
5901 Palisades Ave.
Riverdale, NY 10471

HOWARD A. RUSK INSTITUTE OF REHABILITATION MEDICINE
New York University Medical Center
400 East 34th St.
New York, NY 10016
212-263-7300

INDEPENDENT LIVING RESEARCH UTILIZATION PROGRAM
2323 South Shepherd, Ste. 1000
Houston, TX 77019
713-520-0232
TTY: 713-520-5136
Fax: 713-520-5785
Distributes the *Directory of Independent Living Centers.*

INSTITUTE FOR REHABILITATION AND RESEARCH (RRTC)
1333 Moursund
Houston, TX 77030-3405
713-799-5000
TDD: 797-5790
Fax: 713-799-7095

LONG TERM CARE NATIONAL RESOURCE CENTER
University of Southern California
Los Angeles, CA
213-740-1364

NATIONAL CENTER FOR DISABILITY SERVICES
Henry Viscardi Center
201 I.U. Willits Rd.
Albertson, NY 11507

NATIONAL JEWISH MEDICAL AND RESEARCH CENTER
1400 Jackson St.
Denver, CO 80206
800-222-5864

A.J. PAPPANILOU CENTER ON SPECIAL EDUCATION AND REHABILITATION
University of Connecticut
249 Glenbrook Rd., U-64
Storrs, CT 06269-2064
203-486-5035
Fax: 203-486-5037

RANCHO LOS AMIGOS HOSPITAL
Los Angeles County Hospital
7601 East Imperial Highway
Downey, CA 90242

REHABILITATION INSTITUTE OF CHICAGO
345 East Superior
Chicago, IL 60611

ROOSEVELT WARM SPRINGS INSTITUTE
University of California at Irvine
UCI College of Medicine Foundation
401 Berkeley, Ste. 465
Irvine, CA 92715

SHRINERS BURNS INSTITUTES
Shrine International Headquarters
P.O. Box 31356
Tampa, FL 33631-3356
813-621-3141
Specializes in treatment of burn victims. Call for information on nearest center.

THOMS REHABILITATION HOSPITAL
68 Sweeten Crede Rd.
Ashville, NC 28803
704-274-2400
Fax: 704-274-9482

Periodicals

Subscription prices were current at time of publishing, but please contact the publishers regarding changes. Addresses for agencies and organizations are given in Appendix C; addresses for sources are in Appendix E. Please see *Mealtime Manual* for listing of consumer-focused periodicals on family service, disability, and health.

Activities, Adaptations and Aging. $32 individual, $75 institution. Order through Haworth Press. **Source:** 247.

Advance for Occupational Therapists. Merion Publications, Inc., 650 Park Avenue W., King of Prussia, PA 19406. Free weekly publication sent to occupational therapists and certified OT assistants.

Alzheimer's Disease and Associated Disorders—An International Journal. Quarterly, $78 individual, $98 institution. Order through Lippincott/Raven. **Source:** 330.

American Chronic Pain Association. *ACPA Chronicle.* Quarterly newsletter lists new chapters, articles by professionals and members, book reviews. $10 donation for two years.

American College of Nutrition Journal. Bimonthly, $125 institution. Order through Wiley. **Source:** 575.

American Dietetic Association Journal. Monthly, $90. Order through the American Dietetic Association.

American Journal on Mental Retardation. Monthly, $95 per year in US. Order through the American Association on Mental Retardation.

American Journal of Nursing. Monthly. $23. Source: 41.

American Journal of Occupational Therapy. Monthly, sent to all registered occupational therapists as part of membership. Nonmembers: $25 per year for individuals, $100 for institutions, $110 outside the U.S. Order through the American Occupational Therapy Association, Inc.

American Journal of Physical Medicine and Rehabilitation. Bimonthly, $55 individual, $87 institution. Order through Williams & Wilkins. **Source:** 577.

American Journal of Respiratory and Critical Care Medicine. Contact the American Lung Association.

American Review of Respiratory Diseases. Contact the American Thoracic Society.

Archives of Physical Medicine and Rehabilitation. Monthly, $65 individual, $100 institution. Order through American Congress of Rehabilitation Medicine.

Arthritis and Rheumatism, Official Journal of the American Rheumatism Association. Monthly, $38 student, $75 individuals within U.S., $85 individuals outside U.S., $115 institutions.

Arthritis Care & Research, the Official Journal of the Association of Rheumatology Health Professionals. Quarterly, $42.50 individual, $80 organization. Elsevier Science Publishing Company. **Source:** 185.

Batting the Breeze. Subscription information from Emphysema Anonymous, Inc., P.O. Box 3224, Seminole, FL 34642; 813-391-9977.

This Brain Has a Mouth. Subscription information from This Brain Has a Mouth, Inc., 61 Brighton St., Rochester, NY 14607; 716-473-6764. Publication for people with brain injury and their families.

Canadian Journal of Occupational Therapy. 5 issues per year, $52. Order through Canadian Association of Occupational Therapists.

Caregiving. Monthly, $24. Tad Publishing Co., 114 Euclid, Ste. 270, Park Ridge, IL 60068. Also offers online support. See Appendix F.

Caring Magazine. Monthly, $45 per year, $65 Canadian and international. Order through the National Association for Home Care.

Cognitive Rehabilitation. Six issues per year, multidisciplinary journal. For subscription information, contact Neuroscience Publishers. **Source:** 376.

Continuing Care. Monthly, $39 includes Buyer's Guide. Stevens Publishing Corp., 3630 J.H. Kultgen Freeway, Waco, TX 76706.

Coping: Living with Cancer. Bimonthly, $18. Order through Medic America. **Source:** 352B.

Education and Training of the Mentally Retarded and

Developmentally Disabled. Quarerly, $30. Order through Council for Exceptional Children.

Exceptional Child. Bimonthly for teachers, $40, $44.50 foreign. Order through Council for Exceptional Children.

Exceptional Parent. Monthly, $28 per year. Council for Exceptional Children. P.O. Box 3000, Dept. EP, Denville, NJ 07834. 800-247-8080. Fax: 201-489-1240. (FEN): http://families.com.

Family Therapist Networker. Bimonthly, $20. 7705 13th Street, NW, Washington, DC 20021.

Fine Cooking. 63 S. Main Street, Newtown, CT 06470-9879. Bimonthly, $26 per year. For people who live to cook; gives tips and techniques for easier handling of techniques.

Focus on Geriatric Care and Rehabilitation. 10 issues per year, $85. Aspen Publishers. Practical monthly newsletter edited by practicing geriatric specialists. Each issue focuses on one clinical topic with background, assessment, therapeutic approaches, models of treatment, and caregiving concerns. **Source:** 61.

The Gerontologist and the *Journals of Gerontology* (4 sections). Order through The Gerontological Society of America. Subscription to all publications included in membership, $52 per year.

Headache Quarterly: Current Treatment and Research. Quarterly, $45. International Universities Press, Inc. **Source:** 284.

Home Healthcare Nurse: The Professional Journal for the Community Health Nurse. Bimonthly, $30 individual, $40 institution within US; check for rates outside US. Lippincott/Raven. Subscription orders should be sent to the magazine at P.O. Box 670, Holmes, PA 19043.

Hearing Health. Bimonthly, $14. Voice on hearing issues. Order through Voice International Publishing, Inc., Box V, Ingleside, TX 78362-0500.

Heartline. Montly, $29. Written for consumers. Order through Coronary Club, Inc.

HomeCare® Magazine. Monthly, order through Miramar Communications. **Source:** 363. Guide to home health and rehabilitation products. Website is http://www.homecaremag.com.

Homecare News. Monthly newspaper, $18 per year, $25 Canadian and international. Focus on legislation, regulatory, and legal issues in the home care industry. Order through the National Association for Home Care.

Hospice: The Magazine for Hospice Professionals. Quarterly; annual subscription is included in professional membership dues. For information, contact National Hospice Organization.

Human Factors: The Journal of the Human Factors and Ergonomics Society. Quarterly, free with membership, $135 per volume for non-members.

Hypertension. Monthly, $198. American Heart Association.

In Motion. Bimonthly, $25 individual. Includes membership. Order through Amputee Coalition of America.

Infants and Young Children: Interdisciplinary Journal of Special Care Practices. $72 plus handling per year. Order through Aspen Publishers. **Source:** 61.

Journal of Cognitive Rehabilitation. Bimonthly, $35. Order through Neuroscience Publishers. **Source:** 376.

Journal of Gerontological Nursing. Monthly, $34 individual, $46 institution. Order through SLACK Inc. **Source:** 479.

Journal of Head Injury: A Search for Understanding. Subscription information through the JMA Foundation, Inc., 1900 L St., NW, Ste. 300, Washington, DC 20036. 202-331-8445.

Journal of Head Trauma Rehabilitation. Bimonthly, $105 per year. Aspen Publishers. **Source:** 61.

Journal of Home Economics. Quarterly. Sent to all American Home Economics Association members as a service. $20 per year to non-members. Order through the American Home Economics Association.

Journal of Home Health Care Practice. Quarterly, in-depth focus on a topic. $68 plus $5 shipping and handling. Order from Aspen Publishers. **Source:** 61.

The Journal of Nursing Research. Monthly, $25 individual, $35 institution. Order through the American Journal of Nursing Company. **Source:** 41.

Journal of Pediatrics. Monthly, $59 per year. 11830 Westline Industrial Dr., St. Louis, MO 63146.

Journal of Vision Impairment and Blindness. Large-print, Braille, or cassette, 10 issues a year, $30 individual, $35 institution, foreign add $15 for postage. Order through the American Foundation for the Blind. Circulation Manager, American Foundation for the Blind.

Mental Retardation. Plus *American Journal of Mental Retardation* and *News & Notes.* Bimonthly, $70, $75 outside North America. Order through American Association on Mental Retardation.

Multiple Sclerosis Quarterly Report. Quarterly, $15 per year. Published by the Multiple Sclerosis Society with the Eastern Paralyzed Veterans Association. Order through Demos Publications. **Source:** 164.

National Association for Home Care Report. Weekly policy newsletter, $325 per year, $350 Canadian and international. Order through the National Association for Home Care.

The National Head Injury Newsletter. Quarterly, apply through the National Head Injury Foundation.

National Information Center For Children and Youth With Handicaps (NICHCY) News Digest. Biannual, $8 per year. Box 1492, Washington, DC 20013.

New Directions. Contact the National Jewish Center for Immunology and Respiratory Medicine for subscription information.

The New England Journal of Medicine. Weekly, $79 per year. 10 Shattuck St., Boston, MA 02115.

Occupational Therapy Forum. Weekly, free to registered occupational therapists and certified occupational therapy assistants. Order through Forum Communications. **Source:** 209.

The Occupational Therapy Journal of Research. Bimonthly. For subscription information, contact SLACK Inc. **Source:** 479.

OT Practice. Monthly. Order through the American Occupational Therapy Association, Inc. Subscription included in members' annual dues. Non-member individuals and non-member students, $50 per year; institutions, $85. Member students, $20.

OT Week. Weekly, free to registered occupational therapists and certified OT assistants. $80 per year for non-members. Order through the American Occupational Therapy Association, Inc.

O & P Business News: Linking the Orthotic and Prosthetics Professions. Semi-monthly, 12 issues, $25. Order through JKS

Publications. **Source:** 290B.

The Pulmonary Paper. $14.95. P.O. Box 217, Exeter, NH 03833. Published by group of pulmonary specialists.

Rehab Brief. Monthly, National Institute of Handicapped Research, Office of Special Education and Rehabilitation Services, U.S. Department of Education, Washington, DC 20201.

Rehabilitation Nursing. Bimonthly, $75. Order through Association of Rehabilitation Nurses.

SHHH Journal. Bimonthly. $20 to individuals. Order through Self Help for Hard of Hearing People, Inc.

Team Rehab Report. Free multidisciplinary magazine focuses on equipment and technology for clients with long-term disabilities. Order through Miramar Publications. **Source:** 363. Website: http://www.teamrehab.com.

Topics in Geriatric Rehabilitation. Quarterly journal. Each issue focuses on specific area with interdisciplinary views. $75. Order through Aspen Publishers. **Source:** 61.

Update. Family Survival Project. 425 Bush St., Ste. 500, San Francisco, CA 94108; 415-434-3388.

Update. National Vision Research Institute. Free quarterly.

Wiser Now. Monthly, $24.95 per year. Order through Better Directions, P.O. Box 3064, Waquoit, MA 02536-3064; 800-999-0795 (orders), Fax: 508- 457-5333 (orders). For professionals and caregivers.

Worklife A Publication on Employment and People with Disabilities. Limited number of complimentary subscriptions. Order through the President's Committee for Employment of People with Disabilities.

NEWSLETTERS

With time of the essence, newsletters bring summarized findings to our attention.

AFB News. Free 12-page national newsletter, published five times a year. Order from the American Foundation for the Blind.

American Institute of Cancer Research Newsletter. 1759 R Street, NW, Washington, DC 20009. Quarterly, free.

Bottom Line Personal. Subscription Service Center, Box 50379, Boulder, CO 80321-0379. Biweekly (24 issues per year), $39. Focus is financial, but topics include health, nutrition, planning for medical care, and retirement.

Cancer Smart. Order from Memorial Slan-Kettering Cancer Center, 1275 York Ave., Box 200, New York, NY 10021.

CardiSense. Quarterly, free from Hoechst Marion Roussel. Subscription Service Dept., P.O. Box 748, New York, NY 10159-5433; 800-235-LIFE (5433) for questions regarding subscription. Focus on cardiac health, articles on nutrition, role of exercise, stress, and other factors.

DIRECTIONS: Technology in Special Education. DREAMMS for Kids, Dept. 301, 2763 Tasha Dr., Clearwater, FL 34621-1223; 813-781-7711; E-mail: DREAMMS@aol.com.

The Edell Health Letter. P.O. Box 50162, Boulder, CO 80321-0162. 10 issues, $24. General health topics including nutrition.

Harvard Medical School Newsletter. Monthly, $24 per year. P.O. Box 420234, Palm Coast, FL 32142-0234; 800-829-9171.

Healthline. New England Journal of Medicine Newsletter. 17 issues per year, $18. P.O. Box 52925, Boulder, CO 80321-2929.

The Johns Hopkins Medical Letter: Health After 50. $15 for 12 monthly issues. P.O. Box 420176, Palm Coast, FL 32142. . New health findings especially for older individuals, including topics on nutrition.

Long Cane News. The National Newsletter for Professionals Working with the Visually Impaired and Blind Persons Who Get Around. Biannual, $8 per year. Order through the American Foundation for the Blind.

Mayo Clinic Healthletter and M*ayo Clinic Nutrition Letter.* Monthly, $24 per year in the U.S. Mayo Foundation for Medical Education and Research, 200 First St., Rochester, MN 55905; 800-333-9037.

Mental Medicine Update: Mind/Body Health Newsletter. The Center for Health Sciences. The Institute for the Study of Human Knowledge. Quarterly, $9.95. P.O. Box 176, Los Altos, CA 94023.

Nutrition Action Healthletter. Monthly, $24 per year. Center for Science in the Public Interest. **Source:** 112. Emphasis is on healthy, safe foods, food labeling, often focusing on convenience foods, and giving excellent quick reference charts. CSPI also has wide variety of books, nutrition posters, and audiovisual aids. Website: http://www.cspinet.org.

Parkinson's Disease Update. Monthly newsletter on current medical, social, and psychological aspects of Parkinson's Disease. $40 per year. Order from Medical Publishing Co., P.O. Box 24622-H, Philadelphia, PA 19111; 215-947-6638.

Perspectives in Rehab. Monthly, $79 per year. Each edition summarizes 18 to 20 rehab-related studies from journals with rehabilitation professionals in mind. To order or for more information, call 800-850-7388.

Second Wind. Little Company of Mary Hospital, PEP Pioneers, 4104 Torrance Blvd., Torrance, CA 90503. 213-540-7676 ext. 4499. For people with COPD.

Tufts University Diet and Nutrition Letter. Monthly, $24 per year. 53 Park Place, New York, NY 10007; 800-274-7581. Focus on nutrition, new studies.

University of California at Berkeley Wellness Letter. Monthly, $24 per year. P.O. Box 420291, Palm Coast, FL 32142- 0291; 800-829-9080. Focus on total fitness, which includes at least one article a month on food and nutrition. Excellent tables comparing types of foods, commercially prepared products.

The University of Texas Lifetime Health Letter. Monthly, $24 per year. P.O. Box 420342, Palm Coast, FL 34142-0342; 800-829-9177. Nutrition, wellness, issues on aging.

Sources for Equipment and Materials

When purchasing equipment and materials described in *Meal Preparation and Training: The Health Care Professional's Guide*, check your local resources and facilities. Research the phone book for area home health and hospital equipment suppliers, and department, housewares, hardware, office supply, and specialty stores. These business often have catalogs or computer databases of additional items that may be ordered from jobbers or distributors. When this does not pinpoint the item you require, an inquiry to the manufacturer or distributor usually results in referral to a local or mail-order source, or the agreement to take a personal order. Setting up accounts with the most helpful and expedient self-help and equipment firms reduces the time you must spend in searching out and ordering equipment for clients; frequently there will be a lower professional price as well. Often a local firm will take over the responsibility of filling out forms for insurance or Medicare reimbursement.

Note: The addresses and telephone numbers given here were current at the time of publication. If you have a problem locating a company or product, please write what is required on the suggestion card. I will gladly answer your questions and give, whenever possible, an alternate source or solution.

1. **Abilitations® by Sportime**
   One Sportime Way
   Atlanta, GA 30340
   800-850-8602 (orders)
   800-850-8603 (service)
   Fax: 770-449-5700
   E-mail: orders@sportime.com

2. **Ability Research, Inc.**
   P.O. Box 1721
   Minnetonka, MN 55345
   612-939-0121
   Fax: 612-890-8393
   E-mail: ability@skypoint.com
   http://www.skypoint.com/~ability

3. **Abingdon Press**
   Div. of United Methodist
   Publishing House
   P.O. Box 801
   201 Eighth Ave. South
   Nashville, TN 37202
   800-251-3320

4. **AbleNet®, Inc.**
   1081 Tenth Ave. SE
   Minneapolis, MN 55414-1312
   800-322-0956
   612-379-0956
   Fax: 612-379-9143

5. **Academic Therapy Publications**
   High Noon Books
   20 Commercial Blvd.
   Novato, CA 94949-6191
   800-422-7249
   415-883-3314
   Fax: 415-883-3720
   E-mail: atpuh@aol.com

6. **Academy of Medical Films, The**
   1601 Ygnacio Valley Rd.
   Walnut Creek, CA 94598

7. **Academy Press of America, Inc.**
   8361 Westminster Blvd., Ste. 325A
   Westminster, CA 92683
   714-898-2699
   Fax: 714-897-7215

8. **Accent on Living/Accent Special Publications**
   Cheever Publishing, Inc.
   P.O. Box 700
   Bloomington, IL 61702
   800-787-8444 (credit card orders)
   309-378-2961 (8-4 Central Time)
   Fax: 309-378-4420
   E-mail: acntlvng@aol.com

9. **Access Industries, Inc.**
   Accessiblility Products
   2509 Summer Ave.
   Memphis, TN 38112
   800-925-3100
   901-323-5438
   Fax: 901-323-5559

10. **Access Unlimited**
    570 Hance Rd.
    Binghamton, NY 13903
    800-849-2143
    Fax: 607-669-4595
    E-mail: accessun@specctra.net
    http://www.accessunlimited.com

11. **Access to Recreation, Inc.**
    2509 East Thousand Oaks Blvd.,
    Ste. 340
    Thousand Oaks, CA 91362
    800-634-4351
    Fax: 805-498-8186

12. **Accessible Designs/Adjustable Systems, Inc.**
    94 North Columbus Rd.
    Athens, OH 45701
    614-593-5240
    Fax: 614-593-5451
    TDD: 614-593-7171
    E-mail: ad208@seorf.ohiou.edu

13. **Accessible Work Systems, Inc.**
    2295 CR 292
    Bellevue, OH 44811
    800-344-9301
    Fax: 419-483-4872

14. **Achievement Products, Inc.**
    P.O. Box 9033
    Canton, OH 44711
    800-373-4699
    330-453-2122
    Fax: 330-453-2122

15. **Acor**
    18530 South Miles Pky.
    Cleveland, OH 44128-4238
    800-237-ACOR
    800-225-ACOR (OH)
    Fax: 216-662-4547

16. **Acropolis Books Ltd.**
    415 Wood Duck Ln.
    Sarasota, FL 34236
    800-451-7771
    Fax: 402-423-5839

17. **Action® Products, Inc.**
    22 North Mulberry St.
    Hagerstown, MD 21740
    800-228-7763
    301-797-1414
    Fax: 301-733-2073

18. **ActiveAid®, Inc.**
    One ActiveAid Rd.
    P.O. Box 359
    Redwood Falls, MN 56283-0359
    800-533-5330
    507-644-2951
    Fax: 507-644-2468

19. **Adamo Industries, Inc.**
    WalkerAlls®
    1182 Pallwood Rd.
    Memphis, TN 38122
    800-682-7702
    901-682-1123

20. **Adams, J.A., Co., Inc.**
    Dorset, VT 05251
    800-451-6118
    802-362-2303
    Fax: 802-362-5472

21. **AdaptAbility®**
    Mill St.
    P.O. Box 513
    Colchester, CT 06415-0513
    800-243-9232, Ext. 2104
    203-537-3451
    TDD: 800-688-4889
    Fax: 203-537-2866

22. **Adaptable Design®**
    8658 Rumson Dr.
    Santee, CA 92071
    619-448-7348

23. Adaptations
1758 Empire Central
Dallas, TX 75235-4186
800-688-1758 (M-F, CST)

24. Adaptive Engineering Lab, Inc.
P.O. Box 12930
Mill Creek, WA 98082-0930
800-327-6080
206-806-5568
Fax: 206-806-5569

25. Adaptive Equipment Systems
7128 Ambassador Rd.
Baltimore, MD 21244
800-AES-2370
410-281-1185
Fax: 410-281-0952

25B. Adaptive Mobility Services, Inc.
116 East Gatlin Ave.
Orlando, FL 32806-6908
407-855-8050

26. Addison-Wesley Longman, Inc.
Route 128
Reading, MA 01867
800-447-2226
617-944-3700
Fax: 617-944-9338

27. Advanced Therapy Products, Inc.
P.O. Box 3420
Glen Allen, VA 23058-3420
800-548-4550
E-mail: Atpwork@aol.com

28. Advanced Technology Corp., The
1601 Charlotte
Kansas City, MO 64108
816-421-6688
Fax: 816-221-8371

29. Advantage Bag Co.™
22633 Ellinwood Dr.
Torrance, CA 90505
310-540-8197
Fax: 310-316-2561

30. AJ Press
Now: Shelly Peterman Schwarz
Making Life Easier
933 Chapel Hill Rd.
Madison, WI 53711-2405

31. Alban Institute, Inc., The
4550 Montgomery Ave., Ste. 433
North
Bethesda, MD 20814
800-486-1318
301-718-4407

32. Aldine de Gruyter
200 Saw Mill Rd.
Hawthorne, NY 10532
914-747-0110

33. AliMed®, Inc.
297 High St.
Dedham, MA 02026-9135
800-225-2610 (U.S. and Canada)
617-329-2900
Fax: 617-329-8392

34. Allergy Publications, Inc.
P.O. Box 640
Menlo Park, CA 94026
415-322-1663

35. Altimate Medical, Inc.
P.O. Box 180
262 West 1st St.
Morton, MN 56270
800-342-8968

36. AlumiRamp
90 Taylor St.
Quincy, MI 49082
800-800-3864
517-639- 8777
Fax: 800-753-7267
http://www.inmax.com/alumiramp

37. Amana Refrigeration, Inc.
A Raytheon Co.
P.O. Box 8901
Amana, IA 52204
800-847-3783
Fax: 319-622-2180

38. American Bidet Products
Box 1500
Hollywood, FL 33022-1500
305-981-1111
Fax: 305-983-3333

39. American Book Service
11 Penn Ave., Ste. 300
New York, NY 10001
800-232-5463 (inquiries)
800-232-3044 (orders)
TDD: 212-502-7662

40. American Guidance, Inc.
P.O. Box 4448
Falls Church, VA 22044
800-736-1460
Fax: 212-586-5462

41. American Journal of Nursing Co.
555 West 57th St.
New York, NY 10019.
212-582-8820
800-225-5256

42. American Psychiatric Press
1400 K St. NW, Ste. 101
Washington, DC 20005
800-368-5777
202-682-6231

43. American Source Books
Division of Impact Publishers, See
Source 276

44. American Stair-Glide
Div. of Access Industries, Inc.
4001 East 138th St.
Grandview, MO 64030-2840
800-925-3100
816-763-3100
Fax: 816-763-4467

45. American Walker
900 Market St.
Oregon, WI 53575
800-828-6808

46. Amfit

47. Amigo® Mobility International, Inc.
6693 Dixie Highway
Bridgeport, MI 48722
800-692-6446
517-777-8184
Fax: 517-777-8184

48. Andersen® Corp.
P.O. Box 3900
Peoria, IL 60614
800-426-4261

49. Andrews and McMeel
Universal Press Syndicate Co.
4900 Main St., Ninth Flr.
Kansas City, MO 64112
800-826-4216
816-932-6700

50. Anna-Dote™ Inc.
RD #3, Box 40
40 Pullman Dr.
West Middlesex, PA 16159
800-346-6132
412-346-6132

51. Ansa® Bottle Co., Inc.

52. Apex Dynamics Inc.
829 Pickens Industrial Dr., Ste. 8
Marietta, GA 30062
800-742-0453
770-421-0838
Fax: 770-421-0968
http://www.apexdynamics.com

53. Apex Medical Corp.
800 South Van Eps Ave.
P.O. Box 1235
Sioux Falls, SD 57101-1235
800-328-2935

53B. Apothecary Products
11531 Rupp Dr.
Burnsville, MN 55337
800-328-2742

54. Appleton & Lange
Div. of Simon and Schuster
P.O. Box 120041
Stamford, CT 06912-0041
800-423-1359
203-406-4500
Fax: 203-406-4600

55. Arcoa Industries
Now: ArcMate Manufacturing Corp.
637 South Vinewood St.
Escondido, CA 92029
888-637-1926
760-489-1140
Fax: 760-746-1926

56. Armchair Shopper®, The
P.O. Box 306
Grandview, MO 64030-0306
800-659-7467

57. Arrow Plastics Manufacturing Co.
701 East Devon Ave.
Elk Grove Village, IL 60007
708-595-9000
Fax: 708-595-9122

58. Arrow Star®, Inc.
3-1 Park Plaza, Dept. T
Glen Head, NY 11545
800-645-2833
516-484-3100
Fax: 800-835-2292

59. Arthritis Self Help Products
Aids for Arthritis, Inc.
3 Little Knoll Ct.
Medford, NJ 08055
609-654-6918

60. Asko, Inc.

61. Aspen Publishers, Inc.
Subs. of Wolters Kluwer U.S.
200 Orchard Ridge Dr., Ste. 200
Gaithersburg, MD 20878
800-638-8437
301-417-7500
Fax: 301-417-7550

62. Attainment Co., Inc.
504 Commerce Parkway
P.O. Box 930160
Verona, WI 53593-0160
800-327-4269
608-845-7880
Fax: 800-942-3865

63. Aurora Publishing Co.
P.O. Box 1729
Garden City, KS 67846-1729
800-535-5111

64. Automobility Manufacturing Corp.
128 6th Ave East
Regina, SASK 54N 5A5
Canada
800-470-7067
306-791-9840
Fax: 306-525-0282

65. A/V Health Services, Inc.

65B. Aviano USA
1199 K Ave.
Acaso Camarillo, CA 93102
805-484-8138
Fax: 805-484-9789

66. Avery Publishing Group, Inc.
120 Old Broadway
Garden City Park, NY 11040
800-548-5757
516-741-2155
Fax: 516-742-1892

67. Avon Books
Div. of the Hearst Corp.
1350 Ave. of the Americas, 2nd Flr.
New York, NY 10019
800-238-0658
Fax: 212-977-9401

68. Ayer Company Publications, Inc.
Lower Mill Rd.
North Stratford, NH 03590
603-922-5106
Fax: 603-922-3348

68B. Axess
2421 South Westgate Rd.
Santa Monica, CA 93455
805-922-1426
http://www.axessmed.com

69. BackSaver Products™ Corp.
Div. of Nepsco, Inc.
53 Jeffrey Ave.
Holliston, MA 01746
800-251-BACK
508-429-5940

70. The Bag Lady
Box 531
West Stockbridge, MA 01266
413-637-3534

71. Bandwagon, Inc.
54 Industrial Way
Wilmington, MA 01887
508-658-6252
Fax: 508-657-7023

72. Bantam Doubleday Dell
1540 Broadway
New York, NY 10036-4094
800-223-6834
212-354-6500
Fax: 212-492-8941

73. Barrier-Free Access Systems, Inc.
19 Horseshoe Drive
Northport, NY 11768
516-757-4975
Fax: 516-757-4976

74. Barrier Free Environments Inc.
P.O. Box 30634
Raleigh, NC 27622
919-782-7823

75. Barrier-Free Lifts®
9230 Prince William St.
Manassas, VA 22110
800-582-8732
703-361-6531
Fax: 703-361-7861
http://www.blvd.com./bfl

76. Besam Automatic Door Systems

77. Bauhan, William H.
Box 443
Dublin, NH 03444
New York, NY 10019
800-843-9389
212-261-6500

78. Bausch & Lomb®, Inc.
1400 North Goodman St.
P.O. Box 450
Rochester, NY 14692-0450
800-553-5340

79. Baxter Healthcare Corp.
Chemotherapy Div.
1425 Lake Cook Rd.
Deerfield, IL 60015

80. Beacon Press
25 Beacon St.
Boston, MA 02108
800-788-6262
617-742-2110

81. Beatrice M. Brandtman, Inc.
207 East Westminster
Lake Forest, IL 60045
800-232-7987
800-368-2271
847-615-8890
Fax: 847-615-8894
E-mail: BeasyETS@aol.com
http://www.blvd.com/BeasyTrans

82. Becton-Dickinson® Consumer Products
Becton-Dickinson & Co.
1 Becton Dr.
Franklin Lakes, NJ 07417-1883
800-365-3321
201-847-7100

83. Bed-Check® Corp.
P.O. Box 170
Tulsa, OK 74101
800-523-7956

84. Bernard Food Industries, Inc.
P.O. Box 1497
Evanston, IL 60204
800-323-3663

85. Betterway Publications, Inc.

86. BJB Publishing
16212 Bothell Way SE, Ste. F171
Mill Creek, WA 98012-1219
800-799-3414
206-337-3414

87. Black & Decker
Home Appliance
6 Armstrong Rd.
Shelton, CT 06484
800-231-9786
203-926-3218

88. Boehringer Mannheim Diagnostics
9115 Hague Rd.
P.O. Box 50100
Indianapolis, IN 46250-0100
317-845-2000

89. Borgo Press
P.O. Box 2845
San Bernardino, CA 92406-2845
909-884-5813
Fax: 909-888-4942

90. Brandt Industries, Inc.
4461 Bronx Blvd.
Bronx, NY 10470-1496
800-221-8031
718-994-0800
Fax: 718-325-7995

91. Braun Corporation™, The
1014 South Monticello St.
P.O. Box 310
Winimac, IN 46996
800-THE-LIFT
219-946-6153
Fax: 219-946-4670
E-mail: braun@pwrtc.com
http://www.braunlift.com

92. Braun Inc.
66 Broadway, Route 1
Lynnfield, MA 01940
800-BRAUN-11

93. Broadman & Holman Pubs.
127 Ninth Ave.
Nashville, TN 37234
800-251-3225
615-251-2520
Fax: 615-251-2701

94. Brookes, Paul H.
Now: Paul H. Brookes Publishing Co.
P.O. Box 10624
Baltimore, MD 21285-0624
800-638-3775
410-337-9580
Fax: 410-337-8539
(Imprints: Health Professions Press.)

95. BrooklineBooks
P.O. Box 1047
Cambridge, MA 02288
800-666-2665
617-868-0360
Fax: 617-868-1772

96. Brookstone® Co., Inc.
Corporate Headquarters
17 Riverside St.
Nashua, NH 03062
800-846-3000

97. Brown Engineering Corp.
289 Chesterfield Rd.
Westhampton, MA 01027
800-726-4233
412-527-1800

98. Bruce Medical Supply
411 Waverly Oaks Rd.
P.O. Box 9166
Waltham, MA 02254-9166
800-225-8446
617-894-6262
Fax: 617-894-9519

99. Brunner/Mazel, Inc.
19 Union Sq.
New York, NY 10003
800-825-3089
212-924-3344
Fax: 212-242-6339
(Imprint: Magination Press.)

100. Bruno® Independent Living Aids, Inc.
1780 Executive Dr.
P.O. Box 84
Oconomowoc, WI 53066
800-882-8184
414-567-4990
Fax: 414-567-4341
http://www.bruno.com/

101. Bull Publishing
110 Gilbert Ave.
Menlo Park, CA 94025
800-676-2855
415-322-2855

102. Bullseye Information Services
200 Linden St.
Wellesley, MA 02181

103. Burn Prevention Group
6724 Bluffridge Pky.
Indianapolis, IN 46278-1853

104. Camden House Publications
P.O. Box 1001
Ferry Rd.
Charlotte, VT 05445
800-344-3350
802-425-3961

105. Cardon Rehabilitation Products, Inc.
2045 Niagara Falls Blvd., Unit 5
Niagara Falls, NY 14304-0237
800-944-7868
Fax: 716-297-0411

106. Care Products
158 North Main St.
Florida, NY 10921
800-446-5206
914-651-3332

107. Caring Products International, Inc.
200 First Ave. West, Ste. 200
Seattle, WA 98119
206-282-6040
800-333-5379
Fax: 206-282-6337
and
#8-5850 Bryne Rd.
Burnaby, BC V5J 3J3
Canada
604-436-4650
Fax:604-436-4669

108 Carol Publishing Group
120 Enterprise Ave.
Secaucus, NJ 07094
201-866-0490

109. Carol Wright Gifts
340 Applecreek Rd.
P.O. Box 8533
Lincoln, NE 68544-8533
402-474-5174

110. Cascade Designs®, Inc.
4000 First Ave. South
Seattle, WA 98134
800-827-4548
206-583-0583
Fax: 206-467-9421

111. Center for Healthcare Information
4000 Birch St., Ste. 112
Newport Beach, CA 92660
800-627-2244
714-752-2335
Fax: 714-752-8433
E-mail: chi@hcl.com

112. Center for Science in the Public Interest

113. Ceres Press
Box 87
Woodstock, NY 12498
914-679-5573
E-mail: DGroldbeck@aol.com

114. Channing L. Bete Co.
200 State Rd.
Deerfield, MA 01373-0200
800-628-7733
Fax: 800-499-6464

115. Charles Press Pubs.
P.O. Box 15715
Philadelphia, PA 19130
215-545-8933

116. Charles C. Thomas Publisher
2600 South First St.
Springfield, IL 62794-9265
800-258-8980
217-789-8980
Fax: 217-789-9130

117. Cheney® Co., The

118. Chilton Book Co.
Subs. of Capital Cities/ABC, Inc.
201 King of Prussia Rd.
Radnor, PA 19080
800-695-1214
610-964-4000
Fax: 610-964-4745

119. Chronicle Books
85 Second St.
San Francisco, CA 94105
800-722-6657 (orders)
415-777-7240

120. Chronimed Publishing
P.O. Box 59032
Minneapolis, MN 55459-0032
800-848-2793
612-513-6475
Fax: 800-395-3003
(Imprints include DCI.)

121. Chrysler Motors Corp.
Physically Challenged Resource
Center
P.O. Box 159
Detroit, MI 48288-0159
800-255-9877

122. Churchill Livingstone, Inc.
Subs. of Longman Group
650 Ave. of the Americas
New York, NY 10011
800-553-5426
212-206-5000

123. Clairson International
Closet Maid®
P.O. Box 4400
Ocala, FL 32674
904-351-6100

124. Clinician's View
6007 Osuna Rd. NE
Albuquerque, NM 87109
505-880-0058
Fax: 505-880-0059

125. CMP Adaptive Equipment Supply Co.
60-E South Second St.
Deer Park, NY 11729
516-595-1731
Fax: 516-595-1732

126. Coarc Bags
P.O. Box 217
Mellenville, NY 12544
800-888-4451
518-672-4451
Fax: 518-672-4048

127. College Park Industries, Inc.
17505 Helro Dr.
Fraser, MI 48026
810-728-7950
Fax: 810-728-0067

128. Colonial Garden Kitchens®
P.O. Box 66
Hanover, PA 17333-0066
800-245-3399
Fax: 800-258-6702

129. Columbo USA
67 Emerald St.
Keene, NH 03431
800-542-5943
603-358-0453
Fax: 603-358-0453

130. Columbia University Press
562 West 113th St.
New York, NY 10025
800-944-8648
212-666-1000

131. Columbus McKinnon Corp.
Mobility Products Div.
140 John James Audubon Parkway
Amherst, NY 14228-1197
800-888-0985 x227
Fax: 716-689-5624
http://www.industry.net/cm

132. Communication Skill Builders
Div. of The Psychological Corp.
P.O. Box 839954
San Antonio, TX 78283-3954
800-228-0752
Fax: 800-232-1223

133. Compac Industries Inc.
P.O. Box 29663
Atlanta, GA 30359
404-321-5270

134. CompCare
P.O. Box 12770
Tucson, AZ 85732-2770
502-573-2856

135. Composite International, Inc.
2209 Cloverdale Ct.
Worthington, OH 43235-9868
800-955-4292
Fax: 614-792-5595

136. Conari Press
2550 Ninth St., Ste. 101
Berkeley, CA 94710
510-649-7175
Fax: 510-649-7190

137. Concept Housewares, Inc.
1730 South Amphlett Blvd., Ste. 222
San Mateo, CA 94402
800-255-3129
415-655-7270
Fax: 415-655-7271

137B. Concord Elevator Inc.
107 Alfred Kvehne Blvd.
Brampton, ON L6T 4K3
Canada
800-661-5112 (U.S.)
905-791-5555
Fax: 905-791-2222

138. Constructive Playthings
1227 East 119th St.
Grandview, MO 64030-1117
800-255-6124

139. Consultants for Communication Technology
508 Bellevue Terrace
Pittsburgh, PA 15202
412-761-6062
Fax: 412-761-7336

140. Consumer Care Products, Inc.

141. Consumers Reports Books®
Div. of Consumers Union of U.S., Inc.
101 Truman Ave.
Yonkers, NY 10703
914-378-2000

142. Container Store, The
800-786-7318
Call for nearest store.

143. Contemporary Books, Inc.
2 Prudential Plaza, Ste. 1200
Chicago, IL 60601-6970
800-621-1918 (orders)
312-540-4500
Fax: 312-782-3987

144. Continuum Publishing, Co.
370 Lexington Ave.
New York, NY 10017
212-953-5858

145. Convaid Products, Inc.
P.O. Box 4209
Palos Verde, CA 90274
888-CONVAID
310-539-6814
Fax: 310-539-3670

146. Cool Hands Communication, Inc.
1050 NW First Ave., Ste. 28
Boca Raton, FL 33432
800-428-0578
407-750-9826

147. Cornell University Press
512 East State St.
P.O. Box 6525
Ithaca, NY 14851
800-666-2211
607-277-2211

148. Country Technology, Inc.
P.O. Box 87
Gays Mills, WI 54631
608-735-4718
Fax: 608-735-4859

149. Courage Books
Div. of Running Press Books
125 South 22nd St.
Philadelphia, PA 1910_
800-345-5359
215-567-5080

150. Courage Center
3915 Golden Valley Rd.
Golden Valley, MN 55422
612-520-0257

151. Courage Press
3495 SW Patton Rd.
Portland, OR 97201-1656

152. CRC Press, Inc.
Subs. of Times Mirror Co.
2000 Corporate Blvd. NW
Boca Raton, FL 33431
800-272-7737
407-994-0555

153. Creative Industries
Medical Products Div.
5366 Jackson Dr.
La Mesa, CA 92041
619-469-5012

154. Crestwood Co.
Communication Aids for Children
& Adults
6625 North Sidney Place
Milwaukee, WI 53209-3259
414-352-5768
Fax: 414-352-5679

155. Crow River Industries, Inc.
14800 28th Ave. North
Minneapolis, MN 55447
800-488-7688
612-557-1680
Fax: 612-557-8310

155B. Crown Publications
225 Park Ave. South
New York, NY 10037
212-254-1600

156. Cuisinarts, Inc.
150 Milford Rd.
East Windsor, NJ 08520
800-583-6046

157. Dacor
950 South Raymond Ave.
Pasadena, CA 91109-7202
800-793-0093
818-799-1000
Fax: 818-441-9632
http://www.DacorAppl.com

158. Damaco Freedom on Wheels
5105 Maureen Ln.
Moorpark, CA 93021
800-432-2434
805-532-1832
Fax: 805-532-1836
E-mail: Damacoinc@aol.com

159. Damark® International, Inc.
7101 Winnetka Ave. North
P.O. Box 9437
Minneapolis, MN 55440-9437
800-729-9000

160. Dana Douglas Medical Inc.
9-A Capella Ct.
Nepean, Ont., Canada K1M 2E4
800-267-3552
613-723-1058
E-mail:
76242.2007@compuserv.com

161. Danmar Products, Inc.
221 Jackson Industrial Dr.
Ann Arbor, MI 48103
800-783-1998
313-761-1990
Fax: 313-761-8977
E-Mail: danmarpro@aol.com

162. Davis, F.A., Co.
1915 Arch St.
Philadelphia, PA 19130
800-323-3555
215-440-3001
Fax: 215-440-3016

163. DayLight Technologies, Inc.
P.O. Box 102 CRO
Halifax, Nova Scotia B3J 2L4
Canada
800-387-0896
Fax: 902-422-0798
http://www.up-lift.com

163B. Delta Faucet Co.
55 East 111th St.
Indianapolis, IN 46280
800-345-3358

**164. Demos Vermande Publishing,
Inc.**
386 Park Ave. South, Ste. 201
New York, NY 10016
800-532-8663
212-683-0072
Fax: 212-683-0118

165. DeRoyal/LMB
265 South St., Ste. E
San Luis Obispo, CA 93401
800-541-3992
Fax: 800-541-3992
Fax: 805-781-3443

166. Design Communications, Inc.
P.O. Box 206
Rosenhayn, NJ 08352
609-451-4499
Fax: 609-451-6678

166B. Designs for Comfort, Inc.
2156 New Willow Rd.
P.O. Box 8229
Northfield, IL 60093
800-443-9226
708-446-9190
Fax: 708-446-9224

167. Design Ideas
P.O. Box 2967
Springfield, IL 62708
800-426-6394
Fax: 217-753-3080

167B. Diabetes Self-Management
R.A. Rappaport Publishing, Inc.
150 West 22nd St.
New York, NY 10011-2421
212-989-0200

168. Diction Books
2 Willow Rd.
St. Paul, MN 55127
800-594-4675
612-484-2811

169. Disability Bookshop, The
P.O. Box 129
Vancouver, WA 98666-0129
800-637-2256
360-694-2462
Fax: 360-696-3210

170. Disability Mall
http://disability.com
On-line information and products
crossroads.

170B. Dixie USA, Inc.
P.O. Box 55549
Houston, TX 77255
800-347-3494 (Orders)
713-688-4993
Fax: 713-688-5932
Fax: 800-688-2507 (Orders)

171. Dr. Leonard's® Health Care Products
42 Mayfield Ave.
P.O. Box 7821
Edison, NJ 08818-7821
800-785-0880

172. Doron Precision Systems, Inc.
174 Court St.
P.O. Box 400
Binghamton, NY 13902-0400
607-772-1610
Fax: 607-772-6760

173. Drive-Master Corp.
9 Spielman Rd.
Fairfield, NJ 07004-3403
201-808-9709
Fax: 201-808-9713
E-mail: Drivemastr@aol.com

174. dSi/Driving Systems, Inc.
16141 Runnymeade St.
Van Nuys, CA 91406-2913
818-782-6793
Fax: 818-782-6485
E-mail: dsi2@mail.idt.net

175. Durex Corp.
121 Haven Ridge
Peachtree City, GA 30269
404-728-9654
Fax: 404-728-9653

176. Duro-Med Industries, Inc.
1788 West Cherry St.
P.O. Box 547
Jesup, GA 31598-0546
800-526-4753
912-427-7358
Fax: 800-479-7968

177. Dwyer Products Corp.
418 North Calumet Ave.
Michigan City, IN 46360-5019
800-348-8508
219-874-5236
Fax: 219-874-2823

178. Dycem
P.O. Box 6920
85 Gilbane St.
Warwick, RI 02887
800-458-0060
401-738-4420
Fax: 401-739-9634
E-mail: DYCEM_USA@IDS.NET

179. Dynamic Rehab Videos and Rentals
307 Spruce Ave. South
Thief River Falls, MN 56701
218-681-1624

180. East Hampton Industries, Inc.
81 Newtown Ln.
P.O. Box 5069
East Hampton, NY 11937
800-645-1188
516-324-2224
Fax: 800-323-2248
E-mail: ferrink@aol.com

181. Edmund Scientific Co.
101 East Gloucester Pike
Barrington, NJ 08007-1380
609-573-6289
Fax: 609-573-6295

182. Elder Books
P.O. Box 490
120 Montezuma Ave.
Forest Knolls, CA 94933
800-909-2673
415-488-7002

183. Electric Mobility
#1 Mobility Plaza
Sewell, NJ 08080
800-662-4548
609-468-0270
Fax: 609-468-3426
http://www.emobility.com

184. Eljer Plumbingware
17120 Dallas Parkway
Dallas, TX 75248
972-407-2600
and
3070 Universal Dr.
Mississauga, ON L4X 2C8
416-624-5656

185. Elsevier Science Publishing Co., Inc.
P.O. Box 945, Madison Sq. Sta.
New York, NY 10060-0757
212-989-5800

186. Embracing Concepts, Inc.
40 Humbolt St., Ste. 220
Rochester, NY 14609
800-962-5542
716-654-9090
Fax: 716-654-6108

187. Empire Brushes and Cook's Things, Inc.
Rubbermaid Cleaning Products
1147 Akron Rd.
Wooster, OH 44691
800-359-5359
330-264-6464

188. Empire Publication Services
P.O. Box 1344
Studio City, CA 91614-0344
818-784-8918

188B. Encyclopedia Britannica

189. Ensar Corp.
135 East Hintz Rd.
Wheeling, IL 60090-6036
312-520-1000

190. Eschenbach Optic of America, Inc.
904 Ethan Allen Highway
Ridgefield, CT 06877
203-438-7471
http://www.eschenbach.com

191. Etac USA, Inc.
2325 Parklawn Dr., Ste. J
Waukesha, WI 53186
800-678-3822
414-796-4600
Fax: 414-796-4605

192. Everest & Jennings®
3601 Rider Trail South
Earth City, MO 63045
800-235-4661
314-512-7000
Fax: 800-542-3567
and
Everest & Jennings® Canadian, Ltd.
111 Snidercroft Rd.
Concord, Ont. L4K 2J8
Canada

193. Evlo Plastics
310 Industrial Ln.
P.O. Box 2295
Sandusky, OH 44870-2295
419-626-2430
Fax: 419-626-8183

194. Evo Pen, Inc.
200 East 33rd St., Ste. 280
New York, NY 10016
V/Fax: 212-213-1065
http://www.evo.aluminum,evo.pen,
evo.wood

195. Eye Communications, Inc.
1241 West 9th St.
Upland, CA 91786
800-247-5731
909-949-1494

196. E-Z-On Products, Inc. of Florida
500 Commerce Way West, Ste. 3
Jupiter, FL 33458
800-323-6598
561-747-6920
Fax: 516-747-8779

197. Facts on File, Inc.
11 Penn Plaza
New York, NY 10001
800-322-8755
212-967-8800

197B. Fairview Press
2450 Riverside Ave. South
Minneapolis, MN 55454

198. Fairway King
3 East Main St.
Oklahoma City, OK 73104-2405
800-222-1145
405-528-8571
Fax: 405-235-7483

199. Family Experiences Productions, Inc.
P.O. Box 5879
Austin, TX 78763-5879
512-494-0338
Fax: 512-494-0340

200. Fanlight Productions
47 Halifax St.
Boston, MA 02130
800-937-4113
Fax: 617-524-8838

201. Farberware Inc.
Division of Kidde, Inc.
1500 Bassett Ave.
Bronx, NY 10461-3295
212-863-8000

202. Fashion-Ease
Div. of M&M Health Care Apparel Co.
1541 60th St.
Brooklyn, NY 11219
800-221-8929
718-871-8188

203. Fernanda Manufacturing Co.
120 Marcus Blvd.
Deer Park, NY 11729
516-254-2070

204. Fisher-Price® Co.
7811 Girard Ave.
East Aurora, NY 14052-1879
716-687-3000

205. Flaghouse, Inc.
601 Flaghouse Dr.
Hasbrouck Heights, NJ 07604-3116
800-739-7900
800-265-6900 (Canada)
201-288-7600
Fax: 201-288-7887

206. The Flinchbaugh Co.
390 Eberts Ln.
York, PA 17403
800-326-2418
717-854-7720
Fax: 717-843-7385

207. Flofit Medical, LLC
5455 Spine Rd.
Boulder, CO 80301
800-356-2668
303-530-3666
Fax: 303-530-3758
E-mail: flofit1@flofitmed.com
http://www.flofitmed.com

207B. Flotool International, Inc.
15542 Mosher Ave.
Tustin, CA 92680
800-334-3062
714-850-9212
Fax: 714-850-9748

208. Focal Point Press
P.O. Box 415
Bolinas, CA 94924
415-868-1158

208B. Ford Mobility Motoring Program
P.O. Box 529
Bloomfield Hills, MI 48303-9857
800-952-2248
TDD: 800-TDD-0312
Fax: 810-333-2191

209. Forum Communications
P.O. Box 61090
King of Prussia, PA 19406-0400
800-367-8610
610-337-0381

210. Fox Run Craftsmen
P.O. Box 2727
1907 Stout Drive
Ivyland, PA 18974
800-372-0700 (bulk orders)
215-675-7700
Fax: 215-675-4508
and
20A Voyager Ct. South
Etobicoke, Ont. M9W 5M7
Canada
416-213-9880
Fax: 416-213-9886

211. Frank Eastern Co.
599 Broadway
New York, NY 10012-3258
800-221-4914
NY: 212-219-0007
Fax: 212-2191-0722

212. Frank Mobility Systems, Inc.
1003 International Dr.
Oakdale, PA 15071-9226
412-695-7822
Fax: 412-695-2922

213. Franklin Watts, Inc.
Div. of Grolier, Inc.
Sherman Turnpike
Danbury, CT 06813
800-621-1115
203-797-3500

214. Freedom Designs, Inc.
2241 Madera Rd.
Simi Valley, CA 93065
800-331-8551
805-582-0077
Fax: 805-582-1509

215. **The Futuro Co.®**
Div. of Jung Corp.
5801 Mariemont Ave.
Cincinnati, OH 45227
513-271-3782

216. **Gaggenau USA Corp.**
425 University Ave.
Norwood, MA 02062-2536
617-255-1766
Fax: 617-769-2212

217. **Gale Research, Inc.**
Subs. of The Thomson Corp.
835 Penobscot Bldg.
Detroit, MI 48226-4094
800-877-4523
313-961-2242

218. **Garaventa**
P.O. Box 1
Blaine, WA 98230
800-663-6556

219. **Gaylord Brothers**
Box 4901
Syracuse, NY 13221-4901
800-634-6307
315-457-5070
Fax: 315-457-8387

220. **Gendron, Inc.**
Lugbill Road
P.O. Box 197
Archbold, OH 43502
800-537-2521
Fax: 419-446-2631

221. **General Electric® Co.**
Appliance Park
Louisville, KY 40225
800-626-2000

222. **General Motors® Mobility
Program for Persons with
Disabilities**
P.O. Box 9011
Detroit, MI 48202
800-323-9935
TTY: 800-833-9955
http://www.com/standards/cross-
roads

222B.**Gerber Chair Mates. Inc.**
1171 Ringling Ave.
Johnstown, PA 15902
814-269-9531

223. **Geriatric Resources Inc.**
P.O. Box 1509
Goldenrod, FL 32733-1509
800-359-0390
407-678-1616
Fax: 407-678-5925

224. **Glacierware**
1 Ferry St.
Easthampton, MA 01027
800-6363-8520

225. **Global Business Furniture**
National Order Processing Center
22 Harbaor Park Dr.
Port Washington, NY 11050
800-472-0101
Fax: 800-336-3818

226. **GMR Labs**
1030 East El Camino Real #308
Sunnyvale, CA 94087-3759
800-234-8288
Fax: 408-985-7200
E-mail: roark@gmrlabs.com

227. **Graham-Field, Inc.**
400 Rabro Dr. East
Hauppauge, NY 11788
800-645-8176
516-582-5900
Fax: 516-582-4645

228. **Grandberg Superior Systems**
2502 Thayer Ave.
Saskatoon, SK S7L 5Y2
Canada
306-374-9440
Fax: 306-373-8715

229. **Greatest of Ease Co., The**
2443 Fillmore St., Ste. 345
San Francisco, CA 94115
800-845-1208 (orders)
415-441-6649

230. **Green, Warren H., Inc.
Now: Publishers Service Center**
8356 Olive Blvd.
St. Louis, MO 63132

231. **Greenwood Publishing Group**
88 Post Rd. West
Box 5007
Westport, CT 06881
800-225-5800 (orders)
203-226-3571

232. **Gresham Driving Aids, Inc.**
30800 Wixom Rd.
P.O. Box 405
Wixom, MI 98393
800-521-8930
810-624-1533
Fax: 801-624-6358

232B.**Grey House Publishing**
Pocket Knife Sq.
Lakeville, CT 06039
800-562-2139
203-435-0868

233. **Guilford Press, Inc.**
72 Spring St.
New York, NY 10012-9941
800-365-7006 (orders)
212-431-9800
Fax: 212-966-6708

234. **Gussert Marketing**
329 East Briar Ln.
Green Bay, WI 54301
800-327-2700 Ext. 333 (Credit
Card)

234B.**Hadley-Brickhouse**
Accessible Design Associates, Inc.
150 Herricks Rd.
Mineola, NY 11501
516-294-0555
Fax: 516-294-1976

235. **Hammacher Schlemmer**
Operations Center
9180 Le Saint Dr.
Fairfield, OH 45104-5475
800-283-9400

236. **Handicapped Driving Systems,
Inc.**

237. **Handicaps, Inc.**
4335 South Santa Fe Dr.
Englewood, CO 80110
800-782-4335
303-781-2062

238. Handi-Ramp®, Inc.
Box 475
1414 Armour Blvd.
Mundelein, IL 60060
800-876-RAMP
847-816-7525
Fax: 847-816-7689
E-mail: handiramp@aol.com
http://www.marketzone.com/Handi-
Ramp

239. Handsome Rewards®
19465 Brennan Ave.
Perris, CA 92599
909-943-2023
Fax: 909-943-5574

240. Hanley & Belfus, Inc.
210 South 13th St.
Philadelphia, PA 19107
800-962-1892
215-546-4995
Fax: 215-790-9330

241. Hanover House®
Hanover, PA 17333-0002
717-633-3366
717-633-3377 (Credit card orders
over $15)

242. Hansa America
1432 West 21st St.
Chicago, IL 60608

243. Harcourt Brace Jovanovich
Div. of Harcourt General, Inc.
525 B St., Ste. 1900
San Deigo, CA 92101
800-831-7799
619-699-6526
(Imprints include Saunders.)

244. Harness Designs, Inc.
1511 West University Ave.
Champaign, IL 61821-3132
800-398-5794
217-398-5788
Fax: 217-355-5088

244B. HarperCollins, Publishers, Inc.
10 East 53rd St.
New York, NY 10022
800-242-7737
212-307-7057

245. Harriet Carter
Dept. 17
North Wales, PA 19455
215-361-5151

245B. Hartley and Marks Publishers
P.O. Box 147
Point Roberts, WA 98281
800-277-5887
360-945-2017

246. Hashagen, Werner R.

247. Haworth Press, Inc.
10 Alice St.
Binghamton, NY 13904-1580
800-HAWORTH
Fax: 800-895-0582
http://www.haworth.com

**248. HCF Nutrition Research
Foundation**
P.O. Box 22124
258 Plaza Dr., Ste. 208
Lexington, KY 40522
606-276-3119

249. HDI Publishers
P.O. Box 131401
Houston, TX 77219
800-321-7037
713-682-8700
Fax: 713-956-2288
E-mail: HDIjch@aol.com

250. Health Enterprises, Inc.
90 George Leven Dr.
North Attleboro, MA 02760
800-633-4243
508-695-0727
Fax: 508-695-3061

251. Health Press
P.O. Box 1388
Santa Fe, NM 87504
800-643-2665
505-982-9373

251B. Health Research
P.O. Box 850
62 Seventh St.
Pomeroy, WA 99347
509-843-2385

251C. Health Source Bookstore
1404 K St. NW
Washington, DC 20005
800-713-7122
202-789-7303
Fax: 202-789-7899
E-mail: healthsource@appl.org
http://www.appl.org/healthsource

252. HealthTrac Books, Inc.
P.O. Box 13599
Tallahasee, FL 32317
800-533-5259
904-877-5111

253. Health Valley Foods
16100 Foothill Blvd.
Irwindale, CA 91706-7811
800-423-4846

**254. Healthwares Manufacturing
Corp.**
8665 East Miami River Rd.
Cincinnati, OH 45247
513-353-3691
Fax: 513 353 4315

255. Heartland America®
6978 Shady Oak Rd.
Eden Prairie, MN 55344-3453
800-229-2901
Fax: 800-943-4096

256. Hello Direct, Inc.
5893 Rue Ferrari.
San Jose, CA 95138-1858
800-HI-HELLO or 800-444-3556
E-mail: xpressit@hihello.com
http://www.hello-direct.com
(ordering)

257. Henry Holt & Co.
115 West 18th St.
New York, NY 10011
800-488-5233
212-886-9200

258. Hertz Furniture Systems Corp.
East 55 Midland Ave.
Paramus, NJ 07652-9875
800-526-4677
Fax: 800-942-9290

259. HomeCare® Magazine
23815 Stuart Ranch Rd.
P.O. Box 8987
Malibu, CA 90265-8987
800-543-4116
http://www.homecaremag.com

260. HomeCare Products, Inc.
15824 SE 296th St.
Kent, WA 98402
800-451-1903
206-631-4633
Fax: 206-630-8196

261. Home Decorators Collection
2025 Concourse Dr.
St. Louis, MO 63146-4178
800-245-2217
314-993-1516
Fax: 314-993-0502

262. Home Trends
1450 Lydell Ave.
Rochester, NY 14606-2184
716-254-6520
Fax: 716-458-9245

263. Honeywell Protection Services
1985 Douglas Dr. North
Golden Valley, MN 55422
800-328-5111

264. Horton Automatics
Overhead Door Corp. of Texas
6750 LBJ Freeway
P.O. Box 400150
Dallas, TX 75240
800-531-3111
214-233-6611

265. Houghton Mifflin Co.
222 Berkeley St.
Boston, MA 02116
800-225-3362
617-351-5000

266. Howarth Press
P.O. Box 2608
Falls Church, VA 22042-0608
703-573-8521

266B. Howell, Keith
4850 Rte. 2 Hwy.
Upper Kingsclear, NB E3E 1P8
Canada
506-363-5289

267. The HSM Group, Ltd.
Easy Street® Environments
6031 East Maple Ave.
Tempe, AZ 85283
800-733-8442
602-345-8442
Fax: 602-730-0188

268. Human Kinetics Pubs.
P.O. Box 5076
Champaign, IL 61825-5076
800-747-4457
217-351-5076

269. Human Services Research Institute
2336 Massachusetts Ave.
Boston, MA 02140
617-876-0426
Fax: 617-492-7401
E-mail: JWalkrHSRI@aol.com

270. Hunter House Publishers
P.O. Box 2914
Alameda, CA 94501-0914
800-266-5592
510-865-5282

271. The Hygeia Group
555 Westbury Ave.
Carle Place, NY 11514
516-997-8150

272. Hygenic Corp.

273. IDEA
1393 Meadowbrook Dr.
Pewaukee, WI 53072
414-691-4248

274. IKEA
To locate store near you call:
East Coast: 410-931-8940
West Coast: 818-912-1119

275. Imaginart International, Inc.
307 Arizona St.
Bisbee, AZ 85603
800-828-1376
520-432-5741
Fax: 800-737-1376
Fax: 520-432-5134
E-mail: imaginart@aol.com

276. Impact Publishers, Inc.
P.O. Box 1094
San Luis Obispo, CA 93406
805-543-5911
(Imprints include American Source Books.)

278. Improvements
Quick & Clever Problem Solvers!
Hanover, PA 17333-0084
800-642-2112
Fax: 800-757-9997

279. Independent Living Aids
27 East Mall
Plainview, NY 11803
800-537-2118
516-752-8080
Fax: 516-752-3135

280. InfoVision
12345 A St.
Omaha, NE 68144
800-237-1808
Fax: 402-330-9544

280B. Intellitools®, Inc.
55 Leveroni Ct., Ste. 9
Novato, CA 94949
800-899-6687
415-382-5959 (International)
Fax: 415-382-5950
E-mail: info@intellitools.com
http://www.intellitools.com

281. Interactive Technologies, Inc.
2266 North Second St.
North St. Paul, MN 55109
800-777-5484
612-777-2690
Fax: 612-779-4890

282. International Environmental Solutions
100 Second Ave., Ste. 102
St. Petersburg, FL 33701
813-896-4199
Fax: 813-822-6503

283. ISHK Book Service
The Institute for the Study of Human Knowledge
P.O. Box 176
Los Altos, CA 94203

284. International Universities Press, Inc.
59 Boston Post Rd.
P.O. Box 1524
Madison, CT 06443-1524
800-TELE-IUP
Fax: 203-245-0775

285. Invacare® Corp.
899 Cleveland St.
P.O. Box 4028
Elyria, OH 44036-2125
800-333-6900
216-329-6000
800-668-5324 (Canada)
800-668-5354 (Ontario)
Fax: 216-366-1803
E0mail: selder@invacare.com
http://www.invacare.com

286. Iowa State University Press
2121 State Ave.
Ames, IA 50014-8300
800-862-6657 (orders)
515-292-0140

287. Iron Horse Productions, Inc.
2624 Conner St.
Port Huron, MI 48060
800-426-0354
810-987-6700
Fax: 810-987-6724
E-mail: whlrydr@aol.com

288. Iskra Med
P.O. Box 13427
St. Louis, MO 63138
800-645-1320
314-868-0941
Fax: 314-868-0941
E-mail: imedstl@aol.com

289. J.C. Penney® Co., Inc.
800-222-6161
Call for referral to Catalog
Division nearest you.

289B. J.H. Industries, Inc.
8901 East Pleasant Valley Rd.
P.O. Box 31267
Independence, OH 44131
800-321-4968
216-524-7520 (in OH)
Fax: 216-524-7526

290. J.H. Smith Co., Inc.
330 Chapman St.
Greenfield, MA 01301
413-772-0191

290B. JKS Publications
P.O. Box 3279
Pagosa Springs, CO 81147-3279
800-601-5918
970-264-6161
Fax: 970-264-6165

291. J.L. Pachner
13 Via Di Nola
Laguna Niguel, CA 92677

292. Jaeco Orthopedic Specialities
P.O. Box 75
Hot Springs, AR 71902-0075
501-623-5944

293. Jay Medical® Ltd.
Now: J Medical® Kid Kan
74-77A East Dycrede Pky.
Longmont, CO 80503
800-648-8282
303-442-5529
Fax: 800-300-7502

293B. Jenn-Air® Co.
Division of Maytag
3035 Shadeland Ave.
Indianapolis, IN 46226-0901
800-536-6247

294. Jesana Ltd.
979 Saw Mill River Rd.
Yonkers, NY 10710
800-443-4728
914-376-2894
Fax: 914-376-0021
E-mail: http://www.jesana.com

294B. Joerns Healthcare, Inc.
5555 Joerns Dr.
Stevens Point, WI 54481
715-341-3600

295. Joan Cook
119 Foster St.
P.O. Box 6038
Peabody, MA 01961-6038
800-935-0971 (orders)
508-532-6523 (Service 9-5 E.S.T.)
Fax: 800-933-3732

296. Johns Hopkins University Press
2715 North Charles St.
Baltimore, MD 21218-4319
800-537-5487
410-516-6900

297. Jokari U.S., Inc.
1205 Venture Ct.
Dallas, TX 75006
214-416-5202
Fax: 214-416-5717

298. Jossey-Bass, Inc. Pubs.
S&S Intern.& Business Prof.
Group
350 Sansome St., Fifth Flr.
San Francisco, CA 94104-1342
800-956-7739
415-433-1767

299. Juno Lighting, Inc.
P.O. Box 5065
Des Plaines, IL 60017-5065
800-323-5068

300. K & S Enterprises
P.O. Box 720492
Atlanta, GA 30358

301. Kapable Kids
P.O. Box 250
Bohemia, NY 11716
800-356-1564

302. Kayes Products, Inc.
535 Dimmocks Mill Rd.
Hillsborough, NC 27278
Fax: 800-685 KAYE (5293)

303. Kendall-Futuro® Co.

304. Key Porter Books Limited
70 The Esplanade
Toronto, ON M5E 1R2
Canada
416-862-7777

304B. Kid Kart™, Inc.
732 Cruiser Ln.
Belgrade, MT 59714
800-388-5278
406-388-1080
Fax: 406-388-1081

305. Kingstar International America, Inc.
P.O. Box 10157
Chicago, IL 60610-0157
800-336-6550
312-951-1115

306. Kitchen & Home
Hanover, PA 17333-0072
800-414-5544
Fax: 800-757-9997

306A. Kitchen Aid
Customer Satisfaction Center
P.O. Box 218
St. Joseph, MI 49085
800-541-6390
Fax: 616-541-6390

307. Kohler® Company
Highland Dr.
Kohler, WI 53044
800-456-4537
414-457-4441
http://www.kitchenaid.com

308. Krames Communications
1100 Grundy Ln.
San Bruno, CA 94066-3030
800-333-3032

309. Kroepke Kontrols, Inc.®
104 Hawkins St.
City Island, NY 10464
718-885-1100
Fax: 718-885-1110
E-mail: kroepke@mail.idt.net

310. K-Tel International, Inc.
2605 Fernbrook Ln. North
Minneapolis, MN 55447

311. Kuschall of America
708 Via Alondra
Camarillo, CA 93012-8713
800-654-4768
805-484-3595
Fax: 805-987-9844

312. Kwikset Corp.
516 East Santa Ana St.
Anaheim, CA 92803-4250
714-535-8111

313. LaBac Systems™
3535 South Kipling St.
Lakewood, CO 80235
800-445-4402
303-914-9914
Fax: 303-914-9880

314. Laurel Designs
Now: Innisfree Press

315. LCE, Inc.
P.O. Box 1926
Washington, DC 20036

316. LDC Corp. of America, Inc.
780-B2 Primos Ave.
Folcroft, PA 19032
800-782-6324
610-586-0986
Fax: 610-586-0847
E-mail: dallery@msn.com
http://www.blvd.com/lifestand/index.
html

317. Lea & Febiger
Waverly Books
351 West Camden St.
Baltimore, MD 21201
800-638-1785
Fax: 215-251-2229

317B. Leveron Industries, Inc.
P.O. Box 66295
Auburndale, MA 02166-0003
617-237-8177

318. Liberty Technology
Prosthetics and Orthotics Group
71 Frankland Rd.
Hopkinton, MA 01748
800-437-0024 (orders)
508-435-9061 ext 283 (technical
questions)
Fax: 508-435-8369
E-mail:
msmail.hansonb1@tsod.lmig.
com

319. Life Enhancements
1318 Southdale Center
Edina, MN 55435
800-299-0578
612-920-0525

320. Life Essentials®
345 Burnett Rd.
West Lafayette, IN 47906
800-LIFE-740
317-742-6707
Fax: 317-423-1017

321. Life Spec Cabinet Systems, Inc.
County Rd. 262
Oxford, MS 38655
601-234-0330

322. Lifecare International, Inc.
1401 West 122nd Ave.
Westminster, CO 80234-3421
800-669-9234
303-457-9234
Fax: 303-259000

323. Lifeline International
1421 South Park St.
Madison, WI 53715
800-553-6633
608-251-4778
Fax: 608-251-1870

324. Lifestyle Fascination®, Inc.
1935 Swarthmore Ave.
Lakewood, NJ 08701-8123
800-699-0987
Fax: 908-364-4448

325. Lighter Side® Company, The
4514 Nineteenth St., Court East
P.O. Box 25600, Dept. L9610B
Bradenton, FL 34206-5600

325A. Lighthouse Press
114 R Highland Ave.
Salem, MA 01970
508-740-0648

326. Lighthouse Enterprises
Lighthouse Inc.
3620 Northern Blvd.
Long Island City, NY 11101
800-829-0500

327. Liguori Publications
1 Liguori Dr.
Liguori, MO 63057-9999
800-325-9521
314-464-2500
Fax: 314-464-8449

328. Lillian Vernon® Corp.
Virginia Beach, VA 23479-0002
800-285-5555
TDD/TTY: 800-285-5536

329. LinguiSystems, Inc.
3100 4th Ave.
P.O. Box 747
East Moline, IL 61244-9700
800-776-4332
309-755-2300

330. Lippincott-Raven Publishers
Subs. of Wolters-Kluwer US Corp.
227 East Washington Sq.
Philadelphia, PA 19106-3708
800-777-2295
215-238-4200
Fax: 215-238-4247

331. Little Brown & Co.
A Time Warner Co.
1271 Ave. of the Americas
New York, NY 10020
800-343-9204
212-522-8700

332. Living Media, Inc.
219 Kitchawan Rd.
South Salem, NY 10590

333. Lowell House
Div. of RGA Pub. Group, Inc.
2020 Ave. of the Stars, Ste. 300
Los Angeles, CA 90067
301-552-7555

334. LS&S Group
P.O. Box 673
Northbrook, IL 60065
800-468-4789 (orders)
847-498-9777 (info)
Fax: 847-498-1482

335. Lubidet USA, Inc.
1980 South Quebec St., Ste. 4
Denver, CO 80231-3234
800-582-4338
303-368-4555
Fax: 303-368-0812
E:Mail: lubidet@rmii.com
http://www.lubidet.com

335B. Lucent Technology ACP
Accessible Products Center
14250 Clayton Rd.
Town and Country, MO 63017
800-233-1222

336. Lumex®, Inc.
81 Spence St.
Bay Shore, NY 11706-2290
800-645-5272
516-273-2200
Fax: 800-273-5681

337. Luminaud, Inc.
8688 Tyler Blvd.
Mentor, OH 44060-4348
800-778-9410
216-255-9082
Fax: 216-255-2250

338. The Lumiscope Co., Inc.
400 Raritan Center Parkway
Edison, NJ 08837
201-225-5533
Fax: 201-225-7047

339. Lura Media Inc.
Now: Innisfree Press
136 Ramfort Rd.
Philadelphia, PA 19119
206-365-4116

340. M.C. Distributors
4104 College Ave.
Indianapolis, IN 46203

341. Macmillan Publishing, Inc.
Div. of Simon and Schuster
866 Third Ave.
New York, NY 10022
800-428-5331
212-702-2000

342. Mac's Lift Gate Inc.
2715 Seaboard Ln.
Long Beach, CA 90805-3751
800-795-6227
562-634-5962
Fax: 310-634-4120

343. Maddak®, Inc.
6 Industrial Rd.
Pequannock, NJ 07740
973-628-7600
Fax: 973-305-0841
E-mail: tallete@webspan.net
http://www.maddak.com

344. Maid of Scandanavia® Co.
Div. of Sweet Celebrations, Inc.
P.O. Box 39426
Edina, MN 55439-0426
800-328-6722
612-943-1688 (local)
Fax: 612-943-1688

345. Marvin Windows and Doors
P.O. Box 100
Warroad, MN 56736
800-346-5128

346. MasterMedia Ltd.
17 East 89th St., 7D
New York, NY 10128
800-334-8232
212-546-7650

347. Maxi-Aids
Products for Independent Living
42 Executive Blvd.
P.O. Box 3209
Farmingdale, NY 11735
800-522-6294
V/TTY: 516-752-0521
Fax: 516-752-0689
E-mail: sales@maxiaids.com
http://www.maxiaids.com

348. Maytag® Co.
The Consumer Education
Department
One Dependability Sq.
Newton, IA 50208
515-791-6402
and
Maytag® Co., Ltd.
270 Belfield Rd.
Rexdale, ON M9W 1H7
Canada

349. McBuddy
P.O. Box 541
Whitehall, MT 59759
406-287-3265
406-287-5536

350. McCulloch Products, Ltd.
CPO Box 384
Auckland, New Zealand

351. McGraw Hill Inc.
1221 Ave. of the Americas
New York, NY 10020
800-338-3987
212-512-2000

352. Mechanical Applications, Inc.
6819 Hwy. 90 Blvd., Ste. 580
Katy, TX 77490
713-391-8898
Fax: 713-391-5585

352B. Medic America
Box 682268
Franklin, TN 37068-2268
615-792-2400
Fax: 615-794-0179

353. Medical Economics Co.
5 Paragon Dr.
Montvale, NJ 07645-1742
800-526-4870
201-358-7200

354. Medical Specialties Inc.
4600 Lebanon Rd.
Charlotte, NC 282227
800-334-4143 (orders)
704-573-4040
Fax: 800-694-9060
Voice Mail: 800-582-4040

355. Medicine in the Public Interest

356. Menu Magic®
1717 West Tenth St.
Indianapolis, IN 46222
800-572-5888
317-269-3500

357. Meredith Corp.
Better Homes & Gardens®
1716 Locust St.
Des Moines, IA 50336
800-678-8091
Fax: 515-284-3371

358. Merry Walker Corp.
9804 Main St.
P.O. Box 9
Hebron, IL 60034
815-648-4125
Fax: 815-648-4126

359. Miele® Appliances, Inc.
97 Danbury Rd.
Ridgefield, CT 06877
800-694-4868
vacuums@mieleusa.com

360. Milani Foods
Division of Alberto-Culver USA
Inc.
2525 Armitage Ave.
Melrose Park, IL 60160
800-333-0003
708-450-3189
Fax: 708-450-3354

361. Miles Kimball Co.
41 West 8th St.
Oshkosh, WI 54906-0100
414-231-3800

362. Miller, Inc., G.E.
45 Sawmill River Rd.
P.O. Box 266
Yonkers, NY 10705
800-431-2924
914-445-6060
Fax: 914-446-2631

363. Miramar Communications, Inc.
P.O. Box 8987
23815 Stuart Ranch Rd.
Malibu, CA 90265
800-543-4116
310-317-4522
Fax: 310-317-9644
http://www.homecaremag.com

364. Mirro®/Foley/Wearever/Rema
1512 Washington
P.O. Box 1330
Manitowoc, WI 54221-1330

365. Mobility Products & Design, Inc.
14800 28th Ave. North
Minneapolis, MN 55447
800-488-7688
612-559-1680
Fax: 612-557-8310

366. Mobility Transfer Systems, Inc.
P.O. Box 922
19 Lafayette St.
Randolph, MA 02368-0922
800-854-4687
617-963-4564

367. Modern Education Corp.
Customer Service
P.O. Box 721
Tulsa, OK 74101
918-584-7278

367B. Modern Sponsored Marketing Services
3645 Crook Rd.
Troy, MI 48084
800-243-6877

368. Mosby-Year Book, Inc.
Subs. of Time Mirror Co.
11830 Westline Industrial Dr.
St. Louis, MO 63146
800-426-4545
314-872-8370

369. Motion Control, Inc.
3385 West 1820 South
Salt Lake City, UT 84104
800-621-3347
Fax: 801-972-9072
E-mail: Utah Arm@aol.com

370. Motion Designs
2842 Business Park Ave.
Fresno, CA 93727
800-456-8168
209-292-2171
Fax: 209-292-7412

371. Motovator
22626 South Normandie Ave.
Unit E
Torrance, CA 90502
800-435-2721
310-320-5941

372. Mr. Coffee®
24700 Miles Rd.
Bedford Heights, OH 44146-1399
216-464-4000

372B. Mulholland Positioning Systems, Inc.
P.O. Box 391
215 North 12th St.
Santa Paula, CA 93061
800-543-4769
805-525-7165
Fax: 805-933-1082

373. Nasco
901 Janesville Ave.
P.O. Box 901
Fort Atkinson, WI 53538-0901
414-563-2446
Fax: 414-563-8296
and
Nasco Modesto
4825 Stoddard Rd.
Modesto, CA 95356-9318
209-545-1600
Fax: 209-545-1669

374. National Braille Press, Inc.
88 Stephen St.
Boston, MA 02115-9786
800-548-7323
617-266-6160
Fax: 617-437-0456
E-mail: orders@nbp.org

375. Nationwide Flashing Signal Systems, Inc.
8120 Fenton St., LL110
Silver Spring, MD 20910
V: 301-589-6671
TDD: 301-589-6670
Fax: 301-589-5153

376. NeuroScience Publishers
6555 Carrollton Ave.
Indianapolis, IN 46220
317-257-9672

376B. New Harbinger Publications
5674 Shattuck Ave.
Oakland, CA 94609
800-748-6273
510-652-0215
Fax: 510-652-5472

377. Newmarket Press
Div. of NM Publishing and
Communications
18 East 48th St.]
New York, NY 10017
800-669-3903
212-832-3575

378. Nitty Gritty Productions
Bristol Pub. Enterprises
600 Porterfield Dr.
San Jacinto, CA 92582
800-346-4889
909-654-3406

379. Noble Motion, Inc.
P.O. Box 5366
Pittsburgh, PA 15206
800-234-WALK
412-363-7115
Fax: 412-363-7189

380. Nordicware®
Northland Aluminum Product, Inc.
P.O. Box 16074
Highway 7 at 100
Minneapolis, MN 55416
800-328-4310
Fax: 612-924-8561

381. Norelco®
Div. of Philips Electronics North
America Corp.
1010 Washington Blvd.
P.O. Box 120015
Stamford, CT 06912-0015
800-572-4116
Fax: 203-975-1812

382. Norm Thompson
P.O. Box 3999
Portland, OR 97208
800-821-1287

383. North Coast Medical, Inc.
187 Stauffer Blvd.
P.O. Box 6070
San Jose, CA 95125-1950
800-821-9319
408-283-1900
Fax: 408-283-1950
E-mail: ncmcs@aol.com
http://www.blvd.com/northcoa.htm

384. Northern Speech Services, Inc.
117 North Elm
Gaylord, MI 49735
517-732-3866

385. Norton, W.W., & Co., Inc.
500 Fifth Ave.
New York, NY 10110
800-223-2584

386. NovaCare Sabolich Prosthetic & Research Center
P.O. Box 60509
4301 North Classen Blvd.
Oklahoma City, OK 73146
800-522-4428
Fax: 405-525-4021

387. Nutone®
Madison and Red Bank Roads
Cincinnati, OH 45227-1599
800-543-8687

388. Obus Forme® Ltd.
550 Hopewell Ave.
Toronto, ON M6E 2S6
Canada
416-785-1386
Fax: 416-785-5862

389. Olde Maryland Publishing Co.
10 Jack Frost Ln.
Baltimore, MD 21204
410-823-3460

389B. Oolichan Books
P.O. Box 10
Lantzville, BC V0R 2H0
Canada
Phone/Fax: 250-390-4839

390. Open Sesame™
1933 Davis St., Ste. 279
San Leandro, CA 94577
800-OPEN-911
510-638-0770

391. Optimum Technologies, Inc.
574 Joe Frank Harris Pky.
Cartersville, GA 30190
404-386-3470

392. Optiway Technology Inc.
500 Norfinch Dr.
Downsview, ON M3N 1Y4
Canada
800-514-7061
416-739-8333
Fax: 416-739-6622

392B. Opus Communications
P.O. Box 1168
Marblehead, MA 01945
800-650-6787
617-639-1872

393. Oreck Corp.
100 Plantation Rd.
New Orleans, LA 70123-9989
800-286-8900

393B. Oregon State University
Publication Orders
Extension and Station
Communications
422 Kerr Administration
Corvallis, OR 97331-2119
541-737-2513

394. Ortho-Kinetics, Inc.
P.O. Box 1647
W220 North 507 Springdale Rd.
Waukesha, WI 53187-1647
800-824-1068
414-542-6060
Fax:414-542-4258

395. Otto Bock® Orthopedic Industry, Inc.
3000 Xenium Ln. North
Minneapolis, MN 55441
800-984-8901
800-665-3327 (Canada)
612-553-9464
Fax: 800-962-2549
E-mail: ottobockus@aol.com
http://www.ottobock.com
and
2897 Brighton Rd.
Oakville, ON L6H 5S3
Canada
800-665-3327
Fax: 800-463-3659

396. Oxmoor House®
Div. of Southern Progress Corp.
2100 Lakeshore Dr.
Birmingham, AL 35209
800-633-4910
205-877-6000
Online: OxmoorCS@aol.com

397. Oxo® International
Div. of General Housewares
1536 Beech St.
Terre Haute, IN 47804
800-545-4411

398. Palomino Press
8607 144th St.
Briarwood, NY 11435-3119
718-297-5053

399. Panasonic
Matasushita Consumer Electronics
Co.
Div. of Matasushita Electric Corp.
of America
Executive Offices
One Panasonic Way
Secausus, NJ 07094
201-348-7000

400. Para La Salud
2023 Q St. NW
Washington, DC 20009-1009
202-387-3624
Fax: 202-387-3629

401. Paragon House
370 Lexington Ave.
New York, NY 10017-6503
212-953-5950

402. Parker Publishing
Box 386
Crystal Lake, IL 60039-0386

402B. Parkside Publishing Corp.
205 West Touhy Ave.
Park Ridge, IL 60068
800-221-6364
708-318-0966

403. Parrot Software
P.O. Box 250755
W. Bloomfield, MI 48325-0755
800-PARROT-1
810-788-3223
Fax: 810-788-3224
http://www.parrot.oft.com

403B. Parvin Manufacturing Co.
2031 East 27th St.
Los Angeles, CA 90058
800-648-0770
Fax: 213-585-0427

404. Pathfinder Enterprises, Inc.
P.O. Box 7126
Gainesville, FL 32605
800-289-1763
352-337-0234
Fax: 352-337-0234

404B. Patient Care Products
6845 Laureen St.
Fresno, CA 93710
209-323-6408

405. PCP-Champion®
OTC Professional Appliances
300 Congress St.
Ripley, OH 45167
800-888-0867
NJ: 800-888-9809
CA: 800-888-8201
Canada (Airway Surgical
Appliances): 800-267-3476

405B. Pegasus Products, Inc.
R.R. 1
Carroll, MB R0K 0K0
Canada
800-665-6767
204-483-3151
Fax: 204-483-3141
E-mail: SofPegasus@aol.com

406. Pella® Corp.
102 Main St.
Pella, IA 20519
800-447-3553

407. Penguin Books®
375 Hudson St.
New York, NY 10014
800-526-0275 (orders)
212-366-2607
(Imprints: Dutton, Lodestar, NAL,
Plume, Viking.)

407B. Peoples Medical Society
462 Walnut St.
Allentown, PA 18102
800-624-8773
610-770-1670

408. Permobil, Inc.
6B Gill St.
Woburn, MA 01801
800-736-0925
617-932-9009
Fax: 617-932-0428
E-mail: permobil@aol.com

409. Phoenix Project, NKA, Head Injury Hotline
P.O. Box 84151
Seattle, WA 98124
206-329-1371
206-621-8558
http://www.headinjury.com

410. Pin Dot Products

411. Plenum Publishing Corp.
233 Spring St.
New York, NY 10013-1578
800-221-9369
212-620-8000
Fax: 212-463-0742

412. Porta-Ramps®
5592 East La Palma Ave.
Anaheim, CA 92807
800-654-RAMP
714-970-0683 (CA)

413. Posey® Company, J.T.
5635 Peck Rd.
Arcadia, CA 91006-0020
800-447-6739
Fax orders: 800-767-3933
Fax: 818-443-5064
818-443-3143

414. Power Access Corp.
106 Powder Mill Rd.
P.O. Box 235
Collinsville, CT 06022
800-344-0088
860-693-0751
Fax: 860-693-0641
E-mail: powaccess@aol.com

415. Prairie View Industries, Inc.
P.O. Box 575
714 Fifth St.
Fairbury, NE 68352-0575
800-554-RAMP
402-729-4055
Fax: 402-729-4058

416. Premier Solutions Ltd.
1157 Alameda Dr.
Tempe, AZ 85202
800-526-0982
602-967-4503

417. Prentice Hall Press
Div. of Simon & Schuster, Inc.
160 Gould St.
Needham Heights, MA 02194-2310
617-455-1300

418. Prentke Romich Co.
World Leader, Augmentative
Communication
1022 Heyl Rd.
Wooster, OH 44691
800-262-1933
330-262-1984
Fax: 330-263-4829
E-mail:
INFO@PRENTROM.COM
http://dialup.oar.net/-Pprco/index.html

419. Prevention Plus, Inc.
5775 Wayata Blvd, Ste. 700
Minneapolis, MN 55416
800-887-2282
612-546-7849
E-mail: mmelnikll@aol.com

420. Pride Health Care, Inc.
182 Susquehanna Ave.
Exeter, PA 18643
800-800-8586
717-655-5574
E-mail:
mmiller1@pridehealth.com
http://www.pridehealth.com

**421. Prima Publishing and
Communication**
3875 Atherton Rd.
Rocklin, CA 95765
800-726-0600 (dist. by Random
House)
916-632-4400

422. Prodyne Enterprises
P.O. Box 212
Montclair, CA 91763
714-628-1316
Fax: 714-391-1717

423. Pro-Ed Inc.
8700 Shoal Creek Blvd.
Austin, TX 78757-6897
800-897-3202
512-451-3246
Fax: 800-397-7633

424. Prometheus Books
59 John Glenn Dr.
Amherst, NY 14228-2197
800-421-0351
716-691-0133
Fax: 716-691-0137

425. Production Research Corp.
10225 Southard Dr.
Beltsville, MD 20705
800-772-1123
301-937-9633
Fax: 800-258-8329

426. Publishers Group West
Subs. of Pub. Group, Inc.
4065 Hollis St.
Emeryville, CA 94608
800-788-3123
510-658-3453

427. Putnam Berkley Group, Inc.
200 Madison Ave.
New York, NY 10016
800-631-8571
(Imprints: Jeremy Tarcher, Putnam,
Berkley.)

428. Quartet Technology, Inc.
11 School St.
North Chelmsford, MA 01863
508-251-4432
Fax: 508-251-4915
E-mail: hamer@qtiusa.com
http://www.qtiusa.com

429. R.A.S. International

430. Radio Shack®

431. Rampit, Inc.
P.O. Box 286
Coldwater, MI 49036
800-876-9498
517-278-9015
Fax: 517-278-9023

431B. Rand-Scott, Inc.
401 Linden Center Dr.
Fort Collins, CO 80524
800-467-7967
970-484-7967
Fax: 970-484-3800
E-mail: easypivot@aol.com

432. Random House, Inc.
201 East 50th St.
New York, NY 10022
800-726-0600
212-751-2600
(Imprints: Ballantine, Crown,
Hearst, Knopf, Pantheon, Times
Books.)

433. Random House of Canada
Subs. of Random House, Inc.
1265 Aerowood Dr.
Mississauga, ON L4W 1B9
Canada
905-624-0672

434. Raymo® Products, Inc.
212 South Blake
P.O. Box 248
Olathe, KS 66051-0248
913-782-1515

435. Reader's Digest Association, Inc.
261 Madison Ave.
New York, NY 10016
800-431-1246
212-953-0030

435B. Rebus, Inc.
632 Broadway
New York, NY 10012

436. Redman Inc.
945 East Ohio, Ste. 4
Tucson, AZ 85714
800-727-6684
520-294-2621
Fax: 520-294-8836
E-mail: redman@dakota.com.net
http://www.redmanpowerchairs.com

437. Reese Enterprises, Inc.
P.O. Box 459
16350 Asher Ave.
Rosemount, MN 55068-0459
800-328-0953
612-423-1126
Fax: 612-423-2662

438. Regal® Ware, Inc.
1675 Reigle Drive
Kewaskum, WI 53040
414-626-2121

439. Relaxation Co., The
20 Lumber Rd., Second Flr.
Roslyn, NY 11576
800-788-6670
516-621-2727

440. Research Grant Guides
P.O. Box 1214
Loxahatchee, FL 33470
561-795-6129

441. Research Press
2612 North Mattis Ave.
Champaign, IL 61821
800-519-2707
217-352-3273
Fax: 217-352-1221
and
Research Press of Canada
60 Rankin St.
Waterloo, ON N2V 1V9
519-747-2477
Fax: 519-747-0062

442. Research Products Corp.
1015 East Washington Ave.
P.O. Box 1467
Madison, WI 53701-1467
608-257-8801
Fax: 608-257-4357

443. Resources for Rehabilitation
33 Bedford St., #19A
Lexington, MA 02173
617-862-6455

444. Ricon Corp.
12450 Montague St.
Pacoima, CA 91331
800-322-2884
818-899-7588 (outside U.S.)
Fax: 818-890-3354

445. Rifton Equipment
P.O. Box 901
Rifton, NY 12471
800-777-4244
914-658-8798
E-mail:
sales@commplay.mhs.com-
puserve.com

446. Rival Company, The
Kansas City, MO 64131
816-943-4100

447. Rodale Press Inc.
33 East Minor St.
Emmaus, PA 18098
800-527-8200
215-967-5171

448. Roho®, Inc.
Crown Therapeutics, Inc.
100 Florida Ave.
Belleville, IL 62221-5429
800-850-7646
618-277-9150
Fax: 618-277-6518
E-mail: rohoinc.@rohoinc.com
http://www.rohoinc.com/

449. Rosen Publishing Group, Inc., The
29 East 21st St.
New York, NY 10010
800-237-9932
212-777-3017
Fax: 212-777-0277

450. Routledge, Chapman & Hall
Subs. of Intern. Thomson Org.,
Inc.
29 West 35th St.
New York, NY 10001-2291
212-244-3336
Fax: 212-563-2269

451. Rowman and Littlefield
4720 Boston Way, Ste. A
Lanham, MD 20706
800-462-6420
301-459-3366

451B. Rowoco®
Wilton Industries
2240 West 75th St.
Woodbridge, IL 60517
800-772-7111
708-963-7149

452. Rubbermaid, Inc.
1147 Akron Rd.
Wooster, OH 44691
216-264-6464

453. Rubbermaid® Commercial Products, Inc.
3124 Valley Ave.
Winchester, VA 22601
540-667-8700
Fax: 540-542-8821

454. Rubbermaid® Health Care Products, Inc.
3124 Valley Ave.
Winchester, VA 20601
800-526-8051
540-667-8700
Fax: 540-542-8770

455. Running Press Book Publishers
125 South 22nd St.
Philadelphia, PA 19103-4399
800-345-5359
215-567-5080
Fax: 215-568-2919

456. Rutledge Hill Press
211 Seventh Ave. North
Nashville, TN 37219
800-234-4234
615-244-2700
Fax: 615-244-2978

457. Safety Zone™, The
Hanover, PA 17333-0019
800-999-3030
Fax: 800-338-1635

458. Sage Publications Inc.
2455 Teller Rd.
Thousand Oaks, CA 91320
805-499-0721
E-mail: info@sagepub.com

459. St. Martin's Press
175 Fifth Ave.
New York, NY 10010
800-221-7945
212-674-5151

460. Salton/MAXIM® Housewares, Inc.
550 Business Center Dr.
Mt. Prospect, IL 60056
800-233-9054
and
3088 Walnut Ave.
Long Beach, CA 90807
and
251 South 31st St.
Kenilworth, NJ 07033

461. Sammons Preston, Inc.
A BISSELL® Healthcare Co.
4 Sammons Ct.
Bolingbrook, IL 60440-4989
800-323-5547
708-325-1700
Fax: 800-547-4333
E-mail: sp@mail.sammonspreston.com

462. Sanlex International Corporation
P.O. Box 14717
Dayton, OH 45459
513-297-3011

463. Sanyo Fisher USA Corp.
218 State Rt. 17
4th Floow
Rochelle Park, NJ 07662-3333

464. Sardegna Productions

465. Sassy®, Inc.
Baby Care Products
633 Skokie Blvd., Ste. 404
Northbrook, IL 60062-2826
847-498-9520
Fax: 847-498-0304

466. Science Products
Box 888
Southeastern, PA 19399
800-888-7400
(Imprints of Simon & Schuster,
#477.)

467. Scribners
Rockefeller Center
1230 Ave. of the Americas
New York, NY 10020
(Imprints: Fireside, Free Press,
Pocket, Scribners, Touchstone.)

468. Sears Roebuck
Health Care Catalog
9804 Chartwell
Dallas, TX 75243

469. Self Care Industries, Inc.
P.O. Box 890956
Temecula, CA 92075
Phone/Fax: 909-694-1768

470. Self-Counsel Press, Inc.
1704 North State St.
Bellingham, WA 98225
800-663-3007
360-676-4530
Fax: 360-676-4549
E-mail: selfcoun@pinc.com

471. SeniorNet®
1 Kearny St., 3rd Floor
San Francisco, CA 94108-5501
415-750-5030

472. Serif Press, Inc.
Center for Books on Aging
1331 H St. NW, Ste. 110
Washington, DC 20005-4725
202-737-4650
Fax: 202-783-1931

473. Sharp Electronics
Sharp Plaza
Mahwah, NJ 07430-2135
800-237-4277

474. Sher Company, Inc.
P.O. Box 26886
Philadelphia, PA 19134
Fax: 215-427-0696

475. Signature 2000
Div. of Akron-Cleveland Home
Medical
489 West Exchange St.
Akron, OH 44302
800-227-2152
330-376-2135
Fax: 330-376-0877

476. Signatures®
19465 Brennan Ave.
Perris, CA 92599
909-943-2021
Fax: 909-943-5574

477. Simon & Schuster®, Inc.
Rockefeller Center
1230 Ave. of the Americas
New York, NY 10020
(Imprints: Fireside, Free Press,
Pocket, Scribners, Touchstone.)

478. SK Brown Publishers
2849 Dundee Rd., Ste. 140
Northbrook, IL 60062
708-498-1702

479. SLACK Inc.
6900 Grove Rd.
Thorofare, NJ 08086-9447
800-257-8290
609-848-1000
Fax: 609-853-5991

480. SmileTote, Inc.
12979 Culver Blvd.
Los Angeles, CA 90066
800-826-6130
213-827-0156 (CA)

481. Smith & Nephew, Inc.
Rehabilitation Division
One Quality Drive
P.O. Box 1005
Germantown, WI 53022-8205
800-558-8633
414-251-7840
Fax: 800-545-7758
E-mail: www.easy-living.com
http://www.easy-living.com

482. Solutions
Products That Make Life Easier®
P.O. Box 6878
Portland, OR 97228-6878
800-342-9988 ext110

483. Southside Rehabilitation Products
1815 South Clinton Ave., Ste. 400
Rochester, NY 14618-5799
800-333-0979
716-271-7141
Fax: 716-271-0829

484. Space Tables, Inc.
P.O. Box 32082
8035 Ranchers Rd. NE
Minneapolis, MN 55432-0082
800-328-2580
612-786-9301 (call collect in MN)
800-461-4740 (Canada)

485. Spacewall Northeast, Inc.
567-3 South Leonard St.
Waterbury, CT 06708
800-524-1590
203-597-1328
Fax: 203-597-5570

486. Special Additions
810 DeLong Rd.
Lexington, KY 40515-9504
606-273-1122
Fax: 606-273-8843

487. Special Health Systems
90 Englehard Dr.
Aurora, ON L4G 3V2
Canada
800-263-2223

488. The Speech Bin, Inc.
1925 Twenty-Fifth Ave.
Vero Beach, FL 32960
800-4-SPEECH
561-770-0007
Fax: 888-Fax-2-B (888-329-2246)
Fax: 561-770-0006

489. Spenco® Medical Corp.
P.O. Box 2501
Waco, TX 76702-2501
800-433-3334
254-772-6000
Fax: 254-772-3093
E-mail: spenco@spenco.com

490. Spiegel, Inc.
P.O. Box 182563
Columbus, OH 43218
and
P.O. Box 1496
Windsor, ON N9A 6R5

491. Springer Publishing Co., Inc.
536 Broadway, 11th Floor
NewYork, NY 10012-3955
212-431-4370
Fax: 212-941-7842

492. Springhouse Publishing
1111 Bethlehem Pike
P.O. Box 908
Springhouse, PA 19477-0908
800-346-7844
215-646-8700
Fax: 215-646-8716

493. Stand Aid of Iowa, Inc.
P.O. Box 386
Sheldon, IA 51201
800-831-8580
712-324-5213 (in IA)
Fax: 712-324-5210
E-mail: standaid@rconnect.com
http://www.inmax.com/standaid

494. Stanley® Hardware
Customer Service Dept.
480 Myrtle St.
New Britain, CT 06053
800-622-4393

495. Starcrest of California®
19465 Brennan Ave.
Perris, CA 92599
909-657-2793
Fax: 909-943-5574

496. Starlight Publishing Co.
1893 NE 164th St., Ste. 100
North Miami Beach, FL 33162

497. Suburbanite Industries
P.O. Box 8000
Holliston, MA 01746-8000
800-343-3368
508-429-5100
Fax: 508-429-1289

497B. Sub-Zero Freezer Co., Inc.
P.O. Box 4130
Madison, WI 53744-4130
800-222-7820

498. Sunbeam Appliance Co.
Sunbeam Oster Household
Products
1910 Highway 15 North
Laurel, MS 39441
800-597-5978

**499. Sunrise Medical Guardian®
Products, Inc.**
4175 Guardian St.
Simi Valley, CA 93063
800-423-8034
Fax: 800-579-2828
http://www.quickiedesigns.com
(Divisions include Kid Karts,
Quickee and Guardian.)

500. Sunset Publishing

501. SuperQuad™
P.O. Box 2426
Granite Bay, CA 95746-2426
800-OK-WIJIT

502. Supracor® Systems, Inc.
1135 East Arques Ave.
Sunnyvale, CA 94086
800-787-7226
408-732-1818
Fax: 408-732-2317
http://www.supracor.com

502B. Sure Hands International
982 Route 1
Pine Island, NY 10969-1205
800-724-5305
914-258-6500
Fax: 914-258-6634
E-mail: surehand@warwick.net

503. **Susquehanna Rehab Products**
RD 2, Box 41
9 Overlook Drive
Wrightsville, PA 17368
800-248-2011
Fax: 717-252-1768

504. **Southpaw Enterprises, Inc.**

505. **Tamarack Habilitation Technologies**
1471 Energy Park Dr.
St. Paul, MN 55108-5204
612-644-9950
Fax: 612-644-0240

506. **TASH International, Inc.**
91 Station St., Unit 1
Ajax, ON L1S 3H2
Canada
800-463-5685
905-686-4129
Fax: 905-686-6895
E-mail: tashcan@aol.com

507. **Taunton Trade Co., The**
63 South Main St.
P.O. Box 5563
Newtown, CT 06470-5563
800-283-7252
203-426-8171
Fax: 203-426-7184

508. **Taylor Gifts**
600 Cedar Hollow Rd.
P.O. Box 1770
Paoli, PA 19301-0807
800-829-1133
610-293-3613

509. **Taylor Publishing Co.**
Subs. of Insilco
1550 West Mockingbird Ln.
Dallas, TX 75235
800-677-2800
214-819-8100

510. **Taylor Woodcraft**
P.O. Box 245
South River Rd.
Malta, OH 43758
614-962-3741
Fax: 614-962-2747

511. **TelAssure™**
8045 Big Bend Blvd., Ste. 105
St. Louis, MO 63119
800-821-RUOK
DemoLine: 800-821-DEMO

512. **Teledyne Brown Engineering**
Imperium Products
P.O. Box 070007
Huntsville, AL 35807-7007
800-944-8002
205-726-6749
Fax: 205-726-6739
E-mail:
pam.gardner@pobox.tbe.com
http://www.tbe.com

513. **Telesensory**
455 North Bernardo Ave.
P.O. Box 7455
Mountain View, CA 94039-7455
415-960-0920

514. **Ten Speed Press**
Box 7123
Berkeley, CA 94707
800-841-2665
510-559-1610

515. **T-Fal Corp.**
25 Riverside Dr.
Pine Brook, NJ 07058
201-575-1060

516. **TFH (USA) Inc.**
4537 Gibsonia Rd.
Gibsonia, PA 15044
800-467-6222
412-444-6400
Fax: 412-444-6411

516B. **TherAdapt® Products, Inc.**
17 West 163 Oak Lane
Bensonville, IL 60106
630-834-2461

517. **Theradyne Corp.**
21730 Hanover Ave.
Lakeville, MN 55044
800-328-4014
612-469-4404
800-267-3476 (Central Canada)
800-267-8098 (Canada National)
Fax: 612-469-2200

518. **TheraFin Corp.**
19747 Wolf Rd.
Mokena, IL 60448
800-843-7234
708-479-7300
Fax: 708-479-1515
http://www.inmax.com

519. **Therapet Press**
P.O. Box 1696
Whitehorse, TX 75791

520. **Therapeutic Appliance Group**
P.O. Box 339
Woonsocket, RI 02895
800-457-5535
Fax: 401-762-0252

521. **Therapro**
225 Arlington St.
Framingham, MA 01702
800-257-5376
508-872-9494
Fax: 508-875-2062

522. **Therapy Skill Builders**
Div. of The Psychological Corp.
555 Academic Ct.
San Antonio, TX 78204-2498
800-228-0752
Fax: 800-232-1223

523. **Thermador**
5119 District Blvd.
Los Angeles, CA 90040
800-735-5547
702-833-3600

524. **Thick-It**
See Milani Foods, #360

525. **Thompson Video Productions**
Thompson Medical Specialties
4301 Bryant Ave. South
Minneapolis, MN 55409
800-777-4949
612-823-2058
Fax: 612-823-8652

526. **Three J Productions Ltd.**
2 Pineridge Rd.
White Plains, NY 10603
914-592-6033

527. Tip Top Mobility Inc.
P.O. Box 5009
Minot, ND 58702
800-735-5958
701-857-1182
Fax: 701-857-1181
E-mail: tiptop@dacotah.com

528. Tiresias Press, Inc.
116 Pinehurst Ave.
New York, NY 10033
212-568-9570

529. tlc
Hanover, PA 17333-0080
800-850-9445

530. Toastmaster®, Inc.
1801 North Stadium Blvd.
Columbia, MO 65202
314-445-8666
Fax: 314-876-0618

531. Tommee Tippee Playskool, Inc.
Subsidiary of Hasbro, Inc.
Northvale, NJ 07647

532. Toys for Special Children
385 Warburton Ave.
Hastings, NY 10706
914-478-0960
Fax: 914-478-7030

533. Trademark Medical
1053 Headquarters Park
Fenton, MO 63026-2033
800-325-9044
314-349-3270
Fax: 314-349-3294
E-mail:
trademark@worldnet.att.net

534. Travel Ramp, Inc.
P.O. Box 2015
Alachua, FL 32615
904-462-5267
Fax: 904-462-7744

535. Triad Publishing Co.
P.O. Drawer 13355
Gainesville, FL 32604-1355
904-373-5800

536. Tucker Designs Ltd.
427 Pellerin Dr.
P.O. Box 641117
Kenner, LA 70064
504-464-7479
Fax: 504-464-7480

537. Tumbleforms
145 Tower Dr.
Burr Ridge, IL 60521
800-323-5547
Fax: 800-547-4333

538. Tupperware Inc.
World Headquarters
14901 South Orange Blosson Trail
Orlando, FL 32802-2353
800-858-7221 (U.S.)
800-567-0400 (Canada)
407-826-4568
Fax: 407-826-8864
http://www.tupperware.com

539. Twentieth Century Plastics®
205 South Puente St.
Brea, CA 92821
800-767-0777

540. 21st Century Scientific, Inc.
4915 Industrial Way
Coeurd'Alene, ID 83814
800-448-3680
208-667-8800
Fax: 208-667-6600
E-mail: 21st@wheelchairs.com
http://www.wheelchairs.com

541. Ulti-Mate®
Invacare Corp.
899 Cleveland St.
Elyria, OH 44036
216-329-6000
Fax: 216-365-4558
and
5970 Chadworth Way
Mississauga, ON L5R 3T9
Canada
905-890-8300
Fax: 905-890-5244

**542. Unishape Design Adaptive
Positioning System, Inc.**
1630 30th St., Ste. 208
Boulder, CO 80301
303-443-8348
Fax: 303-443-3136

543. Ultraflo

544. Unipub
3611-F Assembly Dr.
Lanham, MD 20706
800-274-4888
301-459-7666

**545. United States Purchasing
Exchange®**
13571 Vaughn St.
San Fernando, CA 91340
818-895-5555

546. University of California Press
2120 Berkeley Way
Berkeley, CA 94720
800-777-4726
510-642-4247

547. University of Michigan Medsport
P.O. Box 363
Ann Arbor, MI 48106
313-998-7400

548. University of Minnesota Press

549. University of Toronto Press
250 Sonwil Dr.
Buffalo, NY 14225-5516

550. University of Washington Press
P.O. Box 30096
Seattle, WA 98145-5096
207-543-4050

**551. Valhalla Rehabilitation
Publications**
21 Roosevelt Dr.
P.O. Box 195
Valhalla, NY 10595
Voice/Fax: 914-948-1004

552. Van Nostrand Reinhold
International Thomson
Professional Reference Div.
115 Fifth Ave.
New York, NY 10003
800-842-3636
212-254-3232
Fax: 606-525-7778

553. Vandenburg A.D.L.

554. Vantage Industries, Inc.
4530-F Patton Dr. East
P.O. Box 43944
Atlanta, GA 30336
404-691-9500
Fax: 404-691-9149

555. Vantage Mini Vans
5214 South 30th St.
Phoenix, AZ 85040-3730
800-348-8267
602-243-2700
Fax: 348-8267

556. Vector Mobility, Inc.
5030 East Jensen Ave.
Fresno, CA 93725
800-441-0358
Fax: 800-789-3912
http://www.vector.org

557. Velcro® USA, Inc.
406 Brown Ave.
Manchester, NH 03103
800-225-0180
603-669-4893
Fax: 603-669-9271

558. Vermont Country Store®, The
P.O. Box 3000
Manchester Center, VT 05255-3000
802-362-2400
Fax: 802-362-0285

559. Visual Health Information Products
P.O. Box 44646
Tacoma, WA 98444

560. Vitaerobics
41905 Boardwalk
Palm Desert, CA 92211-9028
619-773-5576
Fax: 612-627-1980
E-mail: ump@staff.tc.umn.edu

560B. Volkswagen USA
3800 Hamlin Rd.
Auburn Hills, MI 48326
800-444-VWUS

561. Walk-Away Walker LLC.
P.O. Box 1131
Garden Grove, CA 92842
714-220-0155
Fax: 714-220-0610

561B. Walter Drake® & Sons
Drake Building
Colorado Springs, CO 80940
719-596-3853

562. Warner Books
A Time-Warner Co.
1271 Ave. of the Americas
New York, NY 10020
800-759-0190 (orders)
212-522-7200

563. Washington Products, Inc.
1147 Oberlin Ave. SW
Massillon, OH 44648
330-837-5101

564. Waupaca Elevator Co., Inc.
P.O. Box 246
138 South Osborn
Waupaca, WI 54981
Fax: 715-258-5004
800-238-8739
715-258-5581

565. Wayne State University Press
Leonard North Simons Bldg.
4809 Woodward Ave.
Detroit, MI 48201-7323
800-978-7323
313-577-6120

566. Welbilt® Appliance Corp. of America
P.O. Box 220709
175 Community Dr.
Great Neck, NY 11021
516-773-0300
Fax: 516-773-0966

567. Wellness Reproductions Inc.
23945 Mercantile Rd.
Beachwood, OH 44122-5924
800-669-9208
Fax: 800-501-8120

568. Wells-Engberg Co., Inc.
P.O. Box 6388
Rockford, IL 61125-1388
800-642-3628
815-874-5882
Fax: 815-874-7800

569. Wenzelite™ Medical Supply Co.
220-36th St.
Brooklyn, NY 11232
800-706-WALK
718-768-8002
Fax: 718-768-8020

570. Wheelchairs of Kansas
P.O. Box 320
204 West Second St.
Ellis, KS 67637
800-537-6454
913-726-4885
Fax: 800-337-2447

571. Whirlpool® Corp.
Consumer Assistance Center
200 M-63
Benton Harbor, MI 49022-2692
800-253-1301
616-927-7200
TDD: 800-923-7059
Fax: 616-923-3785
http://www.whirlpoolappliances.com

572. Whitakers
1 Odell Plaza
P.O. Box 1061
Yonkers, NY 10703-9913
800-44-LIFTS
800-924-LIFT (NY)
Fax: 914-423-4200

573. Whitman & Co., Albert
6340 Oakton St.
Morton Grove, IL 60053
800-255-7675
847-581-0033

574. Whitmyer Biomechanix, Inc.
1833 Junwin Ct.
Tallahassee, FL 32308-4449
904-575-5510
Fax: 904-576-4798

575. Wiley, John, & Sons, Inc.
605 Third Ave.
New York, NY 10158-0021
800-225-5945 (orders)
212-850-6000

576. William Morrow & Co., Inc.
Subs. of the Hearst Corp.
1350 Ave. of the Americas
New York, NY 10019
800-843-9389
212-261-6500

577. Williams & Wilkins
351 West Camden St.
Baltimore, MD 21201-2436
800-527-5597
410-528-4000

578. Williams-Sonoma, Inc.
P.O. Box 7456
San Francisco, CA 94120-7456
415-421-4242

579. Wilson Publishing, Inc.
P.O. Box 2190
Glenwood Springs, CO 81602
970-945-5600
E-mail: winco-Medquip@world-net.att.net

580. Winco, Inc.
5516 SW First Ln.
Ocala, FL 34474-9307
800-237-3377
352-854-2929
Fax: 352-854-9544

581. Wingknife, Inc.
P.O. Box 6506
Fort Lauderdale, FL 33316

582. Winsford Products, Inc.
179 Pennington Harbourton Rd.
Pennington, NJ 08534
609-737-3311

583. Woodbine House
6510 Bells Mills Rd.
Bethesda, MD 20817
800-843-7323
301-897-3570
Fax: 301-897-5838
E-mail: woodbine85@aol.com

584. Workman Publishing
708 Broadway
New York, NY 10003
800-722-7202
212-254-8098

585. Worldwide Engineering, Inc.
3240 North Delaware St.
Chandler, AZ 85225
800-848-3433

586. WRF/Aquaplast® Corp.

587. Wy'East Medical
P.O. Box 1625
8850 SE Herbert Ct.
Clackamas, OR 97015
800-255-3126
503-657-3101
Fax: 503-657-6901
E-mail: wyeastmed@europa.com
http://www.wyeastmed.com

588. Y13 Productions
120 West Illinois St., Ste. 5W
Chicago, IL 60610
800-356-8641
312-494-0014
Fax: 312-494-0014

589. Zim Manufacturing Co.
6100 West Grand Ave.
Chicago, IL 60639
312-622-2500

General References

Addresses for publishers, periodicals, and organizations are given in Section Four. Sources are in Appendix E.

BACKGROUND

Barnes, M. R., & Crutchfield, C. A. (1988). *The Patient at Home: A Manual for Exercise Programs, Self-Help Devices, and Home Care Products* (2nd ed.). Thorofare, NJ: SLACK Inc. $22. Instructions for ambulation, transfers, UE/LE exercises, and activities of daily living. Assists therapist and family to work together as a team.

Bucy, D. R. (1996). *Help Yourself: Problem Solving for the Disabled.* New York: Macmillan, Simon & Schuster. $14.95. Listings of professional caregivers, descriptions of assistive equipment, financial and emotional support information.

Case Management Resource Guide. (1992). Newport Beach, CA: Center for Consumer Healthcare Information. Four volumes cover United States (Volume 1: Eastern US; Volume 2: Southern US; Volume 3: Midwestern US; Volume 4: Western US). Has 70,000 entries covering health care resources, including: home care, rehabilitation, mental health, elder care, assistive technology manufacturers, home modification contractors, adaptive transportation resources, referral centers, self-help organizations, and public agencies. $60 per volume, $225 for full set. **Source:** 111.

Christiansen, C. (Ed.). (1994). *Ways of Living: Self-Care Strategies for Special Needs.* Bethesda. MD: American Occupational Therapy Association. #1970. $50 AOTA members, $65 non-members. Framework within which specific self-care issues may be addressed by therapists, contributions by 15 occupational therapists.

Christiansen, C., & Baum, C. (Eds.). (1991). *Occupational Therapy: Overcoming Human Deficits.* Thorofare, NJ: SLACK Inc. $59. Comprehensive core text on human performance, covering cultural influences, performance deficits, sensory, neuromotor, physiological, cognitive, and psychological factors. Environmental assessment, modifications, technological approaches, use of resources.

The Complete Drug Reference. (1992). Yonkers, NY: Consumer Reports® Books. $39.95. Information on more than 5500 prescription and non-prescription medications, written for patients and consumers. How to use and store, side effects, and possible allergic reactions. **Source:** 141.

Consumer's Guide to Therapeutic Services for Children with Disabilities. United Cerebral Palsy Associations. Booklet available from Cambridge, MA: Human Services Research Institute. **Source:** 269.

Cooley, D. A. (1996). *Texas Heart Institute Heart Owner's Handbook.* New York: Wiley, Texas Heart Institute.

DeLisa, J. (Ed.). (1988). *Rehabilitation Medicine: Principles and Practices.* Philadelphia: Lippincott/Raven. $75. Evaluation, therapeutic approaches, major rehabilitation problems, specific disorders.

Eisenberg, M. (1995). *Dictionary of Rehabilitation.* New York: Springer. Multidisciplinary perspective, divided into three parts: core rehabilitation vocabulary, list of national and international associations, and university-related research centers and non-profit research institutes engaged in rehabilitation studies. **Source:** 491.

Falvo, D. R. (1989). *Medical and Psychological Aspects of Chronic Illness and Disability.* Frederick, MD: Aspen.

Galantino, M. L. (1992). *Clinical Assessment and Treatment of HIV: Rehabilitation of a Chronic Illness.* Thorofare, NJ: SLACK Inc. $36. Wellness program addresses all aspects of treatment and rehabilitation for HIV patients. Nutrition, pain management, psychosocial issues, home care.

Goldfarb, L. A., et al. *Meeting the Challenge of Disability or Chronic Illness: A Family Guide.* Baltimore: Paul H. Brookes. $21.

Gregg, C. H., Robertus, J. L., & Stone, J. B. (1989). *The Psychological Aspects of Chronic Illness.* Springfield, IL: Charles C. Thomas. 1989, $54.75.

Guidelines for Occupational Therapy Practice in Home Health. Home Health Task Force. (1995). Bethesda, MD: American Occupational Therapy Association. $18 AOTA members, $23 non-members. Focus is mainly on adult physical disabilities, but guidelines for practice in mental health and pediatric service are also reviewed.

Harrell, M., et al. (1992). *Cognitive Rehabilitation of Memory: A Practical Guide.* Frederick, MD: Aspen. $48. Memory assessment, goal setting, treatment planning, clinical applications.

Hays, R. M., et al. (1994). *Chronic Disease and Disability: A Contemporary Rehabilitation Approach to Medical Practice.* New York: Demos. Principles of assessment and treatment of individuals with disabilities, factors affecting psychosocial and vocational aspects.

Health Information Resources in the Federal Government (#S/N-017-001-00476-6). (1990). Office of National Health Information Center. $3.50 from the Superintendent of Documents, U.S. Government Printing Office. Selected, federally sponsored health information resources useful in responding to health inquiries.

The HomeCare Case Management Source Book. Home Care Magazine, $39.95 plus $4.95 handling. Reference guide to equipment solutions in all areas of daily living, types of equipment available, funding possibilities, and sources for equipment. **Source:** 259.

Kerson, T. S., & Lawrence A. (1985). *Understanding Chronic Illness: The Medical and Psychosocial Dimensions of Nine Diseases.* New York: Free Press, Macmillan, Simon & Schuster. $35. Discusses financial and other sources of assistance in relation to cancer, dementia, epilepsy, stroke, substance abuse, and heart and respiratory failure.

Kurian, George T. (Ed.). *Global Guide to Medical Information.* New York: Elsevier. $85. Periodicals, international and regional organizations, research institutes, national associations, publishers, bibliographies, and conference series.

Moffat, B. C. (1989). *AIDS: A Self Care Manual.* Santa Monica, CA: IBS Press. Check your local library.

NARIC Guide to Disability and Rehabilitation Periodicals. (1991). Silver Spring, MD: National Rehabilitation Information Center.

National Family Caregivers Association. (1996). *The Resourceful Caregiver: Helping Family Caregivers Help Themselves.* St. Louis, MO: Mosby. $9.95. More than 500 resources to help caregivers and those they care for, plus support through hints and quotations. **Source:** 368.

Navarra, T., & Ferrer, M. (1995). *An Insider's Guide to Home Health Care.* Thorofare, NJ: SLACK Inc. $28. Covers roles of all caregivers and potential conflicts between caregivers and patients; discusses cultural problems that can occur in any community; explains how to work as a team for patient's best interests; teaches importance of self-care.

Newman, D. K., & Smith, D. A. (1990). *J. Geriatric Care Plans.* Springhouse, PA: Springhouse Pub. $24.95.

The 1996 Rehabilitation Sourcebook. Reston, VA: American Rehabilitation Association. $50 members, $250 non-members. Lists more than 5000 programs, facilities, state associations, and consultants.

Palder, E. L. (1990). *The Catalog of Catalogs II: The Complete Mail-Order Directory* (1990-1991 ed.). Rockville, MD: Woodbine House. $14.95. Sources for appliances, kitchen utensils, foods.

Professional Guide to Drugs (3rd ed.). (1993). Springhouse, PA: Springhouse Pub. Drugs organized by therapeutic use.

Reaching Out to All People with Disabilities: A Guide for Consumer and Provider Organizations. Knowledge Utilization Program, Institute for the Visually Impaired, Pennsylvania College of Optometry. Available from the National Clearinghouse on Rehabilitation Training Materials or the National Rehabilitation Information Center.

Reed, K. L. (1991). *Quick Reference to Occupational Therapy.* Frederick, MD: Aspen. $39. Facts on diseases, disorders, and dysfunctions, with causes, assessment, and treatment management.

Roggow, P. A., Berg, D. K., & Lewis, M. D. (1993). *The Home Rehabilitation Program Guide* (rev.ed.). Thorofare, NJ: SLACK Inc. $29. Focus on exercises; includes sections on joint protection in arthritis, care of the neck and back, post-mastectomy exercises, relaxation techniques, teaching ADL to LE amputee, crutch walking, use of walkers and canes.

Rorden, J. W., & Taft, E. *Discharge Planning Guide for Nurses.* Orlando, FL: Saunders. 1990, $26.95. Assessment of special risks, flexibility to change dependent on patient's progress, checklist to confirm details.

Schoenberg, J., & Stichman, J. (1990). *Heart Family Handbook.* Philadelphia: Hanley & Belfus. $16.95. Guide for the family of anyone with any heart condition to help make a complete recovery.

Talking with Your Doctor: A Guide for Older People. National Institute on Aging. 32-page guide is free by contacting the NIA Information Center.

Teaching Patients with Chronic Conditions. (1992). Springhouse, PA: Springhouse Pub. Teaching guide with checklists, diagrams, and patient teaching pages that may be photocopied and given to clients. Congestive heart failure, COPD, Parkinson's, Alzheimer's, arthritis, and many others.

Weiss, R., & Subak-Sharpe, G. (Eds.). (1988). *Columbia University School of Public Health Complete Guide to Health and Well-Being After 50.* New York: Times Books, Random House. $24.95. Nutrition, disease-prevention, fitness, etc., with charts and checklists.

REFERENCES ON SELF-HELP AIDS, ACTIVITIES OF DAILY LIVING, AND TECHNOLOGY IN DAILY LIVING

Accent on Living Buyer's Guide. Bloomington, IL: Accent. Annual listing of manufacturers of self-help and hospital equipment. $10. **Source:** 8.

Atkin, G. (1988). *Clothing for People with Special Needs.* College of Human Ecology, Cornell University. $5.75. Manufacturers' garments, patterns to make at home, adaptations for ready-to-wear. Includes apparel for cancer patients. **Source:** 147.

Complete Directory for People with Disabilities. Lakeville, CT: Grey House Publishing. Ask for latest edition. $135. Associations, magazines, newsletters, programs. **Source:** 232B.

Cook, A. M., & Hussey, S. M. (1995). *Assistive Technologies: Principles and Practice.* St. Louis, MO: Mosby. $50.95. Basic information on technologies available, types of disabilities assisted by these technologies, funding sources, and adaptations to user's needs.

Custom Orthotic Seating. St. Paul, MN: Tamarack Habilitation Technologies. $60. Illustrated guide to custom seatings and services. **Source:** 505.

Easy Dressing Fashions. Catalog features women's clothing. Available at any J.C. Penney catalog desk or by calling 800-543-4323. **Source:** 289.

Galvin, J., & Scherer, M. (1996). *Evaluating, Selecting and Using Appropriate Assistive Technology*. Frederick, MD: Aspen. $49. Overview, policies and related legislation, selection, low-tech aids, mobility aids, communication systems, aids for sensory impairments, leisure and recreation devices, interactive technology.

Guidelines for the Use of Assistive Technology: Evaluation, Referral, Prescription. American Medical Association, $5 from the AMA Department for Geriatric Health. Covers patient-physician relationship, matching the client to the device, obtaining funding.

Living in the State of Stuck (2nd ed.). (1996). Cambridge, MA: Brookline Books. $17.95. Addresses the effects of technology on the lives of individuals who were born with or acquired a disability. **Source:** 95.

Mann, W. C., & Lane, J. P. (1991). *Assistive Technology for Persons with Disabilities: The Role of Occupational Therapy #1930* (2nd ed.).Bethesda, MD: American Occupational Therapy Association. $45 AOTA members, $58 non-members. Applications, services, resources, and advances in assistive technology.

Schwarz, S. P. (1995). *Dressing Tips and Clothing Resources for Making Life Easier*. Madison, WI: AJ Press. $18.95 plus $3 postage and handling. Author, who has severe MS, gives tips, techniques, and ways to modify ready-to-wear clothing to make dressing easier. Gives more than 100 resources that carry specially designed or adapted clothing. **Source:** 30.

AUDIOVISUALS ON SELF-HELP EQUIPMENT, ASSISTIVE TECHNOLOGY, AND ADAPTED CLOTHING

Atkin, G. (Producer). *Clothing for People with Special Needs*. Cornell Cooperative Extension, Department of Textiles and Apparel, College of Human Ecology, Cornell University. 19-minute VHS and portfolio of detailed instructions. What to look for in and how to adapt ready-to-wear clothes for the person with a physical limitation, suggestions on purchase of clothing that provides more comfort. Rental, $16; purchase, $65. Comes with one packet as described above. Additional packets are $5.75 each.

Locke, P. *Augmentative Communication Aids* and *Simple-to-Use Technology*. Both videos from AbleNet CAMA Educational Workshop. AbleNet, Inc., Minneapolis, 1995. Demonstrates how to use simple technology to increase independence for people with severe disabilities. Cost is about $10 each. Contact **source** 4 for specifics.

The Tech Act: Dramatic Gains for People with Disabilities. RESNA Press. Video highlights the progress TechAct projects

have made in ensuring availability of assistive technology products for people with disabilities. Available in open- and closed-caption versions, $25 plus $3 shipping and handling.

Also, please see Resources in Chapter 1 and Chapter 6.

COMPUTERIZED INFORMATION SERVICES FOR INDIVIDUALS WITH DISABILITIES

See Appendix C, Section III.

ONLINE

In the fast changing world of the Internet, several websites offer assistance to the health care professional. A few examples are given here.

American Occupational Therapy Association. Home page: http://www.aota.org. AOTA also offers online courses. To find out about planned topics, check: info@online.aota.org.

Caregiving monthly newsletter offers online support with information, tips, links to related websites, and an online support network for caregivers. Website: http://www.caregiving,com.

Disability Mall. Evans Kemp. **Source:** 170. Advertisements by companies that sell products for people with disabilities.

Medline is available to America On-Line (AOL) subscribers, linking them to the National Library of Medicine, one of the largest databases of medical information. It is accessed through the Better Health & Medical Forum or at key word Medline. For information about obtaining AOL software, call 800-827-6364.

NetPractice™—A Beginner's Guide to Healthcare Networking on the Internet. Mary Fran Miller, MS, RRA. Opus Communications, Marblehead, Mass., 1996, 200-page guide to learning your way around the Internet. $37 includes 10 free hours of online service from CompuServe and America On-Line. **Source:** 392B.

Please see additional websites under Sources and Organizations listings.

AUDIOVISUALS

Keep Fit While You Sit. $29.95 from the Disability Bookshop. **Source:** 169.

Swedish Rehab Accessories for Daily Living. 11-minute video from ETAC USA, Inc. Demonstrates aids in chronological sequence as they might be used in a person's daily activities. **Source:** 191.

For a catalog of medical films and videos, write to the Academy of Medical Films. $14.95. **Source:** 6.

The Project for Independent Living in Occupational Therapy (PILOT). Funded by the US Department of Education. Designed to teach students about independent living for people with disabilities. Manual and video illustrate transition needs of individuals with severe physical and/or mental disabilities as they learn to work and live in the community. One section shows use of low-tech aids by a woman with cerebral palsy. Available from the Products Division of the American Occupational Therapy Association.

COURSES

A workshop on simple technology offered through AbleNet® Inc. covers what simple technology is available, where to find it, how to connect a variety of components to make working systems, guidelines for use and selection. Write for a workshop planning packet. **Source:** 4.

Hammel, J. (1996). *Assistive Technology and Occupational Therapy: A Link to Function*. Bethesda, MD: American Occupational Therapy Association. $235 AOTA members, $270 non-members. Self-paced clinical course covers types of assistive technologies, evaluation and intervention, applications, resources. 28 contact hours, 2.8 continuing education units.

Forms and Plans for Making Equipment

The following forms and plans for construction of equipment may be photocopied from the guide and enlarged.

RULES TO REDUCE STRESS

1. I will set priorities that include my own well-being.

2. I will start each day on a positive note. "I am full of energy. I am alive and good will come to me."

3. I will communicate feelings appropriately to those involved rather than keeping them inside, seeking solutions rather than blame.

4. I will set realistic standards within my health and energy capabilities.

5. I will set aside periods of respite for myself and others, knowing that periods of renewal are necessary for enjoying life and maximizing health.

6. I will reach out to those trained to assist should health care and other needs demand it.

7. I will take one half hour each day to read or do something new for my own growth and delight.

8. When I feel stressed, I will release tensions by walking, visualizing, or otherwise removing myself from a circle of worry.

9. I will do something for someone else each day, which can be as small as a big smile, a compliment, or a hello to a person who is alone.

10. Laughter and joy heal, so I will laugh daily and share that laugh with a family member or friend.

PRINCIPLES FOR ALL AMPUTEES

1. Keep your stump clean. Daily washing is important for hygiene.

2. Daily exercise for range of motion and strengthening should continue after you have completed your rehabilitation, as it should for anyone.

3. Stump socks need to be washed frequently, but may take over a day to dry. Keep extras on hand. To protect the skin on your stump, replace socks as they wear thin.

4. Prostheses do need adjustments, repairs, and replacement over a period of time. Bearings and straps wear out, just as with an automobile or other equipment.

5. Any sore should be immediately reported to your nurse or physician. Breakdown on a stump means off-time from work and activities. Causes of breakdown include poor hygiene, poor positioning or fit of your stump in the socket, overwork, and, with a lower extremity prostheses, walking on uneven surfaces.

A special note: If you are an older individual, or have diabetes or peripheral vascular disease, you must also take very good care of your unaffected limb. Daily hygiene and inspection for any signs of skin breakdown and immediate reporting of these to your health care worker will help prevent complications.

RULES FOR WALKING SAFELY

1. When sitting down, make sure the backs of your legs are touching the chair. If possible, reach back with one hand to locate the chair before lowering yourself.

2. To get up, slide all the way to the front of the chair and get both feet under you. Have the less involved leg further back to give that push as you rise. A chair with arm rests is more efficient.

3. All small rugs and throw rugs should be removed. Taping rugs down will not work, because you can still trip on the edges.

4. When walking on carpet, you must pick up affected leg(s) and feet more than on uncarpeted floor because of friction.

5. Do not try stair climbing on your own. It is not worth the risk. Sitting and bumping your bottom down is an alternate in case of emergency. Stair climbing should be taught to you by a physical therapist or other trained health care professional.

6. When going up or down stairs, use the railing. Add a second railing if necessary (for the hemiplegic).

7. The rule for stairs is up with the good, down with the bad; that is, when ascending or going upstairs, the good leg goes first, coming down the bad leg goes first.

8. When sitting down on a regular toilet seat, you will find it is lower than those at a hospital. If you have difficulty, ask a therapist or nurse to have a raised seat installed and/or a safety bar correctly bolted through the wall at the correct place. Do not use a towel bar or soap dish handle.

9. Keep your head up while walking. It is safer and less tiring.

10. Check the rubber tips on your cane, crutches, or walker periodically, and replace them when smooth or dry. They are as important to you as tires on your car, and you would not let those get cracked or smooth.

11. If you do not feel safe or tire quickly while ambulating with a cane, crutch, or walker, talk with your physician and therapist. There may be times that a glider or wheelchair is safer and allows you more independence.

BE GOOD TO YOUR BACK USING PRINCIPLES OF BODY MECHANICS

The following techniques and tips for good body mechanics are designed to help reduce pain in your back. Learn the proper ways under the care of your therapist.

GENERAL SUGGESTIONS

Good posture helps avoid back pain. Make sure several times a day that you are standing correctly.

If you wake up with a painful back, ask a family member or other person to put a bed board between your mattress and box springs. Beds do wear out, and a new mattress might be in order.

WAYS OF WORKING

For jobs that can be done sitting, select a comfortable chair that supports your back and thighs and lets your feet be flat on the floor.

Keep a high stool near your meal preparation area so you may sit and rest when preparing vegetables, cutting, or mixing.

Divide and conquer; carry two light loads rather than putting everything in one. When lifting a bulky object, bend your knees and hold the item close to your body.

Use wheels, rather than carrying heavy items. A dolly, cart, or child's wheelbarrow will roll groceries, laundry, and other things from one place to another.

Select a comfortable chair for sitting and reading, listening to music, or watching television. It should have firm cushions so the weight of your hips and thighs is evenly distributed, and it should completely support your back. Add a back support if it increases comfort.

ON THE ROAD

When traveling in a car, carry a small, rolled towel that you can place behind you to keep the arch in your back. Get out every hour or so to stretch and walk a little.

If you are traveling extensively, pack a folding bedboard in the car to shore up too soft motel or hotel beds.

KEEP THE GOOD TIMES ROLLING

Join an exercise group geared to your level and interests or a pain support group for help in resolving your pain. Aqua aerobics are easy on the joints; exercise in the water reduces gravity.

RULES TO CONSERVE ENERGY

1. I will eliminate all the non-essentials.
2. I will do those tasks that are within my level of energy.
3. will schedule and take a rest between jobs.
4. I will pace myself and not rush. Tomorrow is soon enough for some things.
5. I will wheel loads rather than carrying.
6. Tasks beyond my strength or capability will be delegated to others. For this, I have no guilt, because it makes me able to share and enjoy time with family and friends.
7. I will seek a balanced program of daily tasks, exercise, and rest.
8. Good nutrition is important to keeping up my strength, so I will eat healthy, balanced meals.

TODAY'S PRIORITY ITEMS
1.
2.
3.
4.

MUST DOS
1.
2.
3.
4.

IF TIME AND ENERGY
1.
2.
3.

MAGIC HOUR OF RELAXATION OR RECREATION:

EXERCISES FOR THE DAY:

SOCIAL/PERSONAL ACTIVITY

RULES FOR HANDLING A FIRE

Following rules of safety, such as never wearing loose, flowing clothes or long, loose sleeves when cooking, keeping an eye on what is on the stove, setting a timer if you tend to forget, and always double checking that a burner is off will help prevent fires in the kitchen.

Being prepared in case of emergency is wise, especially if you move slowly. Here are some basic suggestions:

- Keep a small fire extinguisher nearby. (Make sure you are able to use it.)
- Call the fire department even for a small fire. (If fire spreads out of pan and you are alone, call the fire department immediately and then leave the house.)
- Stove top fire: turn off burner if possible without getting burned, smother fire with pot lid or cutting board. Use a potholder to protect hands when picking up lid or board.
- If fire is small, you may throw baking soda (not baking powder) or salt on it but putting on lid or closing oven door is more efficient.
- Keep a one-pound (coffee) can of baking soda next to the stove, identified for fire use only. This puts an extinguisher for small fires right at hand. Change soda every 2 years.
- Oven fire: shut oven door and turn off controls, leave door closed until fire goes out.
- Do not try to carry a burning pan outside, because motion will fan flames. Handle may become too hot to hold so that it is dropped and spills scalding liquid on you.
- Don't try putting out a fire with water, flour, sugar, or other household powders that might explode.

Client Seating Assessment

1 Client Information

Therapist _____ Date _____

Client name _____ Phone _____

Address_____

Disability_____

Age _____ Sex _____ Onset of disability _____

Cognitive status (list any medications) _____

Visual/auditory status _____

Past medical / surgical history _____

2 Wheelchair Evaluation

Describe existing seating or attach instant photograph to fitting form.

Wheelchair frame type (recline, tilt, etc.) and width _____

Seat cushion (width and length) and accessories _____

Back cushion (height) and accessories _____

Head rest / support _____

Arm positioning _____

Foot positioning _____

Belts / harness _____

Sitting posture in wheelchair (check deviations and document with instant photograph)

____ Posterior pelvic tilt   ____ Kyphosis   ____ Leg abduction
____ Anterior pelvic tilt   ____ Lordosis   ____ Leg adduction
____ Pelvic obliquity   ____ Scoliosis convex to: ____ Wind sweeping
　　❑ right ❑ left   　　❑ right ❑ left   ____ Other _____
____ Pelvic rotation   ____ Forward head/neck   _____
　　protracted forward to: 　　hyperextension   _____
　　❑ right ❑ left   _____

3 Function

Type of transfer _____ Amount of assist needed _____

Wheelchair propulsion _____

Activities of daily living _____

4 Sitting Evaluation

Sitting balance
____ Good / Hands-free with ability to weight shift
____ Fair / Hands-free only
____ Poor / Propped with hand support
____ Dependent / Needs external support

Sitting posture on mat table	Fixed	Flexible	Discrepancy: 1"	2"	3"
____ Posterior pelvic tilt					
____ Anterior pelvic tilt	____	____	____	____	____
____ Pelvic obliquity					
❑ right ❑ left	____	____	____	____	____
____ Pelvic rotation protracted forward to:					
❑ right ❑ left	____	____	____	____	____
____ Kyphosis	____	____			
____ Lordosis	____	____			
____ Scoliosis convex to:	____	____			
❑ right ❑ left					
____ Forward head/neck hyperextension	____	____			
____ Leg abduction	____	____			
____ Leg adduction	____	____			
____ Wind sweeping	____	____			
____ Other _____	____	____			
____ Other _____	____	____			

Comments _____
_____
_____
_____
_____
_____

JAY. MEDICAL

Jay Medical, Ltd.
P.O. Box 18656
Boulder, Colorado
80308-8656 USA

(303) 442.5529

(800) 648.8282

© 1991, Jay Medical, Ltd.
XT016

Client Seating Assessment continued

4 Sitting Evaluation
(continued)

Overall body width

Tonal influences/ reflexes in sitting	Seating implications
___ Extensor	Seat to back angle 90° or less
___ Flexor	Evaluate positioning strap placement
___ ATNR	Inhibit head rotation with head support
___ STNR	Inhibit neck flexion/extension with head support
___ Positive support	Foot rest angle important
___ Ankle clonus	Total foot support/positioning straps
___ Other	_____

Comments _____
_____

Sitting length measurements

Hip width _____

Overall body width _____

Leg length (from sacrum to popliteal fossa):

right _____

left _____

5 Supine Evaluation

Supine posture on mat table	Fixed	Flexible	Comments
___ Pelvic tilt			_____
❏ anterior	___	___	_____
❏ posterior	___	___	_____
___ Pelvic obliquity	___	___	_____
___ Pelvic rotation	___	___	_____
___ Kyphosis	___	___	_____
___ Lordosis	___	___	_____
___ Scoliosis	___	___	_____

Supine range of motion

Hip flexion (norm = 0° - 125°) _____

Knee extension with hip at 90° _____

Other _____

Seating considerations

Recline back or leg trough if less than 90°

Foot rest placement

6 Skin Condition

Location	Old Scarring	Redness	Size	Time before redness disappears	Open sore grade 2	3	4	Shape/color
Ischial tuberosities	___	___	___	___	❏	❏	❏	_____
Coccyx	___	___	___	___	❏	❏	❏	_____
Spine	___	___	___	___	❏	❏	❏	_____
Other	___	___	___	___	❏	❏	❏	_____

7 Goal Setting

Determination of goals

❏ Improve posture _____

❏ Pressure relief _____

❏ Accommodate deformity _____

❏ Accommodate joint limitations _____

❏ Relieve pain / increase sitting tolerance _____

❏ Reduce tonal influences _____

❏ Improve functional level _____

❏ Improve head position / visual field _____

❏ Allow for growth / weight gain _____

❏ Improve appearance _____

❏ Meet caregiver goals _____

❏ Meet transportation / vocational / school needs _____

❏ Other _____
_____

JAY. MEDICAL

Jay Medical, Ltd.
P.O. Box 18656
Boulder, Colorado
80308-8656 USA

(303) 442.5529

(800) 648.8282

LOW LAP BOARD - to provide a comfortable, low work surface within the arms of the wheel chair.

Use a plywood board 1/4 to 1/2 inch thick with a semi-circular cut-out to fit around the body.

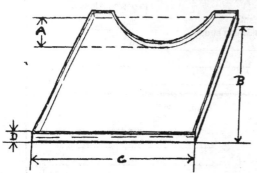

Dimensions: A - approximately 4 and 1/2 inches.

B - depth of the board should fit the person allowing maximum work surface as close to the body as comfortable and not extending more than 6 inches beyond the end of the arm rests.

C - width to fit between the arms of the wheel chair with enough clearance to allow tray to be slid on and off easily.

D - raised edge on all sides, approximately 1/4 inch above surface, to prevent items from sliding off.

Brackets - Back brackets should be as far back as lapboard allows and the front brackets should be at the front end of the arm rests.

For wheel chairs with regular arms.

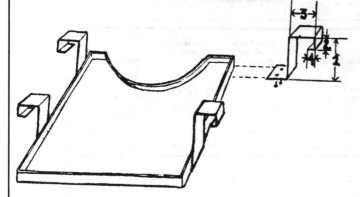

Dimensions:

1. As long as possible to allow level work surface with 1/2 inch clearance above thighs. Measure with braces if they are worn.

2. Thickness of arm rest plus 1/8th inch.

3. Width of the arm rest plus 1/8th inch.

4. Approximately 1/2 inch.

For wheel chairs with desk arms.

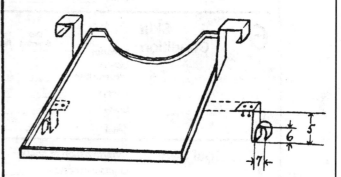

Dimensions:

5. As short as possible to allow level work surface with 1/2 inch clearance above thighs. Measure with braces if they are worn.

6. and 7. To fit around tubing at front of desk arms.

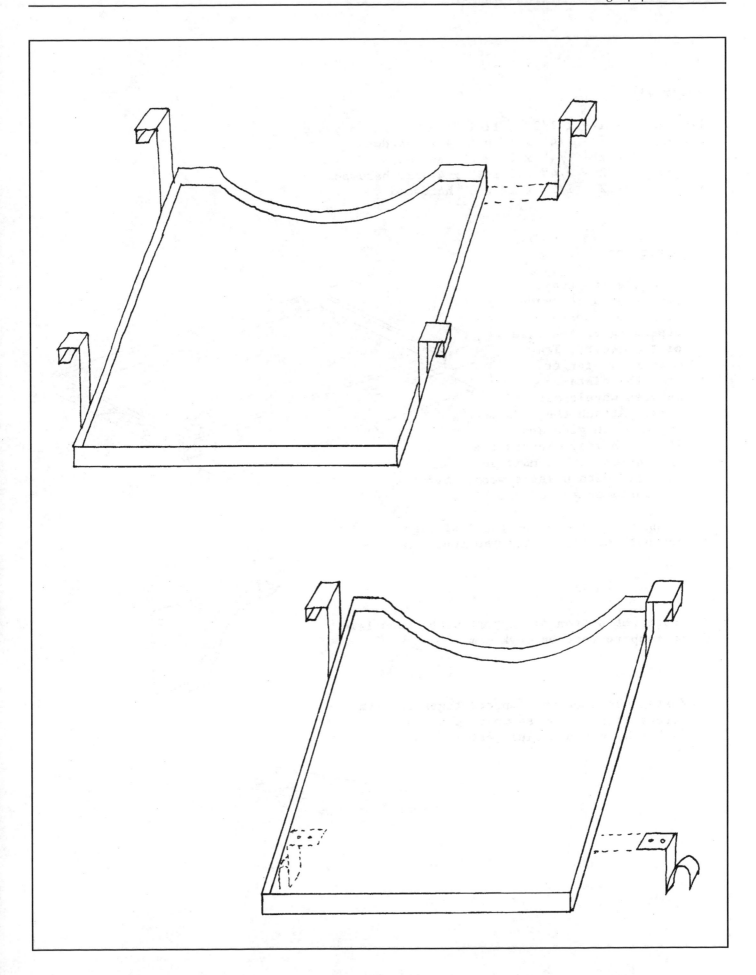

Materials

```
bottom     - 1 - 1 1/2" x 11 1/2" x 21 1/2" plywood
edging     - 2 - 1/4" x 1" x 11 1/2" hardwood
           - 2 - 1/4" x 1" x 22" hardwood
supports  -- 2 - 3/4" x 3 1/4" x 4 1/2" hardwood
hook       - 2 - 1/2" x 2" x 8" hardwood
```

Construction

1. Assemble the tray.
   The tray can be made
   longer or shorter,
   depending on the size
   of the chair. Tray
   must be 4" longer
   than the distance
   between wheelchair
   arms. Attach the
   edging with glue and
   1" wire brads. Recess the
   nail heads with a nail set
   and fill with plastic wood. Sand
   all surfaces and edges.

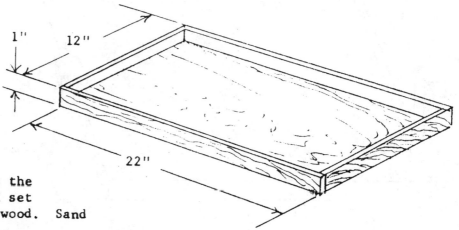

2. Using the patterns on the last page
   cut out the pieces for the supports.

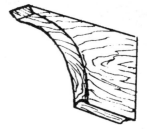

3. Gouge out bottom of support with round file
   or rasp to rest on desk arm.

4. Fasten the hook and support together with
   screws at position shown on pattern.
   (Note: Do not use glue yet)

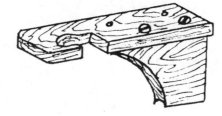

5. Position supports on bottom
of tray.

(a) Measure distance between
wheelchair arms directly below arm rests.

(b) Check wheelchair arms for
alignment. Bent armrests will
affect fitting.

(c) Find center of tray.

(d) Divide measurement (a)
in half. Measure from center
of tray on both sides this
half distance.

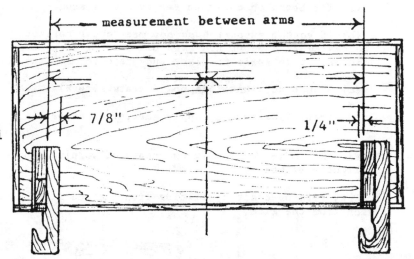

(e) On the side with the hook facing toward the center, measure in 1/4"
and draw a line.

(f) On the side with hook facing away from the center, measure in 7/8"
and draw a line.

(g) Lay pieces along these lines as shown and screw them fast.

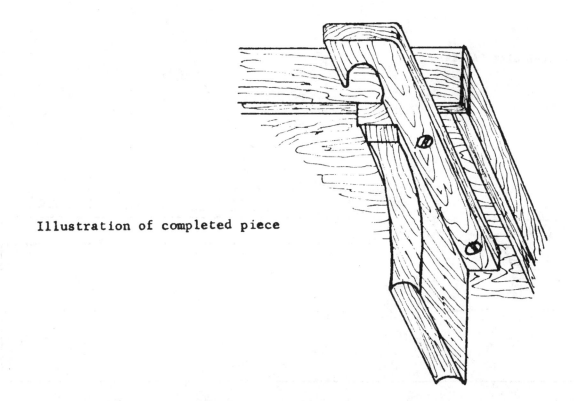

Illustration of completed piece

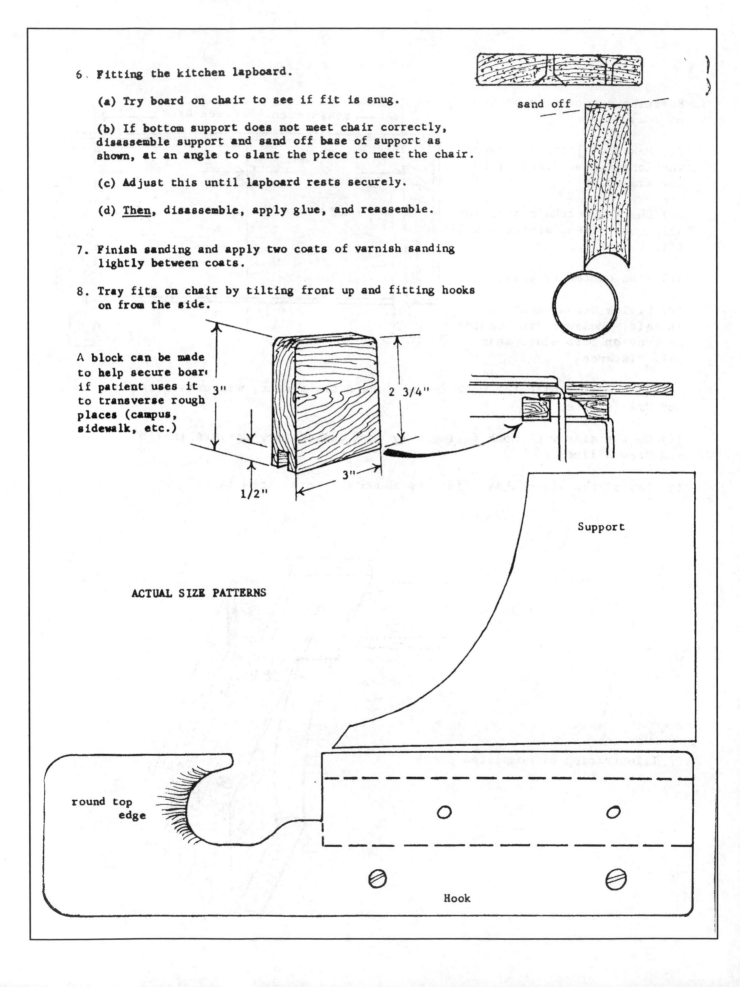

6. Fitting the kitchen lapboard.

   (a) Try board on chair to see if fit is snug.

   (b) If bottom support does not meet chair correctly,
   disassemble support and sand off base of support as
   shown, at an angle to slant the piece to meet the chair.

   (c) Adjust this until lapboard rests securely.

   (d) <u>Then</u>, disassemble, apply glue, and reassemble.

7. Finish sanding and apply two coats of varnish sanding
   lightly between coats.

8. Tray fits on chair by tilting front up and fitting hooks
   on from the side.

A block can be made
to help secure board
if patient uses it
to transverse rough
places (campus,
sidewalk, etc.)

sand off

3"

2 3/4"

3"

1/2"

ACTUAL SIZE PATTERNS

Support

round top
edge

Hook

CERTIFICATE OF MEDICAL NECESSITY FOR DURABLE EQUIPMENT

Date _____

Medicare requires the following information to document medical necessity for the rental/purchase of durable medical equipment. This form must be filled out by the patient's attending physician and is not valid unless signed by the physician.

Patient's Name _____ Age _____ HIC# _____

Patient's Address _____

Diagnosis _____

_____

_____

Method of Treatment _____

Prognosis _____

Months of medical necessity _____ to _____

Complete description of equipment prescribed, include any special features or attachments _____

_____

_____

Medical necessity for special features or attachments _____

_____

_____

Therapeutic value of equipment _____

_____

_____

Physician will supervise equipment use in connection with course of treatment_____

_____

_____

Equipment is necessary to effect improvement or to arrest or retard deterioration in patient's condition_____

_____

_____

Note: Answer the following questions that apply to the piece of equipment.

Is ambulation impaired? _____ If yes, you are prescribing _____

Severity of impairment _____

Is the patient bed confined?_____ Wheelchair confined? _____

Is equipment medically necessary to help patient get in and out of bed? _____

Is the alternative to the use of this equipment wheelchair and bed confinement? _____

Medical condition requiring patient to change body position _____

Is patient highly susceptible to decubitus ulcers?_____

Does patient have decubitus ulcers? _____

Is patient's ability to breathe severely impaired? _____

Is equipment being used to mobilize respiratory tract infections? _____

Comments _____

_____

_____

Physician Name_____ Telephone # _____

Address _____

Physician Signature_____ Date _____

Note: Payment will cease if no reply is received 45 days from the date of this letter.

Effective 10/93   DURABLE MEDICAL EQUIPMENT REGIONAL CARRIER   DMERC 07.01

CERTIFICATE OF MEDICAL NECESSITY: SEAT LIFT MECHANISMS/POWER OPERATED VEHICLES (POV)

SECTION A   CERTIFICATION: ☐ INITIAL ☐ REVISED

PATIENT NAME, ADDRESS, TELEPHONE AND HIC NO.	SUPPLIER NAME, ADDRESS, TELEPHONE, AND NSC NUMBER
(___) ____-____ HICN _____	(___) ____-____ NSC _____

PLACE OF SERVICE ____ REPLACEMENT ITEM ____	HCPCS CODE(S) WARRANTY LENGTH TYPE
NAME AND ADDRESS OF FACILITY IF APPLICABLE (SEE BACK OF FORM):	_____ _____ _____ _____ _____ _____ _____ _____ _____ _____ _____ _____

SECTION B   INFORMATION BELOW TO BE COMPLETED ONLY BY THE PHYSICIAN OR PHYSICIAN'S EMPLOYEE

DIAGNOSIS (ICD9): _____ _____ _____ _____	DOB ___/___/___
I LAST EXAMINED THIS PATIENT FOR THIS CONDITION ON: ___/___/___ PT. SEX ____ (M OR F)	DATE NEEDED INITIAL ___/___/___ REVISED ___/___/___ EST. LENGTH OF NEED: # OF MONTHS: ____ 1-99 (99 = LIFETIME)

ANSWER QUESTIONS 1-5 FOR SEAT LIFT MECHANISMS, ANSWER QUESTIONS 6-14 FOR POWER OPERATED VEHICLES (POV)
Use Y - Yes, N - No or D for Does Not Apply   unless otherwise noted.

SEAT LIFT MECHANISM

[   ] 1.   Does the patient have severe arthritis of the hip or knee?

[   ] 2.   Does the patient have a severe neuromuscular disease?

[   ] 3.   Is the patient completely incapable of standing up from a regular armchair or <u>any</u> chair in his/her home?

[   ] 4.   Once standing, does the patient have the ability to ambulate?

[   ] 5.   Have all appropriate therapeutic modalities to enable the patient to transfer from a chair to a standing position (e.g., medication, physical therapy) been tried and failed? If YES, this is documented in the patient's records.

POWER OPERATED VEHICLE

[   ] 6.   Would the patient be bed or chair confined without the use of a wheelchair?

[   ] 7.   Is the patient unable to operate a manual wheelchair?

[   ] 8.   Can the patient ambulate in the home but the POV is required for movement outside the home?

[   ] 9.   Is the patient capable of safely transferring in and out of the POV?

[   ] 10. Is the patient capable of safely operating the controls of the POV?

[   ] 11. Does the patient have adequate trunk stability to be able to safely ride in the POV?

[   ] 12. Are you a specialist in physical medicine, orthopedic surgery, neurology, or rheumatology?

[   ] 13. Is the patient more than one day's roundtrip from a specialist in physical medicine, orthopedic surgery, neurology, or rheumatology?

[   ] 14. Does the patient's condition preclude a visit to a specialist in physical medicine, orthopedic surgery, neurology, or rheumatology?

I certify the medical necessity of these items for this patient. Section B of this form and any statement on my letterhead attached hereto has been completed by me, or by my employee and reviewed by me. The foregoing information is true, accurate, and complete, and I understand that any falsification, omission, or concealment of material fact may subject me to civil or criminal liability.

PHYSICIAN NAME, ADDRESS	
	PHYSICIAN'S SIGNATURE: _____ ___/___/___ DATE (A STAMPED SIGNATURE IS NOT ACCEPTABLE) ☐ Attending ☐ Consulting ☐ Other ordering UPIN: _____ TELEPHONE #: (___) ____-____

SECTION A: (To be completed by the supplier)

CERTIFICATION TYPE:	Check the appropriate box to indicate if this CMN is the initial certification for this patient or if this is a revised certification.
BENEFICIARY INFORMATION:	Indicate the beneficiary's name, permanent legal address, telephone number and his/her health insurance claim number (HICN) as it appears on the beneficiary's Medicare card and on your claim form.
PLACE OF SERVICE:	Indicate the place in which the item is being used, i.e., patient's home is 12, skilled nursing facility (SNF) is 31, End Stage Renal Disease (ESRD) facility is 65, etc. Refer to your supplier manual for a complete index.
REPLACEMENT:	If the item billed is a replacement for a previously purchased item, place a check mark in the blank.
FACILITY NAME:	If the place of service is a facility, indicate the name and complete address of the facility.
SUPPLIER INFORMATION:	Indicate the name of your company (supplier name), address and telephone number along with the Medicare Supplier Number assigned to you by the National Supplier Clearinghouse (NSC).
HCPCS CODES:	List all procedure codes for items ordered that require a CMN. Procedure codes that do not require a certification should not be listed on the CMN. If the item ordered is purchased equipment, indicate whether the equipment is covered by a warranty. "Y" denotes that there is a warranty and "N" indicates there is no warranty. If it is covered by a warranty, the length and type of warranty must be indicated.

SECTION B: (To be completed by the physician or physician's employee)

DIAGNOSIS:	In the first space, list the ICD9 code that represents the primary reason for ordering this item. List any additional ICD9 codes that would further describe the medical need for the item (up to 3).
EXAMINATION DATE:	Indicate the date (MM/DD/YY) the patient was last seen by the ordering physician prior to the beginning of this certification period.
DOB:	Indicate patient's date of birth (MM/DD/YY).
DATE NEEDED:	Indicate the date (MM/DD/YY) the ordered item was initially needed outside the hospital setting. If this certification is a revised certification, also indicate the effective date of the order change.
EST. LENGTH OF NEED:	Indicate the estimated length of need (the length of time the physician expects the patient to require use of the ordered item) by filling in the appropriate number of months. If the physician expects that the patient will require the item for the duration of his/her life, then enter 99.
QUESTION SECTION:	This section is used to gather clinical information to determine medical necessity. Answer each question within the category of the items ordered, using "Y" for yes, "N" for no, and "D" for does not apply, unless otherwise noted.
PHYSICIAN INFORMATION:	The physician's signature certifies that the item ordered is medically necessary for this patient and that section B was completed or reviewed by the physician. This form must be signed and dated by the physician. Signature and date stamps are not acceptable.
	The physician must indicate whether he/she is the attending, consulting or other ordering physician by putting a check mark in the appropriate box. Indicate other ordering when you are neither the attending or consulting physician. Refer to your supplier manual for more information.
PHYSICIAN NAME, ADDRESS:	Indicate physician's name and complete mailing address.
UPIN:	The physician must indicate his/her Unique Physician Identification Number (UPIN).
PHYSICIAN'S TELEPHONE NO:	The physician must give a telephone number where he/she can be contacted (preferably a number where records would be accessible pertaining to this patient) if more information is needed.

Howard A. Rusk Institute of Rehabilitation Medicine
New York University Medical Center
Occupational Therapy Department

Name: _____

APPLICATION OF ENERGY CONSERVATON TO DAILY ACTIVITIES

BATHING:

1. Use a shower commode chair and a hand-held shower to eliminate the need for standing.
2. Use long handled sponges and soap on a rope to eliminate need for bending.
3. For drying, use a heat lamp, thick bathrobe, or pat dry.
4. Turn on cold water before hot water to reduce steam.
5. Use oxygen at dosage prescribed for exercise.

GROOMING:

1. Sit whenever possible.
2. Organize work space to avoid bending or reaching.
3. Support elbows on table.
4. Coordinate motions of grooming with breathing patterns.
5. Avoid using aerosols or strong scents.
6. Keep grooming needs as simple as possible; short haircuts will tend to decrease upper extremity work.
7. Utilize the barber shop, beauty parlor, home hair care.

DRESSING:

1. Keep well organized, particularly your closet space.
2. Use clothes with front fasteners, clothes which are not tight, slip-on shoes and/or shoes with Velcro closures. Suspenders may be more comfortable than belts, which may constrict the abdomen.
3. Plan ahead. The evening before, organize all clothing for the next day in a convenient place, near your dressing area. Have clothes within arms reach.
4. Sit whenever possible.
5. Use breathing pattern techniques throughout dressing routine.
6. Dress lower body first, as this requires the most energy expenditure.
7. Put on more than one item at a time, such as underwear and pants or skirt.
8. Do not bend. Bring feet up to you or use adaptive equipment as recommended by your Occupational Therapist.
9. Do not rush. Move slowly and methodically.
10. Take rests while you are dressing.

LAUNDRY:

1. Use a laundry cart; do not carry a basket of laundry.
2. Do not wash large loads. Wash small loads throughout the week.
3. Have someone assist you with washing towels and sheets.
4. Avoid scrubbing. Soak very soiled clothes for 20 to 30 minutes or use stain remover before washing.
5. Roll clothes in a towel instead of wringing.
6. Hang clothes on hangers when taking out of the dryer to avoid wrinkles and need for ironing.
7. Do not hang clothes on the line. Always avoid reaching with your hands above your shoulders.
8. Lower ironing board so that you are sitting while ironing. You save 24% of your energy if you sit to iron. Sit on a chair that supports your back and have your feet flat on the floor. Lower ironing board so your wrist is lower than your elbow while ironing.
9. Organize ironing area to avoid bending. For example, place a chair or table within arms' reach to receive the clothes just ironed.
10. Do not bear down on the iron, just guide it.
11. Lift iron as few times as possible.

BEDMAKING:

1. Avoid bending by raising bed on bricks or blocks of wood.
2. Avoid moving the bed by having it away from the walls.
3. If the bed must be moved, have bed on casters or rollers.
4. Do not open sheets up in the air. Place it on the bed and unfold it. Use breathing pattern techniques.
5. Make only one trip around the bed.

MARKETING:

1. Plan ahead. Do frequent shopping to avoid heavy bundles. Plan in advance for the week so that heavy items are purchased on different days.
2. Phone for orders when possible.
3. Have bundles delivered when possible.
4. Use a shopping cart; do not carry heavy bundles.
5. While in the market, use a list to avoid walking down unnecessary aisles.
6. Use breathing pattern techniques.
7. Shop at a relaxed pace, taking rest periods.
8. When at home, store groceries where they will be used first.

MEAL PREPARATION:

1. Plan meals in advance.
2. Store items you use every day on the most convenient shelf to avoid reaching or bending.
3. Store aprons and linens in a convenient drawer.
4. Use breathing pattern techniques.
5. Work at a relaxed pace, taking rest periods.
6. Sit to prepare meals. The height of the working area should allow you to work without raising your hands above the level of your elbows.
7. Slide pots and pans along the counter, do not lift or carry them.
8. When transporting items, use a cart to avoid lifting and carrying. For example, taking items from the refrigerator to the counter or while setting the table.
9. Prepare one dish meals, such as casseroles.
10. Serve food in the baking dish.
11. Soak pots in hot, soapy water to eliminate scouring.
12. Let dishes air dry, rather than wiping them.

HOUSECLEANING:

1. Plan housekeeping tasks throughout the week, to balance heavy and light activites.
2. Clean approximately one room per day.
3. Avoid sweeping, mopping, washing windows, and heavy cleaning.
4. Gather all tools necessary for the task before you begin.
5. Sit while performing tasks, whenever possible.
6. Use breathing pattern techniques.
7. Work at a relaxed pace, take rest periods.
8. Use long handled tools when possible, for example, while dusting or picking up dust from the floor.
9. Dust with two hands.

Please call if you have questions:
Occupational Therapist: _____
Telephone #:_____

Howard A. Rusk Institute of Rehabilitation Medicine
New York University Medical Center
Occupational Therapy Department

JOINT PROTECTION TECHNIQUES AND HINTS

1. Remove scatter rugs so you don't slip and fall.

2. Select chairs that are slightly higher and firmer than a standard chair.

3. Change positions frequently; alternate sitting with standing.

4. Rest often; avoid fatigue. However, keep active for necessary exercise.

5. Stop immediately any activity which produces pain. Do not undertake an activity which cannot be interrupted for rest.

6. Avoid hip and knee flexion contractures by lying on your stomach at night.

7. Avoid twisting of knees when standing up by standing first, then turning.

8. Use both hands during activities to lessen the stress on joints.

9. Always use larger joints rather than smaller joints, i.e., when carrying a tray or plate, rest it on your forearm or palms of hands rather than holding it by the fingers of one hand.

10. Slip a pocketbook over the forearm or use a shoulder bag. Pots can be carried using one hand flat underneath and steadied by the other hand.

11. When lifting objects, place side of one hand on table to assist as object is grasped with other hand. Ex.: lifting a glass or dish.

12. Adjust size of handles for a safe and comfortable grip by wrapping some foam or material around the handle to enlarge it.

13. Adjust the angle of grip to prevent deforming pressure. Ex.: hold a knife with the blade end protruding from the little finger side while pushing the hand away from ulnar deviation. Hold stirring spoons the same way.

14. Sit rather than stand during meal preparation.

15. Use wheeled-vehicles (tea cart) to avoid lifting and carrying: PUSH OR ROLL heavy objects.

16. Avoid holding vegetables; use a board to stabilize the vegetable being cut. Minimize sustained grasp.

17. Store kitchen equipment near the place you will use it first (pans for cooking vegetables near water; baking utensils near flour and sugar).

18. Use lightweight kitchen equipment (aluminum or plastic).

19. Stack only those things that are the same size. Use lazy susans so reaching to the back of cabinets is eliminated.

20. Set the table or make the bed in one trip around.

21. Include exercise while in the kitchen but avoid stress that can cause damage to joints.

    REACH - for shoulder flexion and elbow extension.

    BEND - for flexion and extension of the back, hips, and knees.

22. Avoid increasing flexion deformities in the hands by working with your fingers flat while:

    (a) pushing up from a chair; (b) pushing drawers shut; (c)using a sponge; (d) using a dusting mitt.

23. Use long smooth strokes to help increase motion in the shoulder, elbow, and wrist (ironing, dusting, polishing furniture, vacuuming, washing windows).

24. Press water from a cloth or sponge rather than wring it.

25. When ironing, lower board to a height that is comfortable for sitting; have a chair or table nearby on which to hang or fold and stack ironed clothes.

26. When using a twisting motion always turn hand toward the thumb (turning doorknobs or keys in locks, screwing jar lids on and off, ironing clothes).

Please call if you have any questions or problems.

Ext.: _____   Date: _____

Name: _____

Howard A. Rusk Institute of Rehabilitation Medicine
New York University Medical Center
Occupational Therapy Department

ENERGY CONSERVATION
AND
WORK SIMPLIFICATION TECHNIQUES

The purpose of work simplification and energy conservation is to allow you to use your time and energy more efficiently when performing daily tasks. By adapting the following suggested techniques to your daily lifestyle and home situation, you will be better able to perform your maximum amount of work with minimal expenditure of energy.

General Considerations

1. Use breath control. Exhale with strenuous part of activity (for example, when rising from sitting position).

2. Adopt a moderate pace of working and allow enough time to do things so you don't have to rush at the last minute.
   - Always walk slowly, use breathing control.
   - Use slow, smooth, and flowing movements.

3. Do as much planning ahead as possible.
   - Daily, make a list of things you need to do.
   - Spread activities throughout the day with rest periods in between.
   - Spread heavy and light tasks throughout the week.

4. Break down your activities into steps and figure out the most efficient method of accomplishing the task.
   - Do them the same manner each time; repetition will make you more efficient and save time and energy.
   - Avoid unnecessary trips by carrying all needed equipment at one time, i.e., into the bathroom, setting the table.

5. Organize your work area having most frequently used items easily accessible. Avoid unnecessary bending, reaching, and stretching.

6. Sit for as many activities as possible.
   - Use a chair or stool with back support while performing all activities.
   - Keep your feet flat on the floor or on a footrest for support.

7. Take frequent rests. This will prevent over fatigue and leave you energy for other activities.
   - Always remember to use breath control when resting.

8. Utilize family members to assist with difficult or strenuous tasks.

9. Whenever possible, do not lift or carry equipment. Push objects along or wheel or cart heavy objects.

Please call if you have any questions: _____
                                    Ext.   Date:

Howard A. Rusk Institute of Rehabilitation Medicine
New York University Medical Center
Occupational Therapy Department

BODY MECHANICS PRINCIPLES

1. Use a good base of support; feet should be shoulder distance apart.

2. Keep objects as close to your body and as close to your center of gravity as possible when lifting and carrying. Hold objects in front of your body.

3. Bend at the hips and knees rather than at your waist. Use leg muscles instead of back muscles for lifting and moving.

4. Keep your hips and shoulders parallel. Avoid twisting in your torso. Face the direction of your job.

5. When possible, push before you pull, and pull before you lift. Use your entire body to do these activities.

6. It helps to maintain a slight pelvic tilt when lifting, pushing, pulling, and carrying.

7. Divide loads to avoid one heavy load.

8. Change body positions frequently, sitting and standing.

9. You will tire less if you maintain good posture as you move. Increase your efficiency by using your entire body together as a unit.

10. Use both hands together for lifting, pushing, pulling, carrying, sliding, etc.

11. Use long, rhythmical, sweeping, continuous motions instead of short, jerky ones. Develop a comfortable, regular breathing pattern.

12. Avoid rushing; rest before you get tired and move at a comfortable, easy, relaxed pace.

13. Do not perform unnecessary tasks. Prepare yourself and your activity area before getting started.

14. Wear comfortable and suitable clothes. Wear clothing that allows free leg and arm movements as well as a comfortable breathing pattern. Shoes should provide comfort and support.

RULES TO INCREASE YOUR SAFETY WHEN DRIVING

- Always wear your safety belt, and make sure your passengers do too.

- If you wear a hearing aid, always use it when driving. It's the law. Add extra large mirrors on both sides of the car to give you more visual awareness of traffic patterns.

- If you do not feel like driving, don't go. Ask a friend to drive, call for a transportation service, take a bus, or postpone your errands.

- Do not drive when conditions are at all hazardous.

- Make adjustments in the car, especially if you have lost height, so that you get a clear view over the steering wheel. Add a cushion if necessary.

- Add extra mirrors if there is any limitation in neck motion or peripheral vision. Some models of cars do not have a right hand or passenger's side outside mirror.

- If wearing glasses, avoid frames with wide side pieces that block peripheral vision.

- Do not wear sunglasses or heavily tinted regular glasses for night driving, because they reduce light coming into your eyes.

- Avoid night driving if you are bothered by or cannot adjust to glare, if you think your glasses or windshield are dirty, if you see halos around lights, such as street lights, or cannot walk along the street or in your yard at night as in earlier years.

- Keep glasses as well as the windshield, mirrors, headlights, and tail lights clean for maximum light and minimum glare.

- Avoid dawn and dusk driving, because these are when it is hardest to judge distances.

- Do not drive if taking medications, like analgesics, which may cause confusion, drowsiness, and inability to concentrate. Ask about side effects of any medication, including antihistamines, which may cause blurred vision.

- Pull off the road if you feel weak or dizzy, and wait until you are completely recovered before resuming driving. Consult a physician about the symptoms as soon as possible.

- Keep your car ready for emergencies with flares, flashlight, and a blanket. If your mobility is limited, a cellular phone is a real asset.

PRODUCE/VEGETABLES

asparagus	carrots	kale	peas	squash
avocado	cauliflower	lettuce	peppers	tomatoes
beans	celery	mushrooms	potatoes	zucchini
beets	corn	okra	radishes	
broccoli	cucumber	onions	spinach	
cabbage	garlic	parsley	sprouts	

PRODUCE/FRUITS

apples	berries	lemons	nectarines	pears
apricots	grapefruit	limes	oranges	plums
bananas	grapes	melon	peaches	

BREADS, CRACKERS

bread, white	bread, whole wheat	crackers	rolls, buns

MEATS AND FISH

beef	ham	pork chops	turkey, ground
chicken	hamburger	stew meat	veal
fish	pork	turkey	

JUICES

apple juice	grape juice	orange juice	seltzer	tomato juice
cranberry juice	grapefruit juice	pineapple juice	soda	vegetable juice

FROZEN

beans	ice cream	mixed vegetables	pizza
broccoli	ice milk	pastries	sherbet
cauliflower	orange juice	peas	yogurt

CONDIMENTS

cinnamon	ketchup	pepper	salt substitute
garlic powder	mustard	salt	

DAIRY

butter	cheese, cream	cheese, other	milk	yogurt
cheese, cottage	cheese, Swiss	eggs	ricotta	

CANNED

baby food	fruit	mayonnaise	chicken	vegetable
baked beans	jam, jelly	peanut butter	mushroom	tuna fish
bouillon	kidney beans	soups	oniontomato	

STAPLES

baking powder	cereal, hot	dry milk	pasta
baking soda	cocoa	flour	spaghetti sauce
cake mix	coffee	gelatin	tea
cereal, cold	cookies	oil	vinegar

SUPER SHOPPER CHECKLIST

Most people have a routine when shopping for food. Check the boxes below that best describe what you do before, during, and after each trip to the supermarket. Small changes in your shopping habits may make it easier to prepare meals at home.

	Hardly ever	Sometimes	Most of the time
Before shopping I: Check to see what foods I have on hand. Plan meals to include a variety of foods from each of the major food groups. Plan food purchases to keep amounts of fat, sugars, and sodium moderate. Consider how much money I have to spend on food.			
While shopping I: Read ingredient labels, watching for ingredients that provide fat, sugars, and sodium. Use nutrition labels to help select food products. Use open dating information to ensure freshness. Use unit pricing to compare prices.			
After shopping I: Store food promptly and properly to maintain its nutritive value and quality. Place newer foods in the back of refrigerator, freezer, and cabinet shelves so older foods will be used first. Use perishable foods promptly to avoid waste.			
Shopping for and Making Meals in Minutes Using the Dietary Guidelines, U.S. Dept. of Agriculture, Human Nutrition Information Service. Home & Garden Bulletin No. 232-10.			

Use this form to help you keep track of what you eat each day. Bring it to your next therapy session so you can study it for ways to improve your diet and meet your dietary goals.

	Food Item	Portion Size	Calories from fat	Calories	Cholesterol	Sodium	Fiber
Breakfast							
Lunch							
Dinner							
Snack							
Daily Totals							
Today's Exercise							
Goal							
Today's Summary							

A QUINTET OF RULES AND TWO SEASONING RECIPES TO HELP LOWER SALT INTAKE

1. Choose foods without added salt. An increasing number of low-sodium foods are on the market, including canned and frozen plain vegetables and fruit, lower salt sliced ham and turkey, cheese, soups, tuna, tomato and vegetable juices, even no-salt assorted pickles and snacks as well as seasonings.
2. Put the salt shaker away. Increasingly, you and the family will forget to ask for it.
3. Cook without added salt using non-sodium flavors like herbs and lemon.
4. Avoid sauces and condiments, like soy and chili sauce, and foods in brine like sauerkraut.
5. Read labels when shopping. These two blends season dishes without adding salt:

SPICY BLEND

1 tablespoon dry mustard
¾ teaspoon garlic powder
1 tablespoon onion powder or dried onion
½ teaspoon ground allspice
1 teaspoon ground cumin
⅛ teaspoon ground red pepper (optional)

Mix ingredients well. Store in small tightly covered jar or covered shaker. ¼ teaspoon seasons 4 servings. Try for broiled chicken or fish.

ITALIAN SEASONING MIX

1 tablespoon crushed dried oregano
1 tablespoon crushed dried basil
1 tablespoon dried parsley
¾ teaspoon dried onion powder
¾ teaspoon crushed dried thyme
½ teaspoon garlic powder
½ teaspoon ground pepper (optional)

Mix ingredients well, storing in small covered jar or shaker with a cover. Use for meat loaves, spaghetti sauces, or sprinkle directly on pasta and vegetables then toss well.

This panel appears on the back of every package.

Serving sizes are now more consistent among similar products.

Total calories per serving are indicated, as are the number of these calories derived from fat.

% Daily Value shows how a serving of food fits into an overall daily diet. It is based on a daily intake of 2,000 calories. (There is no daily value for sugars or protein.)

Daily Values, the recommended daily intakes, are provided for both a 2,000 and a 2,500 calorie diet.

THE NEW FOOD LABEL

Nutrition Facts
Serving Size $1/2$ cup (114g)
Servings Per Container 4

Amount Per Serving

Calories 260   Calories from Fat 120

	% Daily Value*
Total Fat 13g	**20**%
Saturated Fat 5g	**25**%
Cholesterol 30mg	**10**%
Sodium 660mg	**28**%
Total Carbohydrate 31g	**11**%
Dietary Fiber 0g	**0**%
Sugars 5g	
Protein 5g	

Vitamin A 4%	•	Vitamin C 2%
Calcium 15%	•	Iron 4%

* Percent Daily Values are based on a 2,000 calorie diet. Your daily values may be higher or lower depending on your calorie needs:

		Calories:	2,000	2,500
Total Fat	Less than		65g	80g
Sat Fat	Less than		20g	25g
Cholesterol	Less than		300mg	300mg
Sodium	Less than		2,400mg	2,400mg
Total Carbohydrate			300g	375g
Dietary Fiber			25g	30g

Calories per gram:
Fat 9 • Carbohydrate 4 • Protein 4

RECIPE/TECHNIQUES CHART

	Swedish turkey meatballs	Stir-fried chicken and vegetables	Spiced orange and apple sauce	Light cinnamon sour cream coffee cake	
Opening can					
Opening box					
Opening jar					
Measuring liquids					
Measuring dry ingredients					
Using measuring spoons					
Preparing vegetables/fruits					
Breaking egg					
Beating egg					
Cutting up meat					
Mixing by hand					
Using electric mixer					
Using food processor or blender					
Transferring batter					
Using stove top					
Setting oven					
Putting pan in oven					
Removing from oven					
Using broiler					
Using electric skillet					
Using microwave					
Recipe					

INDEX

Tear-Out Suggestion Card

From time to time new information that may be of interest or help to you will become available. In order to let you know about it and more fully meet your needs as a homemaker, this tear-out page has been included.

In this third edition of *Health Care Professionals Guide* we've been able to share some of the suggestions that came from readers of the previous edition; we also will be glad to try and answer your questions. Your participation has been valuable and we look forward to hearing from you. Please send suggestions, questions, and comments to:

SLACK Incorporated
6900 Grove Road
Thorofare, New Jersey 08086

Name:
    Miss
    Mrs. _____
    Mr.

Street _____

City _____ State _____ Zip _____

Age: ❑ Under 20   ❑ 20 to 35   ❑ 35 to 50   ❑ 51 to 65   65 to 70   ❑ Over 70

How many do you cook for?   ❑ Myself   ❑ Husband and myself   ❑ Family (give number)_____

Handicap (if any): _____

Suggestions I have found helpful:_____

_____

_____

Other areas and problems I would like to see covered: _____

_____

_____

_____

continue on reverse side

NOTE TO EDUCATORS AND GROUPS: Slides, in color and black and white, illustrating many of the techniques and equipment shown in this guide are available. For information and current costs, send listing of those you desire to the address listed above.

Ideas I would like to share: _____

_____

_____

_____

_____

_____

_____

_____

_____

_____

_____

_____

_____

_____

Mealtime Manual for People with Disabilities and the Aging

Mealtime Manual for People with Disabilities and the Aging **by Judith L. Klinger**, OTR, MA, is a handbook to aid in the preparation of meals for the individual with physical limitations and the aging. A **companion** to *Meal Preparation and Training: The Health Care Professional's Guide*, this manual focuses on hands-on skills that should be used initially during treatment sessions with a health care professional. Eventually these skills can be performed independently by the individual. The book focuses on tasks in the kitchen, including kitchen planning, handling utensils, serving, cleanup, healthy choice of foods, individual tastes, concerns in the kitchen, and shopping.

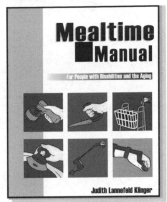

This manual contains information about a wide range of techniques and tools, most of which are readily available to consumers. The physician, visiting nurse service, occupational and physical therapists, home economist, extension service, school, or other local organizations are the primary sources of information for the disabled and the aging; groups that can offer additional help and support are found in the Appendices under Helpful Organizations and Agencies.

Summary of Features

- Much of the equipment described in this book may be found in local stores or through mail-order sources for which addresses are given.
- This guide provides simple aids and techniques to help solve meal preparation problems, including packaging, cutting, mixing, use of a stove, and selection of appliances.
- The manual is user-friendly so that information is easily available to the consumer.

- -

☑ **Yes!** I would like to buy_____ copies of
Mealtime Manual for People with Disabilities and the Aging

Qty.	Title	Order#	Price	Total
_____	Mealtime Manual for People with Disabilities and the Aging	33411	$26.00 ea.	_____

____Bill me (No billing will be done to post office boxes)
____Check Enclosed
____Charge My: ❑ AMEX ❑ Visa ❑ Mastercard
Exp. ____ Account No. _____
Signature _____

NJ Residents
Add 6% Sales Tax _____
Handling Charge _____$4.50_
TOTAL _____

Please Print

Name: _____

Address: _____

City: _____ State: _____ Zip: _____

Phone: (____)_____ Fax: (____)_____

All Prices Are Subject To Change. Shipping Charges May Apply.

SLACK Incorporated, Professional Book Division, 6900 Grove Road, Thorofare, NJ 08086-9447
Call 800-257-8290 or 609-848-1000, Fax 609-853-5991, E-Mail orders@slackinc.com or http://www.slackinc.com